Veterinary Infection Prevention and Control

Veterinary Infection Prevention and Control

Editors

Linda Caveney, LVT, RCST

Barbara Jones, DVM

with

Kimberly Ellis, CVT

⊛WILEY-BLACKWELL

A John Wiley & Sons, Ltd., Publication

Wiley-Blackwell is an imprint of John Wiley & Sons, formed by the merger of Wiley's global Scientific, Technical and Medical business with Blackwell Publishing.

Registered office: John Wiley & Sons, Ltd, The Atrium, Southern Gate, Chichester, West Sussex, PO19 8SQ, UK

Editorial offices: 2121 State Avenue, Ames, Iowa 50014-8300, USA
The Atrium, Southern Gate, Chichester, West Sussex, PO19 8SQ, UK
9600 Garsington Road, Oxford, OX4 2DQ, UK

For details of our global editorial offices, for customer services and for information about how to apply for permission to reuse the copyright material in this book please see our website at www.wiley.com/wiley-blackwell.

Library of Congress Cataloging-in-Publication Data

Veterinary infection prevention and control / editors, Linda Caveney,
Barbara Jones, with Kimberly Ellis.
    p. cm.
  Includes bibliographical references and index.
  ISBN-13: 978-0-8138-1534-3 (pbk. : alk. paper)
  ISBN-10: 0-8138-1534-7
 1. Communicable diseases in animals–Prevention. 2. Nosocomial infections–Prevention.
3. Zoonoses–Control. 4. Veterinary hospitals–Sanitation. I. Caveney, Linda. II. Jones, Barbara, 1981–
III. Ellis, Kimberly.
  SF781.V464 2012
  636.089′44–dc23

                                   2011018166

A catalogue record for this book is available from the British Library.

This book is published in the following electronic formats: ePDF 9780470961445; ePub 9780470961452; Mobi 9780470961469

Set in 10/12 pt Times by Aptara® Inc., New Delhi, India
Printed and bound in Malaysia by Vivar Printing Sdn Bhd

1 2012

Contents

This book has a companion website providing review questions and answers, figures from the book, and additional resources online at www.wiley.com/go/caveney.

Contributors

Audrey Ruple, DVM
Biosecurity House Officer/Oncology Fellow
Colorado State University
James L. Voss
Veterinary Medical Center
Fort Collins, CO

**Nathan Slovis DVM, Dipl. ACVIM, CHT
(Certified Hyperbaric Technologist),
Director**
McGee Critical Care and Medical Center
Hagyard Equine Medical Insititute
Lexington, KY

Barbara Jones, DVM
Appleton, WI

**Kathleen T. Darling, MS, M,
MT(ASCP), CIC**
Infection Control Coordinator
Texas A&M University
Veterinary Medical Teaching Hospital
College Station, TX

Magda Dunowska, LW (vet), PhD
Senior Lecturer in Veterinary Infectious
Diseases (Virology) Institute of
Veterinary, Animal and Biomedical Sciences
Te Kura Mâtauranga Kararehe
Massey University, Palmerston, North New
Zealand

Leslie Hiber, BS, CVT
Infection Control
University of Minnesota
Veterinary Medical Center
St. Paul, MN

Linda Caveney, LVT, RCST
Infection Prevention Specialty Technician
Cornell University Hospital for Animals
Ithaca, NY

Kristina L. Perry, CVT
Equine Medicine/Critical Care Nurse
Colorado State University

James L. Voss
Veterinary Medical Center
Fort Collins, CO

Foreword

There are a select number of defining moments in life that one never forgets. And then, there are those moments that are just simply memorable because the sights and smells of the experience have been forever etched into sensory recall.

It must have been the first day on my very first job back in 1983. . . I was an eager cage-cleaning acolyte of the veterinary profession, and one of my first tasks was to go in and clean up a rather unpleasant mess in an exam room at the veterinary clinic. A Doberman Pinscher had come in to be examined because of severe diarrhea and vomiting, and while in the exam room had provided more than ample evidence of his condition. At the time, I had no idea what parvovirus was, but you only need to be in a room with parvo diarrhea once to know you will never have a problem making *that* diagnosis in the future. As I cleaned up the mess on the floor, I knew nothing of infection control. I didn't really even know what a virus was other than something that gave you a cold.

Now, more than 25 years from that day, I have experienced both the basics and the complexities of infection control in veterinary medicine—from the viewpoints of a practicing veterinarian and a public health professional. In the latter role, I have had the opportunity to speak to human and animal medical professionals and students on issues surrounding infection control, mostly from the perspective of preventing zoonotic diseases. What I convey to them is how cavalier the veterinary profession has historically been with regard to preventing the spread of infection—underestimating the risks to themselves as well as to their patients. Often, veterinary professionals tend to think about infection control mostly in the context of sterile surgery, forgetting that every time we touch an animal, or blow our own noses, we have the potential to spread pathogens.

Several years ago, I investigated an outbreak of salmonellosis among clients and staff of a large veterinary practice. Not only were humans getting ill, but the animals were too, providing a stark reminder that proper infection control provides protective benefit to both humans and animals.

Unfortunately, there are precious few resources for veterinary health professionals to look to for guidance on infection control, especially in the context of preventing nosocomial infections in veterinary practice.

In response to this need, in 2004, Drs. Joni Scheftel and Brigid Elchos, two forward-thinking and motivated public health veterinarians, proposed to the National Association of State Public Health Veterinarians (NASPHV) that the organization should take a lead role in developing guidelines for preventing the transmission of pathogens between veterinarians and their patients—guidance written by vets, for vets. The result was the *Compendium of Veterinary Standard Precautions*, now undergoing its third revision. I have had the honor and privilege of being part of the workgroup that developed that guidance.

Among the concepts in that Compendium (available at http://www.nasphv.org) is that simple precautions must become part of the everyday routine in veterinary medicine, internalized as part of our practice of medicine. The veterinary profession has been fortunate that some of the most serious zoonotic diseases, like brucellosis or canine rabies, have largely been controlled or eradicated in the United States. Yet there are still innumerable opportunities for transmission of pathogens between animals and people.

In addition to the NASPHV Compendium, a text reference such as this is long overdue in veterinary medicine and will help fill a great void in the education of both veterinarians and veterinary technicians. No longer should we be complacent about eating near the fecal microscope, washing our hands after *every* contact with patients, and using other basic infection control techniques. Think to yourselves...would you be happy if your doctor gave you a physical exam right after having his hands in his last patient's mouth, if he hadn't washed his hands? I think we would all be bothered by such a practice.

Yet, we are all guilty of that at various times in veterinary medicine—the nature of the beast, so to speak. The animal world is a dirty place, and we are accustomed to getting dirty with our patients. That does not mean, however, that we should simply accept the potential risk of pathogen transmission. Obvious examples like parvo, *Salmonella*, canine influenza, and methicillin-resistant *Staphyloccus aureus* remind us that nosocomial infections are not merely a nuisance, but are potentially fatal. Preventing transmission in the veterinary setting, whether from environmental contamination, respiratory droplets, or direct contact, should be a priority even when we must wrestle with our patients on the floor, in the kennel, or in the back seat of a client's car.

Infection control isn't just about disinfecting after parvo diarrhea (thankfully, now a rare occurrence) and using good sterile technique in surgery. As you read the chapters in this book, whether a student or a practicing professional, think about how the principles, guidelines, and best practices presented here can be, should be, or already are implemented in your work every day. We can always improve our infection control skills and habits. They are something we must constantly practice, hone, and keep in the front of our minds, until they become second nature.

Bryan Cherry, VMD, PhD, NYS Veterinarian, DYSDOH

Acknowledgments

We wish to acknowledge the professional expertise of the following individuals who offered technical and scientific advice on individual chapters: Chuck Hughes, BS, Head Educator and General Manager of SPSmedical Supply Corp.; Kirsten Thompson, Technical Service Expert of EcoLab; Derek Lashua, Marketing Director, Spectrum Surgical Instrument Corp.; John Caveney, Senior Service Technician, LBR Scientific, Incorp.; Roger Segelken, science writer and editor; and Kayla Kohlenberg, artist/illustrator.

And to Ms. Erica Judisch at Wiley-Blackwell, for all your encouragement, advice, and guidance throughout the entire publishing process of this text-thank you.

Introduction

At a time when cross-species disease transmission is prompting heightened concern among health care professionals and the general public alike, there is practically no science-based and practice-proven information available about infection control in the veterinary setting. What are the risks? What can be done to make animal care safer for patients and caregivers?

Dedicated animal caregivers—whether engaged in the veterinary medical field or dealing with animals in other settings—desperately need authoritative and up-to-date information to confront this growing threat to animal and human health. To the credit of their profession, more veterinary technicians are beginning to take the initiative, learning from best-practice human medicine and adding their specialized knowledge of animal health to design and implementing proactive infection control programs that should be the envy of human-medicine hospitals and clinics.

Now is the time to share that hard-won knowledge with veterinary practice managers, companion animal breeders, stable managers, and animal shelter managers.

Veterinary Infection Control and Prevention is a tool for animal caregivers to use to make informed decisions and develop facility-specific plans. These are the conscientious individuals who will educate staff members on best practice procedures to protect humans and the animals from disease transmission.

Veterinary Infection Prevention and Control

1 What *Is* Infection Control and Biosecurity?

Audrey Ruple, Nathan M. Slovis and Barbara Jones

"First do no harm." This edict reminds all veterinarians that they must consider the possible harm that might be caused by any intervention. Since as early as 1860, this phrase among veterinarians has been an expression of hope, intention, humility, and recognition that acts with good intentions may have unwanted consequences. The vast majority of patients who have access to medical services today are healed. There are some, however, who suffer unintended consequences of care, such as health care–associated infections (HAI). To ensure that such life threatening–life saving care does not result in HAI, modern health care has developed an extensive system for infection prevention. Regardless of the approaches taken, health care facilities must strive for 100% adherence to the institutions' infection control strategies. To achieve this caliber of adherence, proper education of the staff will be necessary.

The focus of this chapter is to educate readers to be proactive when it comes to biosecurity attentiveness to safeguard patients, clients, students, co-workers, animal companions, and the community from potential infectious agent(s). Recognizing the need to establish objectives, expectations, and goals for a successful biosecurity program will in turn lead to quality standards of care delivered by a dedicated and educated team.

DEFINITIONS OF DISEASE CONTROL TERMINOLOGY

It is important to establish a common vocabulary as many of these words have other meanings or uses in veterinary practice. The way these words and phrases are defined here is specifically in the context of how they relate to infection control. The definitions are compiled from those by the Centers for Disease Control (CDC), World Health Organization, Food and Agriculture Organization of the United Nations, and the Occupational Health and Safety Administration. Table 1.1 provides the definitions of disease control terminology used in this book.

EPIDEMIOLOGIC LEVELS OF DISEASE CONTROL ACTIVITIES

Disease control activities against infectious agents occur at four levels: individual, institutional, community, and global.

Veterinary Infection Prevention and Control, First Edition. Edited by Linda Caveney and Barbara Jones with Kimberly Ellis.
© 2012 John Wiley & Sons, Inc. Published by John Wiley & Sons, Inc.

Table 1.1   Definitions of Disease Control Terminology

Alcohol-based hand rubs	An alcohol-containing preparation designed for application to the hands for reducing the number of viable microorganisms on the hands. In the United States, such preparations usually contain 60–95% ethanol or isopropanol.
Antimicrobial soap	Soap or detergent containing an antiseptic agent.
Antiseptic agent	Antimicrobial substances that are applied to the skin to reduce the number of microbial flora. Such substances may include alcohols, chlorhexidine, chlorine, iodine, chloroxylenol, quaternary ammonium compounds, and triclosan.
Antiseptic handwash (or HCW handwash)	FDA product category. An antiseptic-containing preparation designed for frequent use; it reduces the number of microorganisms on intact skin to an initial baseline level after adequate washing, rinsing, and drying; it is broad-spectrum, fast-acting, and, if possible, persistent.
Antiseptic hand rub	Applying an antiseptic hand rub product to all surfaces of the hands to reduce the number of microorganisms present.
Biosecurity	All the cumulative measures that can or should be taken to keep disease from occurring and prevent the transmission of disease. The policies and hygienic practices designed to prevent incidents of infectious disease.
Colonization	Presence of a microorganism on or in a host, with growth and multiplication of the organism but without interaction between host and microorganism; i.e., no clinical signs and no immune response.
Clinical infection	An infection by a microorganism that can be identified through clinical signs and laboratory tests.
Detergent	Detergents (e.g., surfactants) are compounds that possess a cleaning action. They are composed of both hydrophilic and lipophilic parts and generally are divided into three groups: anionic, cationic, and nonionic detergents. Although products used for handwashing or antiseptic handwash in health care settings represent various types of detergents, the term "soap" is used to refer to such detergents in this guideline.
Disinfectant	A chemical agent that can be applied to inanimate objects (surgical equipment, floor, hand surfaces, etc.) that causes the destruction or inhibition of microorganisms, but not necessarily their spores, or some viruses.
Hand antisepsis	Refers to either antiseptic handwash or antiseptic hand rub.
Hand hygiene	A general term that applies to handwashing, antiseptic handwash, antiseptic hand rub or surgical hand antisepsis, or the use of disposable exam gloves.
Handwashing	Washing hands with plain soap and water.
Health care worker	HCW
Infection	The entry and development or multiplication of a microorganism; however, infection does not always cause disease. There are several types of infection: colonization, subclinical, latent, and clinical.
Isolation	An area within the veterinary practice or animal facility that is used to separate animals with a contagious disease from other animals.
Latent infection	An infection that is inactive and is causing no clinical signs, though it continues to be capable of producing clinical signs.
Multiple drug–resistant organism (MDRO)	Microorganisms, predominantly bacteria, that are resistant to one or more classes of antimicrobial agents. Although the names of certain MDROs describe resistance to only one agent, e.g., MRSA, these pathogens are frequently resistant to multiple antimicrobial agents.
Nosocomial infection	An infection produced by a pathogenic agent that was neither present nor incubating at the time the patient was admitted to the veterinary hospital and/or animal facility.

Table 1.1   (*Continued*)

Persistent activity	Persistent activity is defined as the prolonged or extended antimicrobial activity that prevents or inhibits the proliferation or survival of microorganisms after application of the product. This activity may be demonstrated by sampling a site several minutes or hours after application of the product. This property also has been referred to as residual activity. Both substantive and nonsubstantive active ingredients can show a persistent effect if they substantially lower the number of bacteria during the wash period.
Personal protective equipment (PPE)	Specialized clothing or equipment worn by personnel for protection from infectious material.
Plain soap	Plain soap refers to detergents that do not contain antimicrobial agents or contain low concentrations of antimicrobial agents that are effective solely as preservatives.
Reservoir	Any person, animal, arthropod, plant, or place (soil, water) in which an infectious agent normally lives and multiplies. It is the natural habitat of the infectious agent and on which it depends on for survival.
Sanitizer	An agent that reduces the number of microorganisms to safe levels as judged by public health requirements. According to the protocol for the official sanitizer test, a sanitizer is a chemical that kills 99.999% of the specific test bacteria in 30 sections under the test conditions.
Sterilization	A validated process used to render a product free of all forms of viable microorganisms. For any sterilization process, the presence of microorganisms on an individual item can be expressed in terms of probability; although this probability can be reduced to a very low number, it can never be reduced to zero.
Subclinical infection	An infection with no detectable clinical signs, but that is capable of producing clinical signs. Certain subclinical infections can be detected by an immune response.
Surgical hand antisepsis	FDA product category. Antiseptic handwash or antiseptic hand rub used preoperatively by surgical personnel that substantially reduces the number of microorganisms on intact skin; it is broad-spectrum, fast-acting, and persistent.
Surveillance	Ongoing systematic collection, collation, analysis, and interpretation of data and the dissemination of information to those who need to know in order that action may be taken. The data chosen to be collected depends on the needs of the individuals, practices, institutions, or facilities; for example, specific Salmonella isolates in a tertiary equine hospital to monitor for nosocomial infections.
Transmission	Any mechanism by which an infectious agent is spread from a source or reservoir to an individual.
Waterless antiseptic agent	An antiseptic agent that does not require use of exogenous water. After applying such an agent, the hands are rubbed together until the agent has dried.
Zoonosis	Any infectious disease that can be naturally transmitted from vertebrate animals to humans.

The first level, the individual, is predominantly the domain of the primary provider. A variety of prevention strategies can be targeted to individuals through their primary provider, normally a veterinarian providing wellness and general health services. One example is the use of chemoprophylaxis (antibiotics) to help prevent surgery-site infections.

The second level is that of the institution, which is the domain of the infection-control practitioner or the organization health official. This level would include veterinary hospitals, pet boarding facilities, human health care facilities, nursing homes, other human residential facilities, and schools. Programs to prevent the spread of fecal, respiratory, and blood-borne pathogens to health care workers or patients are examples of control strategies targeted at the institutional level.

The third level is targeted to the community (in general) and is predominately the domain of public health agencies (local, state, and national levels). The removal of dead animal carcasses after a hurricane is an example of a control measure targeted for the community.

The fourth level is related to global strategies. For a number of important pathogens, it has become evident that global control strategies are critical to disease occurrence within the United States. Examples of this are the global strategies for bovine spongiform encephalopathy and avian influenza.

Although some control measures are specific for each one of these levels, substantial overlap can occur. For instance, immunization programs operate at all four levels (Osterholm et al., 2000).

TARGETED ELEMENTS FOR DISEASE PREVENTION

The transmission of infectious agents requires three elements: a source (or reservoir) of the infectious agent, a susceptible host with a portal of entry receptive to the agent, and a mode of transmission for the agent. Identification of areas or processes in which transmission of pathogens is likely to occur (control points) and implementation of measures aimed at minimizing the possibility of such transmission, while allowing for reasonable flow and function within the veterinary hospital or animal facility, are important components of biosecurity (Dunowska et al., 2007; Lappin, 2003; Morley, 2002). During the assessment and development of the prevention and control activities targeted to infectious diseases, the weakest link in the chain of infection (agent, transmission, host) needs to be considered for each specific pathogen. In some situations, control of the agent in a specific reservoir may be the best way to reduce disease occurrence. Chlorination of water is an example of destroying an agent in its reservoir or eliminating a possible mode of transmission.

Strategies aimed at the level of transmission need to be tailored to the type of transmission involved. An example of a control activity targeted to airborne transmission is the isolation of the infected animal to a facility where there is no shared airspace or where no other animals are currently housed on the premises. The control of vector-borne transmission can be targeted toward destroying the vector and toward the use of repellents, such as in the case of vesicular stomatitis or West Nile virus outbreaks.

In many instances, the best way to prevent disease occurrence is through modification of the host, such as developing or boosting immunity through active or passive immunization. Other control activities targeted to the host may include improving the nutritional status of a neglected animal or providing chemoprophylaxis (antibiotics) against a variety of agents. Even simple bathing and grooming of animals can help with identification of external parasites and skin conditions. Every effort should be made to minimize the contact between animals with a history or clinical signs suggestive of infectious contagious disease, or those with confirmed contagious disease, and the remainder of the patients or animals at a boarding facility (Traub-Dargatz et al., 2009). Chapter 5 describes strategies for disease prevention in animal facilities.

EVALUATION OF RISK, FEASIBILITY, COST, AND EFFECTIVENESS

Before implementing disease prevention and control strategies, several issues need to be considered, including risk, feasibility, cost, and effectiveness.

Risk Assessment

Risk assessment deals with the probability for potential disease exposure. Epidemiologic studies or analysis of surveillance data can serve to define animals at risk and can also quantify risk within different populations. Information that is needed for making the optimal decisions regarding the risk posed would include history of the arriving animal, history regarding contact of the arriving animal with other animals having contagious disease, pertinent laboratory testing performed prior to arrival, physical findings on initial examination of the new arrival, and pertinent laboratory tests results if available at arrival or soon thereafter (Traub-Dargatz et al., 2009). To help better understand the risks of the animal to disseminate a disease, there is a need for knowledge of the past disease status and exposure status in order to best implement targeted control measures for contagious disease. One method to accomplish this is by the having the owner/authorized caretaker/transporter sign a form and state the past history of the animal in relation to exposure to a specific disorder. The reason for such self-certification is to establish risk level. Without this type of information, those receiving the animal would have no mechanism to gather critical information for those animals that have no overt signs of disease at the time of presentation to the facility. The animal could have had exposure to a contagious disease agent that would pose a substantial risk to other animals in the facility if not managed accordingly (Traub-Dargatz et al., 2009).

Another strategy is an admittance-based system. An admittance-based alert system notifies infection control and clinical personnel about re-admitted or transferred patients with a history of infection or colonization. This system allows for review of policies and procedures to be instituted prior to the arrival of the patient with the infectious disease. This provides for routine assessment of education and training among personnel and can improve infection prevention measures at the facility level (Morley, 2002).

Risk adjustments require collection of pertinent information (i.e., *Salmonella* in hospitalized patients, surgery-site infections, etc.) about the total population being monitored so that objective data can be used to help direct decisions being made regarding risk assessments. These risk adjustments are important because policies and procedures will need to be updated based on these findings.

Feasibility

In developing control programs, the feasibility of a policy also needs to be assessed. Feasibility or practicality of the policy is dependent not only on the sociodemographic factors but also on the operating needs of the facility. For instance, equine facilities that buy and sell horses on a routine basis might accept the risk of contagious disease outbreaks, such as *Streptococcus equi*, as the norm, instead of isolating newly arrived horses for a period of time required. Animal control shelters face many challenges and risk factors with overcrowding, stress and decreased immune status of animals, and continually changing populations. The risk for infectious disease cannot be totally eliminated, but steps to minimize introduction and spread are addressed regularly (Petersen et al., 2008).

Cost

Cost and availability of resources also need to be considered when developing control strategies. Implementing and maintaining even the most basic biosecurity program requires trained personnel and an adequately staffed facility with appropriate supervision. Outbreak investigations have indicated an association between infections and understaffing; the association was consistently linked with poor adherence to hand hygiene (Harbarth et al., 1999; Fridkin et al., 1996; Vicca, 1999). The understaffing of human nurses facilitates the spread of MRSA in intensive-care settings through relaxed attention to basic control measures (Vicca, 1999).

Effectiveness

Finally, control strategies need to be evaluated for their effectiveness. For example, the effectiveness of the control strategy is a critical issue in evaluating ways to curb salmonellosis in equine care facilities. Cost-effectiveness models are often used in making recommendations for population-based vaccine programs. Challenges to prevention include measurement of outcomes that may be complicated by diagnostic limitations. An example of this is the diagnosing of ventilator associated pneumonia in humans.

PREVENTION INTERVENTIONS

Prevention strategies for infectious diseases can be characterized by using the traditional concepts of primary, secondary, or tertiary prevention. Primary prevention is defined as the prevention of infection by personal and community-wide efforts. Secondary prevention includes measures available to individuals and the population for detection of early infection and effective intervention. Tertiary prevention consists of measures available to reduce or eliminate the long-term impairment and disabilities caused by infectious diseases (Osterholm et al., 2000).

Primary Prevention

An example of primary prevention is immunoprophylaxis, which can be classified as active or passive. Active immunization involves the administration of all or part of the microorganism, live or inactivated (canine distempter vaccine is a modified live virus), or a product of the microorganism (toxoid) to alter the host by stimulating an immune response aimed at protecting against infection. Active administration is also used in postexposure situations, including immunization after exposure (e.g., tetanus). Some vaccines may be given in conjunction with an antitoxin in the postexposure setting. Passive immunization involves the administration of preformed antibodies, often to specific agents, after exposure. The common forms of passive immunization may be hyperimmunized plasma for a foal with failure of passive transfer or botulism hyperimmunized plasma. Human rabies immunoglobulin used for postexposure to a possible rabid animal is another example of passive immunization.

A second type of primary prevention is antimicrobial prophylaxis, often referred to as chemoprophylaxis. Use of effective chemoprophylaxis requires that the infectious agent be susceptible to the antimicrobial used. When used as a primary prevention, the medication may be used before or after exposure in order to prevent infection. Examples of chemoprophylaxis in the postexposure setting include treating with azithromycin for *Rhodococcus equi* infections or metronidazole for *Clostridium perfringens* enterocolitis. Prophylaxis against surgical wound infections with broad-spectrum antimicrobials coverage before surgery is an example of chemoprophylaxis in a hospital setting. In many situations, chemoprophylaxis is used because the likelihood of exposure to pathogenic organisms is present, even though proper documentation of exposure is not clear.

Secondary Prevention

Secondary prevention activities entail chemoprophylaxis for active infections and involve the identification of early or asymptomatic infection with subsequent treatment so that infections are eradicated and the sequels are prevented. Although most secondary prevention programs involve intervention at the individual level through the use of chemoprophylaxis, such programs often operate within the context of a population-based or institutional-based screening effort. Most hospital infection control policies include the judicious use of antimicrobials, and many hospitals actually have a committee that establishes policy or outlines issues related to the judicious use of antimicrobials. This may include the exclusion of specified antimicrobials on food animal species, the consideration of reserving certain antibiotics for particular infectious etiologies or presentations, avoidance of use of certain drugs that are considered "big guns" in the human public health realm to avoid the development of antimicrobial resistance in specific populations of bacteria or viruses, and the establishment of minimum therapeutic doses, acceptable routes of administration, or application of minimum inhibitory concentration (MIC) result information from antimicrobial sensitivity testing of culture specimens, when available. An example of secondary prevention would be the use of procaine penicillin or ceftiofur on horses that test positive for *Streptococcus equi* on a nasopharyngeal screening wash during a farm outbreak of the disease.

Tertiary Prevention

Tertiary prevention efforts involve measures to eliminate long-term impairment and disabilities from existing conditions. Since most infectious diseases are treatable, tertiary prevention activities are less common. This concept is applicable to control some viral infections that are chronic and cannot be eradicated. The use of antimicrobial prophylaxis against possible other opportunistic agents is an example of tertiary prevention activity (Osterholm et al., 2000).

INFECTION CONTROL: STANDARD OPERATING PROCEDURES

Infection control plans, protocols, procedures, and policies are an essential component of disease prevention management (hereafter referred to as plans). These plans must be written, posted, and continually enforced by a designated staff member in order to be effective in preventing infection transmission between patients, between patients and the environment, and between patients and personnel caring for those patients.

There are many considerations to take into account when setting up or modifying an infection control plan, and different areas may need to be emphasized depending on the individual needs of the practice, institution, or animal facility. To be effective, an infection control plan must first identify which infectious agents need to be controlled, which in turn is dependent on the demographics of the patients (small animals vs. dairy), the type of practice or facility (small private practice vs. tertiary referral hospital), location (both geographically and rural vs. urban), public health concerns, and cost of control.

A comprehensive infection control plan encompasses preventing transmission of infectious disease, minimizing contamination of the environment, decontaminating the environment, surveillance for the infectious agents being controlled for, protection of personnel and optimizing overall health of patients and personnel (Elchos et al., 2008; Traub-Dargatz et al., 2009). This section discusses general considerations of the patient, environment, employee, and surveillance in setting up a comprehensive infection control plan, as well as information on writing an infection control plan, education, training and enforcement, and finally compliance.

The Patient

General Considerations

The patient (in this case, an animal with an appointment for a wellness check or disease state or an animal that is hospitalized) is usually the source of an infectious agent in situations relevant to hospitals, clinics, and animal facilities. If the patient is not properly identified, handled, or treated, the result can be contamination of the environment (leading to potential for nosocomial infections), direct transmission of disease to other patients, or infection of personnel in the case of zoonotic agents. Although this section will discuss infection control in regards to the patient, it is important to mention animals that are not patients, for example, employee pets or companions of patients that are brought to visit the clinic, hospital, or animal facility. It is rarely, if ever, appropriate to allow pets to visit a hospital, clinic, or farm, and the infection control plan should address this potential point of contention with personnel or owners to avoid any misinterpretations. Apparently healthy pets affect infection control from several standpoints:

1. They can harbor subclinical infections or act as carriers for an infectious agent.
2. They can act as fomites for environmental infectious agents.
3. They can spread infectious agents from one part of a building or farm to another as they visit different areas.
4. They can acquire an infection from the hospital, clinic, or farm.

It is important to have a written policy regarding personnel bringing pets to work with them. There are situations in which pets can and should be allowed in a hospital, clinic, or farm visit setting, such as teaching situations at tertiary universities or when personnel cannot leave their pets home that day. In cases where a pet does come into a clinical setting, there should be guidelines for where the pet will be housed during the day (office vs. ICU) and how to minimize the pet's interaction with the patient setting.

Regarding the patient, the infection control plan should start before the animal walks into the clinic and should take into account the history, health status, work-up, housing requirements, diagnostics, surveillance, discharge, and exposure incidents.

Patient History

Receptionists and other administrative personnel should be trained to identify patients with potential infectious disease so they can advise owners of precautions that should be taken before bringing their animals into the waiting room. The following situations should be specifically addressed:

- **Open wounds:** Animal owners should be advised to bandage any wound, if possible, before bringing the patient into the hospital. If a wound is not able to be bandaged, provisions should be made to cover the wound in some way or have a gurney available to bring the animal into the hospital to minimize contamination of the environment.
- **Coughing patients:** Patients with a history of cough of unknown origin should be kept separate from other animals. These patients should not be allowed into the waiting area and should be taken immediately into an isolation area. Examples of possible diseases include *Bordetella bronchiseptica* or equine *Streptococcus equi* var. *equi*. In addition to the risks of environmental contamination and patient-to-patient contact, there is also a concern for zoonotic potential of many upper respiratory pathogens. Although viruses like influenza type A subtypes are known to regularly cross the host species barrier, even respiratory pathogens, such as *Bordetella bronchiseptica,* have the potential to cause zoonotic disease in humans (Gueirard et al., 1995; Hewlett, 1995).
- **Diarrhea:** A patients with clinical signs including diarrhea should be considered to have an infectious gastrointestinal disease until proven otherwise. Many of the gastrointestinal pathogens can be difficult to remove from the environment and can also be highly contagious. For example, *Clostridia difficile* is an emerging concern and has caused serious nosocomial infections in several veterinary teaching hospitals. Dr. Weese and colleagues studied a single veterinary hospital and identified *Clostridium difficile* at sites in both the small- and large-animal clinics; these sites were geographically associated with patient nosocomial infections (Weese et al., 2008). The list of gastrointestinal pathogens of concern for infection control protocols and policies includes *Salmonella*, parvovirus, *Clostridium*, *Escherichia coli*, coronavirus, *Giardia*, canine distemper virus, and many others. In addition, there are reports of nosocomial infections with antibiotic-resistant strains of many of the bacterial gastrointestinal pathogens, such as *Salmonella typhimurium*, in patients and humans (Wright et al., 2005).
- **Neurologic disease:** The list of diseases that cause neurologic signs is potentially endless, and the variation of signs associated with lyssavirus species (rabies) alone necessitates infection control protocols for patients with neurologic signs due to the potential for transmission to other patients as well as humans. Animals infected with rabies can present with signs ranging from ataxia to aggression, and there is not always a clear history of exposure.

The above signs should be identified before the animal is admitted or seen in a veterinary clinic, hospital, or ambulatory setting by the personnel responsible for setting up appointments or admitting emergencies to a referral center. Personnel, usually receptionists or administrative assistants, should undergo training in how to identify signs of potential contagious or zoonotic diseases from the patient's history or clinical signs, in addition to how to implement the infection control protocols in individual cases.

Patient Vaccination

Although vaccination recommendations are a routine part of every veterinary practice, infection control protocols need to specifically address public (owner) education for diseases with vaccinations available. Owners should be given information on recommended vaccinations based not on geographic prevalence of infectious diseases, but on a pet's future exposure risks, such as traveling or boarding. An example of this is giving the canine influenza vaccine if a dog is going to be shown in an American Kennel Club show. The infection control protocol should include vaccination recommendations for all species that the veterinarian and staff see on a routine basis.

Vaccination is a critical control point for prevention of infectious diseases. Vaccination is not only relevant from the standpoint of preventing zoonotic infections, but also from the standpoint of preventing infections between individuals, be they dogs, cats, horses, or food production animals. This concept has been used successfully in rabies programs in several countries, such as the United States. This strategy has been used for control of many viral diseases, such as rabies (lyssavirus), and some bacterial diseases, like *Brucella melitensis* (Blasco, 2010) and *Bacillus anthracis*.

This is an often underused and underappreciated area of infection control, but it provides one of the best infection control strategies—prevention of disease. Infection control through prevention of infection is far easier, more economical, and more beneficial than handling a patient infected with a contagious or zoonotic disease.

Patient Classification

Animals arriving at veterinary hospitals or other types of facilities should be classified by their relative infectious disease risk level. More specific information regarding animal health can be ascertained prior to or at the time of admission to the facility in order to screen for infectious diseases.

The general population of animals in a facility should be housed in groups that are matched according to age, use, and reason for admission. This organizational system places animals with similar disease risk together to minimize the potential for pathogen transmission between animals by co-mingling or inadvertent transfer of pathogens by hospital personnel. The relative risk level will help determine where the animal is to be housed and the necessary precautions required to prevent transfer of disease. Table 1.2 provides an example of this type of housing by risk classification at an equine facility.

Patient Exposure Incidents

Guidelines for dealing with exposure incidents need to be written down to prevent improper handling of an incident. There are two exposure types to consider: human exposure to zoonotic agents and patient exposure to contagious agents. Infection control, after a patient or human is exposed to an animal with a contagious or zoonotic disease, starts with training people to recognize potential exposures and then dealing with those exposures immediately. Bites by unvaccinated animals, especially to employees or other personnel, are usually outlined in infection control protocols due to the concern of rabies. A comprehensive infection control plan must outline protocols for handling all situations in which a person or patient has been exposed to a potential or known zoonotic or contagious agent.

The Environment

Practice Type

Different considerations for infection control need to be made based on the practice type. The practice type could be defined as a retrofitted clinic or purpose-built veterinary clinic or

Table 1.2 Risk Classification of Equine Patients

Code category	Risk assessment level	Classification of patients
Green	Low risk	<ul><li>Ophthalmic patients</li><li>Orthopedic patients, excluding joint ill foals</li><li>Surgical patients not requiring inhalation anesthesia</li><li>Patients in stages of recovery that have been upgraded from **Caution Level Yellow**</li><li>Any patient presenting with conditions that do not warrant a higher level caution</li></ul>
Yellow	Medium risk	<ul><li>Colic patients</li><li>Inpatients presenting to medicine from surgery</li><li>Surgical patients requiring inhalation anesthesia (excluding orthopedic cases)</li><li>Immunocompromised patients</li><li>Newborn foals</li><li>Nurse mares</li><li>Patients in stages of recovery that have been upgraded from **Caution Level Orange**</li><li>Recipient mares that are under quarantine, unknown disease status. These mares will be identified with a "**yellow**" tag.</li></ul>
Orange	Medium-high risk	<ul><li>Newborn foals less than 24 hours old, presenting with diarrhea with no farm history of problems.</li><li>Joint ill foals younger than 7 months of age</li><li>Patients with bone infections</li><li>Patients that have **one** of the following, of **unknown** origin: Fevers greater than 102°F Low WBC (<4800) Loose manure</li><li>Recipient mares that are testing negative, despite having been exposed to a horse that tested positive for an infectious disease. These mares will be identified with an "**orange**" tag.</li></ul>
Red	High risk	<ul><li>Patients positive for infectious disease</li><li>Suspect neurological patients for infectious disease</li><li>Patients older than 24 hours of age, presenting with diarrhea</li><li>Patients that have **two** of the following, of **unknown** origin: Fevers greater than 102°F Low WBC (<4800) Loose manure</li><li>Recipient mares that test positive for infectious disease. These mares will be identified with a "**red**" tag. These mares may be upgraded upon testing negative for infectious disease.</li></ul> The **only** time a **CODE RED** patient may be upgraded is if a suspect neurological patient is determined not to be positive for infectious disease. Otherwise, all patients classified as **CODE RED** will stay at this classification until discharge.

Adapted from source: Slovis N, Biosecurity Procedures for McGee Critical Care and Medical Center, Hagyard Equine Medical Insititute, Lexington, KY.

hospital; an ambulatory versus hospital-based practice; or by the species treated (i.e., only feline or equine practice). A university small-animal hospital would need to consider the species being treated (dogs, cats, birds, and exotics) and, in addition, must take into consideration the flow of traffic between surgeries, diagnostics, ICU, day appointment areas, and areas where humans congregate (computer stations). Whereas a private practice small-animal clinic that treated dogs and cats only would need to consider fewer species, but would potentially have less ideal traffic flow for infection control.

Facility, Equipment, Flow

Ideally, veterinary clinics or hospitals would be purpose-built with infection control principles taken into consideration during the design phase. In purpose-built clinics, patient and personnel flow patterns, materials used, ventilation systems, cleaning systems, location of cages or kennels, and isolation design are a few of the elements that need to be considered to enable the design of an infection control program to be as complete and efficient as possible. Flow patterns are an integral part of most clinic and hospital designs, but designing the flow patterns to minimize environmental contamination, minimize patient interaction, and provide personnel with convenient access to hand sanitation devices is often not the first consideration.

There are several things to consider when choosing materials used in different aspects of the building, such as permeability and ease of cleaning. The location of kennels should be designed to minimize interaction of patient-to-patient contact and also to minimize potential environmental contamination during periods when the patients need to be out of their kennels or cages, such as during treatments or going outside for walks. Isolation areas are easiest to design in purpose-built hospitals but can be designed for existing buildings with careful planning.

The Employee

Health/History and Vaccination

Employee health is an essential component of an infection control protocol and should be included in written infection control documents. The employee health section of the infection control protocol should include vaccination recommendations, exposure incident policies, and guidelines for reporting changes in health status. It is important to discuss the critical nature of staff health with all employees because collection of employee health information is on a voluntary basis.

Employees should be assured that any disclosure of health information is confidential and will only be used to help protect their health. For example, pregnancy changes the immune system in such a way that the individual is more susceptible to infection from a variety of agents, including *Toxoplasma* spp. If any staff member declines to disclose his/her health status or to take recommendations, it is recommended to have a signed waiver on file. Employee health records should always be kept confidential.

Employee Vaccination

Vaccination for rabies and tetanus should be recommended to all employees that come into contact with animals or biological specimens. For employees in contact with birds or swine, it is also recommended that they be vaccinated for influenza every year. Although the Occupational Safety and Health Administration (OSHA) has no specific requirement for veterinary or animal facility employers to offer rabies or tetanus vaccination, OSHA's General Duty Clause states that employers "shall furnish to each of his employees employment and a place of employment which are free from recognized hazards that are causing or are likely to cause death or serious physical harm to his employees" (U.S. Department of Labor, 1970). This clause is broad enough to cover vaccination for disease with a known risk for the veterinary and certain animal-contact professions (e.g., wildlife rehabilitation), such as rabies.

The CDC also supports employee vaccination. The CDC's *Morbidity and Mortality Weekly Report* (Manning et al., 2008) on Human Rabies Prevention states that vaccination should be offered to veterinarians, their staff, and animal handlers. Rabies titers should be checked every two years. Even if personnel refuse to be vaccinated, it is necessary to discuss the type and amount of risk associated with their job and how the infection control protocol addresses that risk.

Personal Protection

Personal protection against infection is a critical component in preventing spread of infectious disease between patients and between patients and personnel, and it can also be seen as the last barrier of protection against zoonotic diseases. This portion of the infection control plan should include sections on actions that personnel should routinely take as well as equipment that should be routinely used to prevent infection.

Protective action includes topics such as hand hygiene, personal items, and barrier precautions. Each area should include explicit, detailed, step-by-step instructions. For example, the hand hygiene section should include specific information on when hands are to be washed, what should be used to wash the hands, and an outline of an acceptable hand-washing procedure. Hand hygiene and barrier precautions are discussed in detail in Chapter 5.

Exposure Incidents

OSHA defines an exposure incident under the toxic and hazardous substances subpart as "a specific eye, mouth, other mucous membrane, non-intact skin, or parenteral contact with blood or other potentially infectious materials that results from the performance of an employee's duties" (OSHA, 1992). OSHA uses this definition for blood-borne pathogens, but it is relevant to exposure to infectious agents as well. A bite, scratch, or saliva in a cut all meet the requirements of the definition of exposure to an infectious agent.

Incident reporting is important not just from a legal standpoint and potential mandatory reporting of bite incidents and zoonotic disease exposure; it is an important component of tracking where and how incidents are happening in order to intervene in problem areas.

Surveillance

Surveillance within a clinic or hospital allows for the detection of nosocomial and zoonotic agents for use in prevention of transmission (i.e., place patient in isolation) as well as providing a means to quantify how well infection control programs and intervention are working. The parameters used in surveillance vary upon the institution or clinic, but most often include tracking all antibiotic-resistant cases, enteric pathogens, reportable disease pathogens, and *Salmonella* spp. in large-animal facilities. In addition, surveillance allows a determination of whether the incidence of pathogens of concern is increasing, as well as whether individual cases are related through a common patient. Common bacteria used in surveillance data include *Salmonella* spp., *Clostridium difficile*, and *Staphylococcus aureus*. Surveillance systems need to be set up to be monitored by one infection control person to maximize the likelihood of recognizing a trend or potential relatedness of cases.

A surveillance component to your infection control program is essential in order to gauge the effectiveness of your biosecurity policies. Data collected through the surveillance process will provide information regarding your current protocols as well as providing early warning regarding potential contagious disease threats. The type of surveillance program your facility will employ needs to be determined based on several factors, including cost, efficiency, and the number of high-risk cases routinely housed in your facility.

Passive Surveillance

One type of surveillance method employed in most veterinary teaching hospitals is passive surveillance (Benedict et al., 2008). Using this method, data regarding infection rates are collected through medical records or obtained from diagnostic lab results from samples that were submitted for other purposes (i.e., fecal flotation or cultures from patient sources). This approach takes very little effort as one employee can be in charge of compiling data as they are received from the lab, but it is not necessarily an effective way of detecting potential problems regarding nosocomial spread of disease.

Active Surveillance: Laboratory Diagnosis

One type of surveillance employed by veterinary hospitals is active surveillance. This can take several forms, but most commonly involves collecting a sample or samples from hospitalized patients for the express purpose of detecting an agent or agents of concern. It is not reasonable to collect samples from every hospitalized patient in order to detect every possible infectious agent. In order for active surveillance to be used effectively in a veterinary hospital, you must target the high-risk population of interest and determine what agent or agents are of greatest concern. For example, fecal shedding of *Salmonella* spp. in hospitalized equine patients can lead to outbreaks of nosocomial salmonellosis (Ekiri et al., 2009). If your practice routinely hospitalizes equine patients, taking fecal samples from these patients at the time of admission and then regularly throughout hospitalization may be of benefit to your practice. This would allow you to take additional precautions with patients that are known to be shedding *Salmonella* as well as rapidly detect nosocomial transmission of *Salmonella*.

Active Surveillance: Clinical Diagnosis

Another type of active surveillance involves the use of clinical rather than laboratory diagnosis of potential nosocomial infections. These diagnoses can be lumped into defined categories such as postoperative surgical site infection or gastrointestinal disorders. Clinicians could then define a nosocomial event as having occurred based on predetermined clinical signs. For instance, surgical site infection could be defined as redness and swelling at the incision site, or gastrointestinal disorders could be defined as vomiting and/or diarrhea that begin during hospitalization. An increased number of these syndromic events may warrant further investigation and a laboratory analysis to determine the cause of the problem, but syndromic surveillance can be used as an effective form of detection of nosocomial events.

Environmental Surveillance

Environmental surveillance is another detection method employed in most veterinary teaching hospitals (Benedict et al., 2008). It has been documented that environmental contamination with contagious agents has contributed to nosocomial outbreaks in veterinary hospitals (Morley, 2004). As such, culturing the hospital environment regularly may help to insure that a minimum amount of environmental contamination is present. Veterinary teaching hospitals generally take environmental samples for the detection of *Salmonella* monthly. An alternative to taking environmental samples for one specific agent is to count the total number of bacteria present on hospital surfaces using either swabs or contact plates (Morley and Weese, 2008). In order for this to be an effective form of surveillance, it would need to be done routinely because bacteria can be found on most surfaces, and a baseline normal number of bacteria would need to be determined for each hospital surface cultured.

WRITING THE INFECTION CONTROL PLAN

Before writing an infection control plan, a staff member should be designated as the head of infection control. This individual is responsible for implementing the infection control program, updating the protocols on at least an annual basis, handling incident reporting, collecting and disseminating data, keeping records, and monitoring compliance.

As outlined by the National Association of Public Health Veterinarian's Compendium of Veterinary Standard Precautions (Elchos et al., 2008), an effective infection control plan should meet the following criteria:

- Reflect the principles of infection control as previously discussed
- Be specific to the facility and practice type
- Be flexible so that new issues can be addressed easily and new knowledge incorporated
- Provide explicit and well-organized guidance
- Clearly describe the infection control responsibilities of all staff members
- Include a process for the evaluation of infection control practices
  Provide contact information, resources, and references, specifically reportable disease list, public health contacts, local rabies codes and environmental health regulations, OSHA requirements, websites, and client education materials

An essential component of infection control is the need for continual updating of the documented policies. Emerging and re-emerging diseases, such as the influenza virus and antibiotic-resistant bacteria, require that the infection control policies be updated on at least an annual basis to take into account new information about transmission, prevention, and control of those agents. The infection control procedures should also include specific instructions for data collection of those agents relevant to the practice type, such as antimicrobial resistance, zoonotic diseases, or nosocomial infections.

EDUCATION, TRAINING, AND ENFORCEMENT

Without staff education, training, and enforcement, a written infection control policy will not be effective. Education and training help ensure consistency in use of the procedures and also allow for a thorough review process of all policies decided upon. In addition, documented policies demonstrate due diligence on the part of the practice and can be useful from a legal liability standpoint should there be an occurrence of nosocomial or zoonotic infection (Morley and Weese, 2008).

CONCLUSION

Every veterinary facility, large or small, should have a biosecurity program that describes the prevention methods employed to protect the patients, staff, and owners. There is no one plan that fits all facilities, but the risk of disease transmission can be minimized by employing basic hand hygiene and prevention strategies.

Regular reassessment of protocols is necessary to keep up with the continual emergence of new infectious diseases. Once a biosecurity program is developed, a large amount of time will be spent in the areas of education and compliance. A biosecurity program is only successful when, as a whole, the entire unit has a "by in" to the program. This in turns creates compliance and with that you have a strong foundation with accountability.

REFERENCES

Benedict KM, Morley PS, Van Metre DC. 2008. Characteristics of biosecurity and infection control programs at veterinary teaching hospitals. *J Am Vet Med Assoc* 233(5):767–773.

Blasco JM. 2010. Control and eradication strategies for brucella melitensis infection in sheep and goats. Presented at the International Scientific Conference for Brucellosis in South Eastern Europe and the Mediterranean Region. *Prilozi* 31(1):145–165. Available at: http://www.manu.edu.mk/prilozi.

Dunowska M, Morley PS, Traub-Dargatz JL, VanMetre DC. 2007. Biosecurity, in DC Sellon, M Long, eds. *Equine Infectious Diseases*, Saunders, Philadelphia, pp 528–539.

Ekiri AB, et al. 2009. Epidemiologic analysis of nosocomial *Salmonella* infections in hospitalized horses. *J Am Vet Med Assoc* 234(1):108–119.

Elchos BL, et al. 2008. Compendium of veterinary standard precautions for zoonotic disease prevention in veterinary personnel. *J Am Vet Med Assoc* 233:415–432.

Fridkin SL, et al. 1996. The role of understaffing in central venous catheter-associated bloodstream infections. *Infect Control Hosp Epidemiol* 17(3):150–158.

Gueirard P, et al. 1995. Human *Bordetella bronchiseptica* infection related to contact with infected animals: persistence of bacteria in host. *J Clin Microbiol* 33:2002–2006.

Harbarth S, et al. 1999. Outbreak of *Enterobacter cloacae* related to understaffing, overcrowding, and poor hygiene practices. *Infect Control Hosp Epidemiol* 20:598–603.

Hewlett EL. 1995. Bordetella species, in GL Mandel, JE Bennett, R Dolin, eds. *Principles and Practice of Infectious Diseases*, Churchill Livingstone, New York, pp 2078–2084.

Lappin MR. 2003. Prevention of infectious diseases, in RW Nelson, CG Couto, eds. *Small Animal Internal Medicine, 3rd ed.*, Mosby, St. Louis, MO, pp 1250–1258.

Manning SE, et al. 2008. Human rabies prevention–United States 2008: recommendations of the Advisory Committee on Immunization Practices. *MMWR Recomm Rep* 57(RR-3):1–28.

Morley PS. 2002. Biosecurity of veterinary practices. *Vet Clin North Am Food Anim Pract* 18:133–155.

Morley PS. 2004. Surveillance for nosocomial infections in veterinary hospitals. *Vet Clin North Am Equine Pract* 20:561–576.

Morley PS, Weese JS. 2008. Biosecurity and infection control for large animal practices, in BP Smith, ed. *Large Animal Internal Medicine, 4th ed.*, Elsevier, New York, pp 1524–1550.

[OSHA] Occupational Safety and Health Administration. 1992. Bloodborne pathogens. Toxic and Hazardous Substances. Regulations standard 1910.1030(b). Available at: http://www.osha.gov/pls/oshaweb/owadisp.show_document?p_table=standards&p_id=10051.

Osterholm MT, Hedberg CW, Moore KA. 2000. Epidemiology of infectious diseases, in GL Mandell, JE Bennett, R Dolin, eds. *Principles and Practice of Infectious Diseases, 5th ed.*, Churchill Livingstone, Philadelphia, pp 161–163.

Petersen CA, Dvorak G, Steneroden K, Spickler AR. 2008. *Maddie's Infection Control Manual for Animal Shelters for Veterinary Personnel, 1st ed.*, Center for Food Security and Public Health, Ames, IA.

Traub-Dargatz JL, Morley PS, Acteo HW, Slovis NM. 2009. Criteria for determination of infectious contagious disease risk level of large animal patients and on-farm new arrivals. American College of Veterinary Internal Medicine Convention Round Table Discussion, Montreal.

U.S. Department of Labor. 1970. Occupational Safety and Health Act of 1970, General Duty Clause. Available at: http://www.osha.gov/pls/oshaweb/owadisp.show_document?p_table=OSHACT&p_id=3359.

Vicca AF. 1999. Nursing staff workload as a determinant of methicillin-resistant *Staphylococcus aureus* spread in an adult intensive therapy unit. *J Hosp Infect* 43:109–113.

Weese JS, Clooten J, Kruth S, Arroyo L. 2008. Prevelence and risk factors for *Clostridium difficile* colonization in dogs and cats hospitalized in an intensive care unit. *Vet Microbiol* 129:209–214.

Wright JG, et al. 2005. Multidrug-resistant Salmonella Typhimurium in four animal facilities. *Emerg Infect Dis* 11(8):1235–1241.

2 Microbiology Review

Kit T. Darling and Barbara Jones

Infection prevention requires an understanding of the agents that cause infectious disease in order to know how to efficiently and adequately intervene in a specific infectious process. This chapter will provide background information on the various pathogenic organisms and review the process of obtaining samples for diagnostic purposes.

THE SCIENCE OF MICROBIOLOGY

Microbiology is the study of microorganisms that cannot be seen with the naked eye. Bacteria, fungi, viruses, and protozoa are included in the science of microbiology. The majority of these microorganisms are nonpathogenic. This chapter will focus on pathogenic microorganisms that invade, establish, and grow in the host tissue, causing infection. The information provided will include the application of microbiology, bacteria, fungi, viruses, protozoa, and prions.

SPECIMEN SELECTION, COLLECTION, AND TRANSPORT

Proper specimen selection, good technique in specimen collection, and proper transport are important in obtaining results that can aid in the diagnosis of infection in the animal. Poor technique may lead to contamination and overgrowth of the causative organism. The following are some basic principles for specimen selection, collection, and transport:

1. Whenever possible, obtain specimens before antimicrobial therapy has begun. If antimicrobial therapy has been started prior to obtaining the specimen, inform the laboratory as to which antimicrobial agent the patient is receiving.
2. Specimen must be obtained aseptically.
3. Specimen must be obtained from a site that is representative of the disease process.
4. Sufficient quantity of material must be obtained.
5. To prevent contamination of the specimen, all specimens should be placed or collected in a sterile container.

Veterinary Infection Prevention and Control, First Edition. Edited by Linda Caveney and Barbara Jones with Kimberly Ellis.
© 2012 John Wiley & Sons, Inc. Published by John Wiley & Sons, Inc.

6. The specimen must be collected at the proper time in the course of the disease. The best specimens are collected during the acute phase of the infection and before the initiation of antimicrobial therapy.
7. Aspirates, body fluids, and tissues are the best specimens.
8. Swabs can be used for collecting specimens from pustules, ears, conjunctiva, soft-tissue infections, deep-draining tracts or wounds, and the reproductive tract.
9. The preferred swabs have plastic shafts and are calcium alginate, rayon, or Dacron.
10. Specimens are placed in transport systems to maintain the organism in an environment in which it is viable, has the appropriated aerobic or anaerobic conditions, and will prevent overgrowth of contaminates.
11. Urines may be refrigerated to preserve viability and prevent overgrowth, whereas other specimens that may have anaerobes or other fastidious organisms should be held at room temperature.
12. Label the specimen with patient identification information and complete the submission form with the patient's identification, date, source or site of the specimen, tests requested, and other relevant clinical information (Songer and Post, 2005).

LABORATORY DIAGNOSTICS

The specific diagnostic tests for the identification of microorganisms vary greatly but usually include direct exam under a microscope, isolation of the organisms, biochemical reactions, and detection of organisms by immunologic or molecular procedures. Figure 2.1 illustrates a flowchart for processing microbiology specimen.

The specimen is inoculated broth (liquid media) and agar (solid media). Broth allows the recovery of organisms that are fastidious and also allows for the recovery of a small number of organisms. The inoculation of the specimen on agar allows for the isolation of organisms into separate colonies. Initially, most specimens are inoculated on blood agar and MacConkey agar. Identification of the bacteria is done by visual examination of the colony morphology, color, and hemolysis; gram staining the colony; inoculation into biochemical reagents; and analysis of those reactions. Figure 2.2 shows the identification of bacteria.

Often veterinary practices choose to send specimens for culture and identification to microbiology laboratories that have the appropriate equipment and expertise. Most bacteria optimal growth temperatures are 35–37°C, with the exception of *Campylobacter jejuni,* which grows at 42°C. Most fungi grow at 25–30°C. Most bacteria grow aerobically (with oxygen, usually room air), whereas some require CO_2 or anaerobic conditions (without oxygen). Most gram-positive bacteria do not grow on MacConkey agar.

In addition to the identification of the organism, antimicrobial susceptibility testing is important in determining which antimicrobial might be used to treat the infection in the animal. The most common testing method in veterinary medicine is disc diffusion or Kirby-Bauer. This method is flexible, simple, and relatively low cost. Another method often used, especially if the specimen is processed by a reference laboratory, is the dilution susceptibility test. Broth microdilution is widely used and can be semiautomated. In this method, microtiter plates contain several antimicrobials agents tested against a single isolate. The minimum inhibitory concentration of the antimicrobial completely inhibits the bacterial growth. Standardized reference methodology for testing of human and animal pathogens in the United States is provided by the Clinical and Laboratory Standards Institutes (CLSI). Interpretation and understanding of antimicrobial susceptibility testing are important in selecting the appropriate antimicrobial therapy.

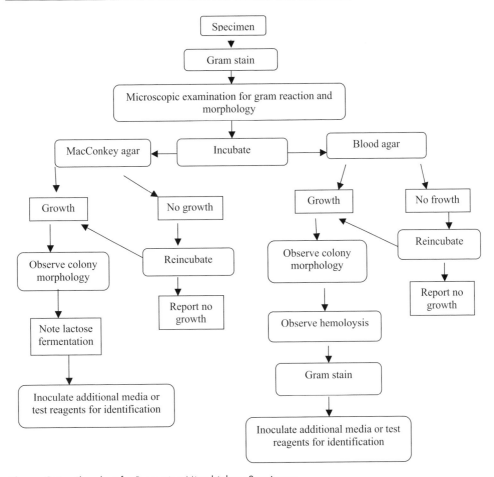

Figure 2.1   Flowchart for Processing Microbiology Specimens

BACTERIA

Bacteria are divided into two groups: gram positive and gram negative. Gram-positive bacteria stain blue because of a thick uniformed cell wall composed of peptidoglycan and techoic acids. Gram-negative bacteria stain pink to red because the cell wall is a more complex structure with an outer membrane and periplasmic space with a small amount of peptidoglycan (Quinn and Markey, 2003).

In addition to differentiating whether a bacteria is gram-positive or gram-negative, the morphology or shape of the bacteria also helps in its identification. Bacteria may be rods or cocci, and the arrangement may include single, pairs, or clusters.

Gram-Positive Bacteria

The gram-positive cocci include *Staphylococcus* and *Streptococcus*. The gram-positive rods include *Bacillus, Clostridium, Corynebacteria, Mycobacteria, Corynebacteria, Actinomyces, Listeria, Rhodococcus*, and *Erysipelothrix*.

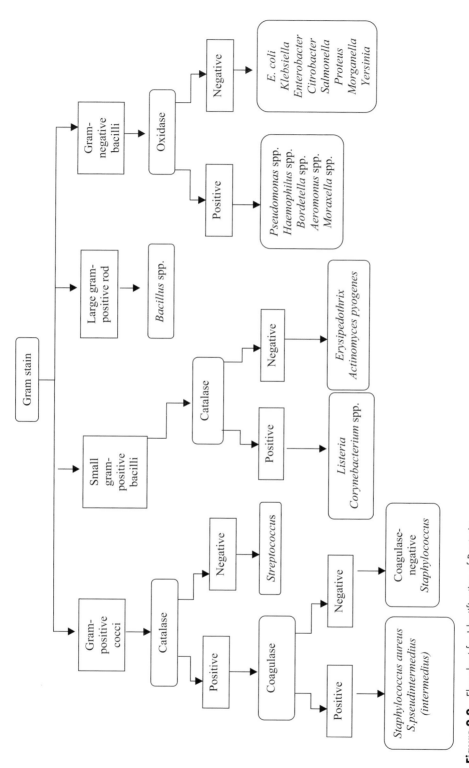

Figure 2.2 Flowchart for Identification of Bacteria

Staphylococcus

Staphylococci are gram-positive cocci that occur in grapelike clusters, pairs, or singly. The colonies are white to off-white or yellow, with a smooth surface and consistency that resembles butter. They are catalase positive and coagulase positive or negative. *S. aureus* and *S. intermedius* are beta hemolytic on blood agar, whereas other species are not. *Staphylococcus* is found on the skin of animals and humans and on mucous membranes as well as in the environment. They are opportunistic pathogens. Animals and humans may be colonized or have active infections of *Staphylococcus*. They cause a variety of suppurative infections in animals. Methicillin-resistant *S. aureus* emerged as a problem in human medicine and is now a concern in veterinary medicine.

Streptococcus

Streptococci are gram-positive cocci in chains that are catalase negative, non-spore-forming, and nonmotile. The colonies are small and shiny. They may exhibit alpha (incomplete hemolysis, greenish area), beta (complete hemolysis, clear area), or gamma (no hemolysis) hemolysis on blood agar. In the 1930s, Rebecca Lancefied developed a grouping technique based on species-specific carbohydrate cell wall antigens. The groups are A through H and K through V. The animal pathogenic streptococci are A, B, C, D, E, G, L, and V. There are a few streptococci that cannot be grouped (Songer and Post, 2005). *S. pneumoniae*, alpha hemolytic streptococcus, is sensitive to optochin. *Enterococcus*, found in the gastrointestinal tract, is bile esculin positive. This organism has emerged as a pathogen of several domestic animals and causes enteritis, septicemia, respiratory disease, mastitis, and urinary tract infections.

Actinomyces

Actinomyces are gram-positive, non-spore-forming, non-acid-fast rods and are facultatively anaerobic. Most species will produce mycelium, and angular branching is common. *Actinomyces* are slow-growing, small, nodular, white colonies (Hendrix and Sirois, 2007). *A. bovis, A. suis,* and *A. viscosus* are most often associated with disease in domestic animals

Arcanobacterium

Arcanobacterium is a gram-positive, pleomorphic (irregular), non-spore-forming rod that is catalase positive. The colonies are small and hemolytic. The following species may cause disease in animals (Songer and Post, 2005):

1. *A. haemolyticum*: equine vaginitis
2. *A. phocae*: seal septicemia
3. *A. pluranimalium*: deer lung abscess; porpoise splenic abscess
4. *A. pyogenes*: bovine mastitis, liver abscesses, endocarditis, endometritis, abortion; caprine mastitis; porcine septic arthritis, endocarditis; poultry osteomyelitis, nephritis; ovine abortion, endometritis, pneumonia

Corynebacterium

Corynebacteria are catalase-positive, urease-positive, non-spore-forming, non-acid-fast, pleomorphic gram-positive rods that are usually nonmotile. They may appear as "Chinese letter" (Tighe and Brown, 2008). The following are species that cause disease in animals:

1. *C. pseudotuberculosis*: goat and sheep caseous lymphadenitis. Infected animals should be isolated and possibly cull chronically infected animals. Fomites may transmit the organism. Thorough disinfection of any item that comes into contact with the animal is necessary.
2. *C.* renale: sheep, cattle, and pig urinary tract infections

Rhodococcus

The only pathogen in this genus is *Rhodococcus equi*, which is an aerobic, catalase-positive, gram-positive, pleomorphic coccobacillus. Colonies will appear salmon pink to red and mucoid with no hemolysis. The organism is a cause of foal pneumonia and was previously known as *Corynebacterium equi*.

Norcardia

Members of the genus *Norcardia* are non-spore-forming, aerobic, nonmotile, catalase positive, and they reduce nitrates and oxidize sugars. They are pleomorphic and take the form of cocci, rods, or diptheroids. They may produce hyphae or branching filaments. *Norcardia* is weakly acid fast. It is a slow grower, and plates should be held for 7–10 days. Depending on the species, colonies are small, dry, granular, and may vary in color from white to pink to orange to tan (Engelkirk and Duben-Engelkirk, 2008).

Mycobacteria

Members of the genus *Mycobacterium* are aerobic, acid-fast, non-spore-forming, nonmotile, catalase-positive, gram-positive rods. They may stain irregular and appear beaded. Some members are slow growers requiring 7–14 days or longer. They are difficult to grow and require specialized media. If *Mycobacterium* is suspected, it is best to send the specimen to a reference laboratory that has the specialized media and conditions to safely handle these organisms.

Listeria

Listeria species are non-spore-forming, catalase-positive, oxidase-negative, motile, gram-positive coccobacillus. Colonies are small, transparent, and smooth. The three species that are important pathogens in animals are *L. monocytogenes, L. ivanovii,* and *L. innocua*.

Erysipelothrix

Erysipelothrix is a straight or slightly curved thin rod. It is gram positive but may appear as gram negative because it decolorizes easily. The organism may be single, in short chains, in pairs in the form of "V," or in groups. The colony is small, transparent, circular, and alpha hemolytic on blood agar. The colony may be in three different forms: smooth, intermediate, and rough. The organism is catalase negative, oxidase negative, and nonmotile. *E. rhusiopathiae* is found in tonsils and intestines in many species. It may cause septicemia, especially in swine, sheep, and fowl. This organism is resilient in the environment. For disinfectants to be effective in killing the organism, organic matter must be removed.

Bacillus

All members of the *Bacillus* genus form spores. Most of these organisms are catalase positive and motile. Even though they are gram positive, they may stain gram variable and appear as parallel-sided rods with endospores. They are medium to large colonies, grow only on blood agar, have a grainy or mucoid appearance, and may be hemolytic.

Clostridium

Clostridium is an anaerobic, spore-forming, large, gram-positive rod. They also may appear on gram stain as gram variable or gram negative. The spores may or may not be visible on gram stain. They can be differentiated by their biochemical reactions and toxin production. The animal pathogenic clostridia include the following (Songer and Post, 2005):

1. Neurotoxic: *C. botulinum, C. tetani*
2. Histotoxic: *C. perfringens, C. septicum, C. chauvoei, C. novyi*
3. Enteric: *C. difficile, C. perfringens, C. sordelli, C. colinum, C. spiroforme, C. piliforme*

Gram-Negative Bacteria

Many members of the family *Enterobacteriaceae* are pathogens in humans and animals. All of its members are gram-negative coccobacilli or bacilli, non-spore-forming, catalase negative (except *Shigella dysenteriae*), oxidase negative (except *Pleisomonas shigelloides*), reduce nitrate to nitrites, and grow on MacConkey agar (Engelkirk and Duben-Engelkirk, 2008). Media and tests that can be useful in the identification of these organisms are triple-sugar agar or Kligler iron agar, decarboxylase test, IMViC (indole, methyl red, Voges-Proskauer and citrate) reactions, decarboxylase, urea production, and nitrate reduction tests. Members of *Enterobacteriaceae* look alike on gram stain.

Escherichia

Member of the genus *Escherichia* are straight, medium-to-long, gram-negative rods occurring singly or in pairs. These organisms are aerobic, oxidase negative, catalase positive, produce acid and gas from D-glucose, and have both oxidative and fermentative metabolism. They ferment lactose. *E. coli* is the most significant pathogen in this genus and inhabits the intestinal tract of most vertebrates with colonization occurring shortly after birth. *E. coli* associated with gastrointestinal disease may be enterotoxigenic, enteropathogenic, enterohemorrhagic, or necrotoxigenic. Septicemia and nonenteric localized disease may occur with *E. coli*. This organism may occur as a pathogen of the urinary tract, or opportunistic *E. coli* may invade the body to produce localized or systemic effects. *E.coli* is large, smooth, mucoid colonies on blood agar with variable hemolysis. On MacConkey agar, the colonies are hot pink to red (Hendrix and Sirois, 2007).

Klebsiella

The genus *Klebsiella* is nonhemolytic on blood agar, shiny gray colonies that ferment lactose. They are indole-negative, nonmotile, Voges-Proskauer-positive, citrate-positive, urea-positive, gram-negative rods. These organisms are common in nature and are found in water, sewage, and soil. The most common pathogen is *K. pneumoniae*, which causes a variety of infectious processes, including bovine mastitis, equine metritis, pyometria, cystitis, pneumonia, and neonatal septicemia. It causes various infections in a number of species. *K. pneumoniae* appear as large, sticky, white, nonhemolytic colonies on blood agar and as large, mucoid, pink colonies on MacConkey agar.

Enterobacter

Enterobacter are gray, shiny, nonhemolytic, gram-negative rods that ferment lactose. Members of this genus are motile, indole negative, citrate positive, Voges-Proskauer positive, and urease negative. They can cause urinary tract infections, mastitis, septicemia, and wound infections in a variety of animal species.

Citrobacter

The members of the genus *Citrobacter* are shiny, gray, lactose-fermenting, nonhemolytic, gram-negative rods. They are usually motile, Voges-Proskauer positive, citrate positive, and may or may not be urease positive. These organisms are opportunistic pathogens.

Proteus

The members of genus *Proteus* are small, gram-negative rods and appear colorless or white on MacConkey agar because they are non-lactose fermenting. Most *Proteus* swarms on blood agar. They are oxidase negative, urease positive, reduce nitrate to nitrite, and produce hydrogen sulfide. This organism can cause urinary tract infections.

Morganella

Morganella are gram-negative rods that are motile, oxidase negative, indole positive, methyl red positive, urease positive, and nitrate positive, but they do not swarm on blood agar. *Morganella morganii* is a flat colony and non-lactose fermenting.

Salmonella

The genus *Salmonella* has approximately 2500 serovars (Songer and Post, 2005) The organism is a motile, gram-negative rod. It is nonfermenting, produces H_2S, methyl red positive, and utilizes citrate. Salmonella are non-lactose fermenting except for *S. enterica* ssp. *arizonae* and *S. enterica* ssp. *diarizonae* (Songer and Post, 2005) Enrichment broth and selective and differential media are used to isolate *Salmonella*. Tetrathionate broth is the enrichment broth frequently used, and selective media include xylose lysine deoxycholate (XLD) and Hektoen enteric (HE) agar. On XLD or HE agar, the colonies will have black centers due to H_2S production. Immunoassays may be used to detect somatic (O) and flagellar (H) antigens. Serovar-specific antigens are commercially available, and some laboratories use polymerase chain reaction (PCR) methods to identify *Salmonella*. *Salmonella* is a pathogen of the gastrointestinal tract.

Yersinia

Yersinia is a non-lactose-fermenting, oxidase-negative, catalase-positive, methyl red gram-negative rod. All are motile with the exception of *Y. pestis*. *Yersinia* is pinpoint, gray-white, translucent colonies at 24 hours. At 48 hours, they are gray-white to light yellow and opaque. *Y. pestis* is slow growing, raised, irregular and has a "fried egg" appearance that becomes more pronounced with age. *Y. pestis* often will grow better at 28°C.

Gram-Negative Bacilli: Nonfermenters

These organisms do not ferment glucose, may or may not grow on MacConkey agar, and are oxidase and nitrate variable.

Pseudomonas

Members of the genus *Pseudomonas* are straight or slightly curved gram-negative bacilli. They are aerobic, non-spore forming, motile by one or more polar flagella, oxidase positive, and catalase positive. Most species are nitrate positive. *Pseudomonas* grows well in wet areas. *P. aeruginosa* is a significant pathogen in humans and animals. The colony may have a blue-green appearance. Some may produce a red or brown pigment. Some strains produce a mucoid or runny appearance.

Burkholderia

More than 20 species make up the genus *Burkholderia.* Two of these are animal pathogens *B. mallei* and *B. pseudomallei.* Both of these species are classified as select agents and must be reported to the CDC. If these organisms are suspected in samples, biosafety level 3 precautions should be used. Members of the genus *Burkholderia* are non-spore forming, catalase positive, and grow on MacConkey agar. They would be isolated from blood or tissue. Selective medium facilitates their isolation.

Bordetella

Bordetella is most commonly isolated from respiratory samples that may include nasal or tracheal swabs, transtracheal washes, and lung tissue. They are transmitted from one host to another by aerosol. All members of this genus are catalase positive, and optimum growth is 35°C to 37°C. Most grow on blood agar and MacConkeys with the exception of *B. pertussis.* The species are differentiated by their appearance and growth on blood agar and MacConkey agars, oxidase production, urease reaction, nitrate production, citrate use, and motility.

Actinobacillus

Actibacilli are pleomorphic and appear as dots and dashes on gram stain. Some species are hemolytic on blood agar, and others are not. The colonies may be waxy or sticky. They are usually oxidase positive, catalase variable, and nitrate positive.

Mannheimia

The genus *Mannheimia* was formerly a member of the genus *Pasteurella*. All members of *Mannheimia* ferment mannitol and do not ferment D-mannose. They grow on blood agar and are smooth, grayish colonies with variable beta hemolysis. Like *Pasteurella*, they are nonmotile, gram-negative coccobacilli or rods. Oxidase is usually positive, and nitrate is reduced to nitrite.

Pasteurella

Pasteurella will grow on blood agar and will grow better on chocolate agar. This gram-negative organism has variable morphology and colony morphology on blood agar. It is most frequently isolated from the affected tissue. Knowing from which animal the species has been isolated is helpful in identification because many have unique host predilections.

Brucella

Members of *Brucella* are gram-negative coccobacilli or small rods. They are motile, oxidase positive, catalase positive, reduce nitrate, and are urease positive except for *B. ovis*. They are negative for idole, methyl red, and Voges-Proskauer. They may be transmitted by aerosol and have been classified as a potential bioterrorism agent. *Brucella* may survive in the environment for long periods of time under appropriate conditions. They may survive for 125 days in soil, 1 year in feces, and 6 months in carcasses and tissue. The organism is susceptible to most disinfectants, including, 1% bleach, 70% alcohol, phenoics, iodophors, gluteraldehyde, and formaldehyde. It can be inactivated by moist heat (121°C for longer than 15 minutes) and dry heat (160–170°C for 1 hour or more) (Songer and Post, 2005).

Francisella

The pathogen and potential bioterrorism agent *F. tularensis* is a small, pleomorphic, gram-negative coccobacillus. The organism may be grown on glucose cysteine blood agar, chocolate agar, buffered charcoal-yeast agar, modified Thayer-Martin medium, and thioglycolate broth. The colonies are smooth and gray. On blood-based media, the colony will be surrounded by a characteristic green zone of discoloration. Because of the risk for airborne transmission, many laboratories avoid trying to grow this organism. Serology using tube agglutination, microagglutination, or enzyme-linked immunosorbent assay (ELISA) may be used as a diagnostic test.

FUNGI

Some infectious processes may be caused by fungi. Like with bacteria, the proper specimen selection, collection, and transport are important for accurate identification. With a basic knowledge of mycology (study of fungi), many fungal infections can be presumptively diagnosed in the veterinary clinic. This requires minimal equipment and reagents, including a microscope, 10% potassium hydroxide (KOH) in glycerol, india ink, stain [such as lactophenol cotton blue, Diff-Quik, or gram stain (fungi will stain blue)], glass slides, cover slips, and a book with an atlas of medical mycology. The specimens are the same types as the bacteria with the addition of hair clippings, nail clippings, and skin scrapings. The same guidelines that were stated in the bacteria section apply to the collection of fungi specimens. The specimens should be collected, if possible, before the administration of antifungal agents. Figure 2.3 illustrates a flowchart for processing fungal specimens.

Fungal identification is done by microscopic examination of clinical material and/or isolates obtained by fungal cultures. Initially, wet mounts are done on the clinical specimen. The specimen is placed on a glass slide, and one to two drops of 10% KOH are added. The specimen may be incubated at room temperature for 30 minutes or gently heated on a slide warmer or

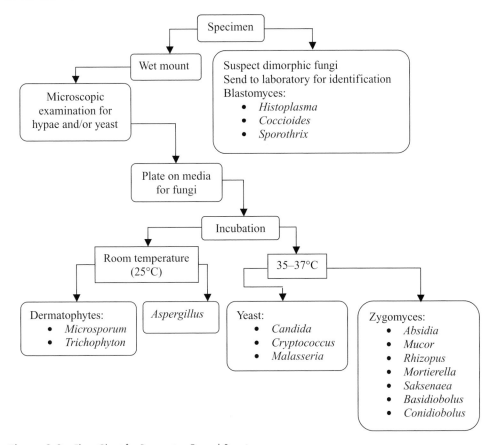

Figure 2.3   Flow Chart for Processing Fungal Specimens

passed several times through the flame of a Bunsen burner. Then, the slide is examined under the microscope. One of the previously mentioned stains may be used to enhance the visibility of the fungi morphology.

The most common media used for fungi is Sabouraud dextrose agar. Other types of media that may be used are brain heart infusion agar with or without blood and/or antibiotics added, Sabhi agar with or without antibiotics, potato dextrose with or without antibiotics, and dermatophyte test media. Mycosel may also be used for the isolation of dermatophytes. Antimicrobial agents are often added to fungal media to inhibit the growth of bacteria that otherwise might overgrow the fungi. Plates are incubated at 25–30°C for up to 6 weeks. If dimorphic fungi are suspected, then 5% blood is incorporated and the plates should be incubated at 35–37°C.

Yeast may be identified both by morphology and physiologic reactions. Several commercial yeast identification systems are available.

Other methods used to identify mycoses may include histological examination of biopsy material and latex agglutination and enzyme immunoassay tests for fungal antigens.

The fungal pathogens of veterinary importance include the dermatophytes, yeasts, and dimorphic and opportunistic fungi. Table 2.1 shows a summary of the most common pathogenic fungi of veterinary importance.

Table 2.1 Most Common Pathogenic Fungi of Veterinary Importance

Organism	Species affected	Disease or lesion	Specimens
Microsporum		Ringworm	Fresh hairs and skin scrapings from edge of lesion
M. canis	Dogs, cats		
M. gallinae	Poultry		
M. gypsem	Horses, dogs, cats, other		
M. nanum	Pigs		
Trichophyton			
T. equinum	Horses, donkeys		
T. mentagrophytes	Most animal species		
T. verrucosum	Cattle		
Candida	Many animal species	Lesions, infections of oral and intestinal mucosa	Affected tissue or scraping from tissue
Malassezia pachydermatis	Dogs	Chronic otitis	Ear swabs
Cryptococcus neoformans	Cattle	Mastitis	Affected tissue, lung, brain
Coccidioides immitis	Horses, cattle, sheep, dogs, cats, captive feral animals	Granulomas, often in bronchial and mediastinal lymph nodes and lungs; lesions in brain, spleen, liver, kidney	Affected tissue
Histoplasma capsulatum	Dogs, cats, horses, sheep, pigs, people	Granulomas in lungs, lesions of intestine, liver, spleen, lymph nodes	Affected tissue
Blastomyces dermatitidis	Dogs, cats, people	Granulomas in lungs, skin	Affected tissue
Sporothrix schenkii	Horses, dogs, cattle, pigs, fowl, people	Subcutaneous nodules or granulomas, may involve bone and visceral organs	Pus, granulomas
Aspergillus	Many animal species and birds	Lesions	Deep scrapings or affected tissue

Dermatophytes

The dermatophytes are a group of septate fungi that invade keratinized tissue, including hair, nails, and superficial layers of skin. Lesions may exhibit crusty debris and be characterized by a spreading area of pruritus. The lesion may be single or multifocal and have variable hair loss. The most common dermatophytes of veterinary importance are from genus *Microsporum* and *Trichophyton*. The most significant are *Microsporum canis, M. gallinae, M. gypseum, M. nanum, Trichophyton metagrophytes, T. equinum*, and *T. verrucosum*.

Yeasts

The yeasts that are the most important animal pathogens are *Candida* species (especially *Candida albicans*), *Cryptococcus neoformans*, and *Malassezia pachydermatis*. Antibiotic therapy and immunosuppression can disturb the resident flora on mucosal surfaces causing overgrowth of yeast and may lead to tissue invasion.

Candida

The genus *Candida* has more than 200 species. They are normal inhabitants of the alimentary, upper respiratory, and genital mucosa of animals. Primarily they are associated with infections of the mucous membranes and skin; however, they can invade most organs of the body. *Candida albicans* is the most common pathogen of this genus. This organism grows aerobically at 25–37°C on a variety of media, including Sabouraud dextrose agar. The colonies are circular, creamy, white, and opaque. On gram stain, *C. albicans* may appear as budding yeast or in the form of pseudohyphae or hyphage. The germ tube test is a presumptive test to differentiate *C. albicans* from other *Candida* species. The test is done by placing several colonies from nonselective fungal media in animal serum and incubating at 37°C for 3 hours. Under the microscope, the germ tubes appear as short hyphal segments without constriction (Songer and Post, 2005).

Cryptococcus neoformans

Cryptococcus neoformans grows as yeast in infected tissue and the environment. This organism is an opportunistic yeast, and diagnosis can be established by fungal isolation, cytology, histology, and serology. India ink may be used to stain impression smears of lesions. Upon examination of the smears, there will be encapsulated yeast cells that are round or oval with thin, dark walls. The buds are on narrow bases. *Cryptococcus* can grow on a variety of media and appear as a mucoid colony that is cream, tan, or yellowish in color. *C. neoformans* is the only species that has the ability to grow at 37°C.

Malassezia

Malassezia species are normal cutaneous flora of animals and humans. *Malassezia pachydermatis* is the species of veterinary importance and is associated with otitis externa and dermatitis. Cytology is most useful for diagnosis, and the yeast will have a slightly elongated oval or bottled-shaped morphology with a thick wall and unipolar budding. Finding 10 yeasts per high-power field is considered diagnostic (Songer and Post, 2005).

Dimopthic fungi

The dimorphic fungi occur in two forms: the mold form and the yeast form. They exist in the environment as the mold form and will grow on Sabouraud dextrose agar incubated at 25–30°C. They have a white, cottony appearance that turns brown with age. These organisms will grow as yeast on brain heart infusion agar incubated at 37°C and appear as cream to tan, wrinkled, and waxy. The most common dimorphic fungi in domestic animals are *Blastomyces dermatitdis*, *Histoplasma capsulatum,* and *Coccidioides immitis* and enter the host through the respiratory tract. Another dimorphic fungus, *Sporothrix schenckii*, causes infections in horses, cats, dogs, and humans. This fungus may cause chronic cutaneous or lymphocutaneous disease.

VIRUS

Viruses do not reproduce without a host cell and are described as intracellular parasites. A virus particle consists of nucleic acid, either RNA or DNA, and a protein coat called the capsid. Some viruses have an outer envelope. Figure 2.4 provides a diagram of the virus classified by nucleic acid replication and viral families.

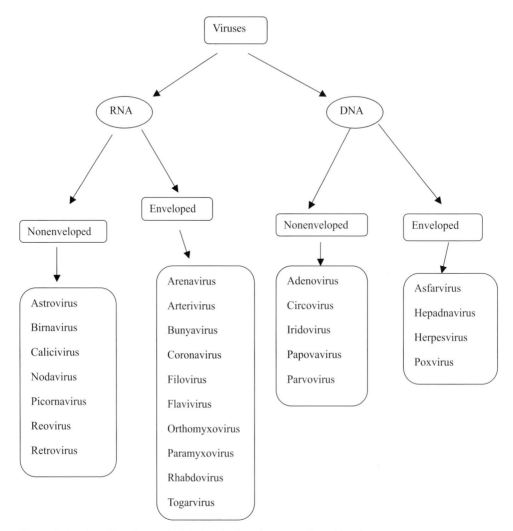

Figure 2.4 Virus Classification by Nucleic Acid Replication and Viral Families

Viruses range in size from 20 to 300 microns (Quinn and Markey, 2003). Usually, viruses are host and tissue specific. Viral infections may produce clinical signs in the acute or chronic stage or no clinical signs in a subclinical infection. There are more than 200 viral diseases of veterinary importance that affect animals. Table 2.2 contains some of the common viral diseases of veterinary importance.

Laboratory diagnosis requires examination of the appropriate specimen along with the correlation of clinical signs. Ideally, clinical specimens should be collected as early as possible (3–7 days after the onset of symptoms) before secondary bacterial or fungal infections become established.

The collection and type of specimen are dependent on the laboratory procedure used to diagnose the viral infection. The laboratory procedure may be virus isolation (cell culture), antigen or antibody detection, molecular procedure, or histology or cytology. Contact the laboratory for information about what type of specimen to collect, pertinent information needed about the

Table 2.2 Common Viral Diseases of Veterinary Importance

Species	Virus	Disease/Consequences of infection	Enveloped
Canine	Canine adenovirus 1	Infectious canine hepatitis	No
	Canine adenovirus 2	Infectious canine tracheobronchitis	No
	Canine distemper virus (paramyxovirus)	Highly contagious respiratory and neurologic disease	Yes
	Canine parainfluenza virus (paramyxovirus)	Respiratory infection	Yes
	Canine parvovirus 2	Highly contagious enteric disease	No
	Canine herpesvirus 1	Upper respiratory tract or external genitalia infection, fatal for neonatal pups	Yes
Feline	Feline calicivirus	Upper respiratory tract infection	No
	Feline coronavirus	Feline infectious peritonitis	Yes
	Feline herpesvirus 1	Feline viral rhinotracheitis	Yes
	Feline immunodeficiency virus (retrovirus/lentivirus)	Affects immune system	Yes
	Feline panleukopenia virus	Feline infectious enteritis	No
	Feline leukemia virus (retrovirus)	Feline leukemia virus	Yes
Equine	Equine adenovirus A	Mild respiratory infection	No
	Equine influenza A (orthomyxovirus)	H7N7 causes acute respiratory disease	Yes
	Equine herpesvirus 1 & 4	Equine rhinopneumonitis Equine herpesvirus abortion	Yes
	Equine encephalitis virus (EEEV, WEEV, VEEV) (togavirus)	Mild fever and depression to fatal febrile encephalomyelitis	Yes
	Equine infectious anemia (retrovirus-lentivirus)	Equine infectious anemia	Yes
Bovine	Bovine adenovirus	Mild respiratory and enteric disease	No
	Bovine leukemia virus (retrovirus)	Bovine leukemia virus	Yes
	Foot and mouth disease (picornavirus)	Highly contagious disease with fever and vesicles on epithelial surfaces	No
	Bovine herpesvirus 1, 2, & 5	Infectious bovine rhinotracheitis and pustular vulvovaginitis	Yes
All mammals	Rabies (rhabdovirus)	Central nervous system disease	Yes

animal and the specimen, and the appropriate conditions for transport of the specimen. Some ELISA and latex agglutination test kits are available to run in veterinary clinics for some viral diseases.

PROTOZOA

Protozoa are unicellular eukaryotic organisms that are classified on the basis of their means or motility. The zoonotic parasitic organisms that are of significance in the veterinary field are

Giardia lamblia (also known as *Giardia intestinalis*), *Cryptosporidium parvum*, and *Toxoplasma gondii.*

Giardia

Giardia is a flagellated trophozoite with a "tear drop" shape, having two nuclei at the anterior end and tumbling motililty. The cyst is approximately 13 microns long and oval, with two to four nuclei. They can be diagnosed by direct microscopic observation of the trophozoite or cysts in the feces; either stained preparations or unstained wet mounts can be used. Several samples may be needed because shedding can be intermittent. Concentration method (i.e., zinc sulfate fecal flotation) is most commonly used. ELISA test can be used to detect *Giardia* antigens, and immunofluorescence can be used to visualize the organism.

These protozoal parasites are found most commonly in untreated or contaminated water, which is where Beaver Fever, the other common name for Giardiasis, comes from.

Cryptosporidium

Cryptosporidium is an obligate intracellular coccidian parasite. Mature oocysts are 4–5 microns in diameter and contain four flat, motile sporozoites. *Cryptosporidium parvum* is diagnosed after fecal flotation in sucrose or zinc sulfate solutions. Oocysts appear red after acid-fast staining. Repeat sampling may be necessary as the oocysts are not shed continuously. It can also be diagnosed with fresh intestinal scrapings.

The oocyst stages of *C. parvum* are found widespread in the environment and are extremely resistant in this state. They may survive for 2–6 months in a moist environment. The sporulated oocysts are shed in feces and are immediately infectious.

Toxoplasma

Toxoplasma is an obligate intracellular parasite. The major forms of the parasite are oocysts containing the sporozoites, which are shed in the feces; tachyzoites, rapidly multiplying form found in the tissues; bradyzoites, slowly multiplying form found in the tissue; and tissue cysts, walled structures often found in the muscle and central nervous system, containing the dormant form of the parasite bradyzoites.

In cats, active infections can be diagnosed by fecal flotation for oocysts. *Toxoplasma* oocysts are ovoid and 10–12 microns in diameter. It is difficult to differentiate *Toxoplasma* oocysts from *Hammondia*, *Isospora*, and *Besnotia* (CFSPH, 2007). Toxoplasmosis is often diagnosed by serology through means of ELISA tests, indirect fluorescent antibody (IFA) test, complement fixation, latex agglutination, and modified agglutination tests. IgG and IgM titers may distinguish between recent and older infections.

In all species, tachyzoites or bradyzoites may be found in aqueous humor in ocular disease, cerebrospinal fluid in neurologic disease, and in impression smears or biopsies from a variety of other tissues (CFSPH, 2007). On impression smears, the organism appears crescent-shaped and will stain with any Romanowsky stain. In thin sections, tachyzoites are found to stain similar to host cells, having an oval to round shape. Tissue cysts are usually ball-shaped, with silver-positive walls. Bradyzoites from tissue sections stain strongly with periodic acid Schiff stain (CFSPH, 2007).

Oocysts excreted in feces sporulate in the environment. This takes 1–5 days under perfect conditions but can take up to several weeks. The oocyst then contains two sporocytes, each with four sporozoites. The oocysts are highly resistant to environmental conditions and can remain infectious for as long as 18 months in water or warm, moist soils (CFSPH, 2007).

PRIONS

Prions are small infectious proteins that cause certain diseases in animals and humans. They cause fatal spongiform encephalopathies (disease of the brain). The brain becomes sponge-like and is filled with amyloid proteins, which replace the neurons that are normally present. Diseases caused by prions occur sporadically and are significantly influenced by the genome of the affected animal. These diseases are slow progressive neurodegenerative and have long incubation periods. Some diseases caused by prions in animals include bovine spongiform encephopathy, scrapie in sheep and goats, and chronic wasting disease in deer and elk. As a group, these diseases are called transmissible spongiform encephalopathies. Unlike viruses, they are devoid of nucleic acid. Prions are nonimmunogenic and extremely resistant to many chemicals, irradiation, and heat. They are stable at a wide range of pH and can last in the environment for years. Hamster-associated scrapie prions have been shown to survive in soil for at least 3 years. Diagnosis must be done at a USDA-approved state veterinary diagnostic lab. All transmissible spongiform encephalopathies are reportable. The following information on known transmissible spongiform encephalopathies gives important details that are points for infection control.

Bovine Spongiform Encephalopathy

Bovine spongiform encephalopathy (BSE), commonly known as mad cow disease, is a transmissible, chronic, fatal, neurodegenerative disease of the family *Bovidae*. An epidemiologic study of the United Kingdom epidemic suggests that transmission occurs by ingestion of meat and bone meal feed that contains neurologic tissue; however, there is some evidence that offspring of infected individuals are at increased risk through an unknown mechanism. Although BSE shows no evidence of horizontal transmission, it is considered potentially zoonotic through consumption of contaminated meat products.

BSE primarily affects the central nervous system; however, there is also limited involvement of the distal ileum and the retina. Incubation is 2–8 years, with a mean incubation of 4–5 years. Dairy and dairy crossbreeds are more prevalent than the beef breeds. The disease is fatal within a few weeks to a few months after onset of clinical signs. Clinical signs are those indicative of central nervous system disease and include behavior changes, gait changes, and abnormal posture.

There are no antemortem diagnostic tools for BSE and no gross lesions observable on postmortem examination. Currently, BSE can only be diagnosed on histologic samples of the central nervous system, particularly the mid-brain, and ELISA, immunohistochemistry, and immunoblot of the disease isoform of the prion protein in unfixed, fresh, or frozen brain tissue. A whole-brain sample with brain stem or medulla taken as soon after death as possible is required for histopathological examination. There have been three BSE cases in the United States, the last one in 2006; however, Canada had a confirmed case of BSE on May 15, 2009 (CDC, 2011a; OIE, 2002; WHO, 2002).

Chronic Wasting Disease

Chronic wasting disease (CWD) is a transmissible spongiform encephalopathy of cervids, specifically white-tailed deer, elk, moose, and mule deer in North American captive and wild cervid populations. In contrast with other transmissible spongiform encephalopathies, CWD is thought to be transmitted through direct animal-to-animal contact or through environmental contamination. Saliva from clinically infected deer has been shown to be infectious and provides a mechanism for environmental contamination as well as direct contact transmission. The incubation period is 18–24 months before clinical signs appear. Clinical signs include the behavioral changes seen in other transmissible spongiform encephalopathies, but progressive weight loss is the most obvious clinical sign. Antemortem diagnosis can be done with a tonsil biopsy; however, postmortem diagnosis through immunohistochemistry, immunoblotting, and ELISA is more common (CDC, 2011b; USGS, 2007).

Scrapie

Scrapie is a transmissible spongiform encephalopathy of sheep and goats. The primary route of transmission is thought to be from the ewe to her offspring, but it can also be transmitted through contact with the placenta or placental fluids. Incubation period is usually 2–5 years, and sheep can live for 1–6 months after clinical signs appear. Clinical signs include the behavioral and gait changes seen in BSE but also include pruritis. Scrapie can be diagnosed antemortem with a biopsy of the third eyelid lymphoid tissue, but it is also diagnosed through histopathologic examination (USDA factsheet, 2004).

Transmissible Mink Encephalopathy (TME)

Transmissible mink encephalopathy (TME) primarily occurs as outbreaks in the United States and other countries among ranch-raised mink, most likely caused by feed contaminated with an unknown agent (CFPSH, 2008). The unknown contaminant is currently thought to be a variant BSE prion (Baron, 2007). The last outbreak in the United States was in 1985. The incubation period is 6–12 months, and clinical signs include difficulty eating, changes in grooming, ataxia, and self-mutilation. Diagnosis is the same as other transmissible spongiform encephalopathies.

Feline Spongiform Encephalopathy

Feline spongiform encephalopathy (FSE) has been seen in housecats and captive wild felids and is caused by the same infectious prion strain as BSE. Transmission is thought to occur orally through ingestion of contaminated bovine tissue. Although the incubation period in housecats is unknown, the incubation period in cheetahs is thought to be 4–8 years. Clinical signs are initially behavioral (timidity or aggression), rapidly progressing to ataxia and hyperesthesia. Sample collection and diagnosis is the same as for BSE. High-risk bovine tissues have been banned from cat food since 1990, and bovine meat is no longer fed to captive wild felids. FSE has not been identified in the United States.

CONCLUSION

Microbiology is the study of microorganisms that are invisible to the naked eye. Clinical microbiology is the study of pathogens such as bacteria, fungi, viruses, protozoa or parasites, and prions that cause disease or infection. Proper specimen selection, collection, and transport are important in obtaining useful results that can aid in the diagnosis of infection in animals. Antimicrobial susceptibility testing assists in determining appropriate antimicrobial therapy to treat the infection. This chapter provides information about fundamental knowledge of microorganisms, basic laboratory techniques used in their identification, and significance as a pathogen.

REFERENCES

Aspinall V. 2006. *The Complete Textbook of Veterinary Nursing*, Elsevier, Philadelphia.

Baron T. 2007. Phenotypic similarity of transmissible mink encephalopathy in cattle and L-type bovine spongiform encephalopathy in a mouse model. *Emerg Infect Dis* 13: 1887–1894. Available at: http://www.cdc.gov/EID/content/13/12/pdfs/1887.pdf.

[CDC] Centers for Disease Control and Prevention. 2011a. National Center for Emerging and Zoonotic Infectious Diseases (NCEZID), Division of High-Consequence Pathogens and Pathology (DHCPP), United States Department of Health and Human Services. BSE (Bovine Spongiform Encephalopathy, or Mad Cow Disease). Available at: http://www.cdc.gov/ncidod/dvrd/bse/.

CDC. 2011b. National Center for Emerging and Zoonotic Infectious Diseases (NCEZID), Division of High-Consequence Pathogens and Pathology (DHCPP), United States Department of Health and Human Services. Chronic Wasting Disease (CWD). Available at: http://www.cdc.gov/ncidod/dvrd/cwd/.

[CFSPH] The Center for Food Security and Public Health, Iowa State University. 2007. Feline Spongiform Encephalopathy. Available at: http://www.cfsph.iastate.edu/Factsheets/pdfs/feline_spongiform_encephalopathy.pdf.

CFSPH. 2008. Mink Spongiform Encephalopathy. Available at: http://www.cfsph.iastate.edu/Factsheets/pdfs/transmissible_mink_encephalopathy.pdf.

Engelkirk PG, Duben-Engelkirk J. 2008. *Laboratory Diagnosis of Infectious Diseases*. Lippincott Williams & Wilkins, Baltimore, MD.

Hendrix CM, Sirois M. 2007. *Laboratory Procedures for Veterinary Technician, 5th ed.*, Mosby Elsevier, St. Louis, MO, pp 114–150.

[OIE] World Organization for Animal Health (OIE). 2002. Bovine Spongiform Encephalopathy. http://www.oie.int/eng/maladies/fiches/a_B115.htm.

Quinn PJ, Markey BK. 2003. *Concise Review of Veterinary Microbiology*. Blackwell Publishing, Ames, IA.

Rovid-Spickler A, Dvorak G. 2007. Technical fact sheets for zoonotic diseases of companion animals, in G Dvorak, A Rovid-Spickler, JA Roth, eds., *Handbook for Zoonotic Diseases of Companion Animals, 1st ed.*, CFSPH, Ames, IA.

Songer JG, Post KW. 2005. *Veterinary Microbiology: Bacterial and Fungal Agents of Animal Diseases*, Elsevier Saunders, St. Louis, MO.

Tighe MM, Brown M. 2008. *Mosby Comprehensive Review for Veterinary Technicians, 3rd ed.*, Mosby Elsevier, St. Louis, MO, pp 98–111 and 126–133.

United States Animal Health Association-Committee on Foreign and Emerging Diseases. 2008. *Foreign Animal Diseases, 7th ed.*, Boca Publications Group, Boca Raton, FL, pp 185–188.

United States Department of Agriculture (USDA). Animal and Plant Health Inspection Service (APHIS). 2004. Scrapie Factsheet. http://www.aphis.usda.gov/animal_health/animal_diseases/scrapie/downloads/fs_ahscrapie.pdf

[USGS] United States Geologic Survey. 2007. Chronic Wasting Disease Factsheet 2007-3070. Available at: http://www.nwhc.usgs.gov/publications/fact_sheets/pdfs/cwd/CWDFactsheet2007.pdf.

[WHO] World Health Organization. 2002. Fact Sheet No. 113, Bovine Spongiform Encephalopathy. Available at: www.who.int/mediacentre/factsheets/fs113/en.

3 "Links in the Chain" of Disease Transmission

Madga Dunowska

INTRODUCTION

Infectious agents have been a part of our lives since the start of documented history and undoubtedly have played an important role in the history of humanity. Examples of the power of unseen, microscopic enemies are many and include the devastation of the smallpox epidemic in the Americas brought by Spanish conquerors, an outbreak of Spanish flu of 1918 that killed more people than the First World War, and the impact of human AIDS on health and welfare of many communities (Chastel, 2007; Fenner, 1993; Morens et al., 2008). An outbreak of rinderpest in Africa at the end of nineteenth century killed nearly 90% of all hoof-cloven animals in the entire continent (Blystone, 2001). The above examples illustrate the efficiency with which the microscopic pathogens can spread through a population.

Transmission of infectious agents from one host to another is a complex and multistep process. It occurs through a chain of events and requires a number of conditions to be fulfilled. Understanding how infectious agents spread from one host to another, under what circumstances they are likely to cause disease, and how they are maintained within individual hosts and within populations is a prerequisite for any successful control program. In other words, in order to break a link in a chain of disease transmission, we need to first understand what constitutes "the links." In a sense, the old saying "know your enemy" could not be more true than when it comes to the fight against invisible enemies such as microbes. The better we understand the offenders themselves and the ways that they use to survive and perpetuate themselves, the better we are able to effectively choose the best links to break, and the more successful our control strategies become.

Infectious diseases in animals and humans are caused by a variety of pathogenic agents, including viruses, bacteria, fungi, and helminths (internal parasitic worms), as shown in Table 3.1.

Members of all four kingdoms vary significantly in their basic properties, such as size, complexity, or nutrient requirements. However, all can cause diseases with similar clinical signs, and definite diagnosis often requires laboratory confirmation. For example, diarrhea in any animal species (including humans) has a variety of infectious and noninfectious causes (Foster and Smith, 2009). Infectious causes of diarrhea include infection with a number of viruses (rotaviruses, parvoviruses, coronaviruses), bacteria (*Salmonella, Escherichia coli*), or parasites (*Cryptosporidium, Giardia*). It is important to understand the actual pathogen(s) involved

Veterinary Infection Prevention and Control, First Edition. Edited by Linda Caveney and Barbara Jones with Kimberly Ellis.
© 2012 John Wiley & Sons, Inc. Published by John Wiley & Sons, Inc.

Table 3.1 Basic Biological and Physiochemical Characteristics of Different Types of Infectious Pathogens

	Approximate diameter (μm)	Growth on nonliving media	Contain DNA and RNA	Binary fission	Multicellular
Viruses	0.02–0.3	No	No	No	No
Bacteria (including Mycoplasma, Rickettsia, and Chlamydia)	0.05–2	Yes	Yes	Yes	No
Protozoa	3–several cm	Yes	Yes	Yes	Yes
Parasitic Helminths	Macroscopic (typically visible with a naked eye)	No*	Yes	No	Yes

*Some, such as *Strongyloides* spp. have a free-living stage in their life cycle.

(i.e., when controlling an outbreak of infectious disease) or potential pathogens involved (i.e., when designing a biosecurity program for a specific establishment) so that control measures can be tailored to the known characteristics of pathogen(s) in question. Chapter 2 reviewed the characteristics of various pathogenic microorganisms.

This chapter provides a short overview of common steps necessary for transmission of pathogens from one host to another, with an emphasis on diversity of strategies employed at each step by different pathogens. The focus of the chapter has been narrowed for the most part to microscopic pathogens, such as bacteria and viruses, with fewer examples of other infectious agents, such as pathogenic fungi or parasites. However, general principles described can be easily extrapolated to a variety of infectious diseases.

DEFINITIONS OF KEY TERMS

It is important to establish a common vocabulary that will be used throughout this chapter. These terms may have other meanings or uses in the veterinary field, but the way these words are defined here is specific to the context in this chapter. Table 3.2 provides a table of definitions of disease transmission terminology.

COMMON LINKS IN THE CHAIN OF DISEASE TRANSMISSION

There is a great variability of infectious agents able to cause disease in a variety of domestic and wild animal species. Each of these agents has some unique characteristics that set it apart from others. However, most infectious agents also have some common features that can be exploited in design of effective control strategies against more than one pathogen (see Figure 3.1). Transmission of infectious pathogens between hosts can occur via a variety of routes, as shown in Table 3.3.

Transmission patterns are closely linked to the individual pathogen's biology. Similarly to the variability in characteristics of different infectious agents, there is also a great variability in the way those pathogens transmit from one host to another. However, although specific details can vary, most pathogens have to follow the same basic general steps to enable them to establish infections in susceptible hosts. These basic common steps include entry, replication

Table 3.2 Definitions of Disease Transmission Terminology

Infectious disease	A disease that is caused by an infectious agent. Infectious agents include a variety of pathogenic viruses, bacteria, fungi, or parasites.
Contagious disease	A disease caused by an infectious agent, which can be transmitted from one host to another. Not all infectious diseases are contagious.
Virulence	Ability of the pathogen to cause disease in a given host. More virulent pathogens cause more severe disease.
Infectious period	Time during which an infectious agent can be transmitted from one host to another. It may or may not be accompanied by disease.
Incubation period	Period between the time of infection and development of clinical signs of disease.
Maintenance host	Infected host (reservoir host) that typically develops only mild or no signs of clinical disease following infection with a pathogenic agent, but can spread this agent to other susceptible hosts.
Dead-end host	Infected host that may develop disease (often severe) following infection with a pathogenic agent, but is unable to transmit the agent to other animals; it constitutes the "dead end" of the chain of transmission.
Reproductive number (R_0)	Expected number of secondary infections resulting from introduction of one infected individual to a fully susceptible population.
Subclinical infection	Infection without any overt clinical signs, also referred to as "asymptomatic infection."
Arboviruses	Viruses that are biologically (not just mechanically) transmitted by an arthropod vector. Infection and replication in the arthropod is a necessary step in the life cycle of arboviruses. They are typically transmitted by bites of infected arthropods.

and spread within the host (either locally or systemically), and exit to enable infection of the new host. The cycle of infection can be divided into an incubation period, disease (may be subclinical), and recovery (or death). In addition, most pathogens have to be able to survive in the outside environment for long enough to enable a chance exposure of a new susceptible host and subsequent establishment of a new infection. Figure 3.1 shows the steps in the transmission of disease.

Route of Entry

Respiratory and gastrointestinal tracts are the most common routes of entry for pathogenic microorganisms. Other possible routes include entry through skin abrasions, wounds, conjunctiva, urogenital tract, or placenta. Some pathogens use exclusively one route of entry, whereas others can use several different ones. For example, arboviruses such as West Nile virus, equine encephalitis viruses, or African horse sickness virus are transmitted via bites of infected arthropod vectors (mosquitoes or midges). See Figure 3.2 for an example of arthropod vector. Animals infected with these viruses are not directly infectious to in-contact animals (Bunning et al., 2002; Wilson et al., 2009). Other pathogens can use several different routes to enter the host. For example, equine arteritis virus (EAV) can establish infection in a new host via a respiratory route (airborne transmission), via a veneral route either by natural service or through contaminated equipment used for artificial insemination (fomites), or via transplacental infection of a fetus (Balasuriya et al., 1999; Guthrie et al., 2003; Holyoak et al., 2008).

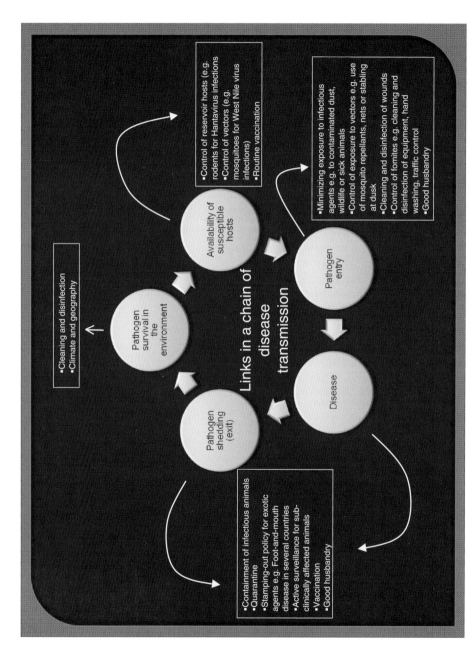

Figure 3.1 "Links in the chain of disease transmission": Critical steps in transmission cycles of infectious pathogens and examples of actions that can facilitate breakage of the transmission cycle.

Table 3.3 Common Transmission Pathways of Infectious Pathogens

Transmission pathway	Description	Examples
Direct contact	Transmission via direct contact between the infected animal and a susceptible host. The level and nature of contact required varies for different pathogens.	Mammalian influenza viruses (airborne) (Tellier, 2006), FIV (bite) (Hosie et al., 2009), FeLV (grooming) (Lutz et al., 2009), canine distemper virus (airborne) (Beineke et al., 2009), rabies virus (bite) (Hampson et al., 2009)
Indirect contact	Transmission of pathogens without direct contact with an infectious individual, commonly via fomites or infectious aerosols.	Examples listed under individual headings (airborne, fecal–oral, fomites, and water-borne).
Airborne	Transmission via infectious droplets or aerosols, usually via respiratory route, either by direct or indirect contact. Fragile pathogens require direct contact (e.g., mammalian influenza viruses). Environmentally stable pathogens can be spread as infectious aerosols by wind over large distances (e.g., FMD virus).	Mammalian influenza viruses (Tellier, 2006), FMD virus (Gloster et al., 1982) feline calicivirus (Radford et al., 2009), feline herpesvirus (Thiry et al., 2009), equid herpesviruses, equid rhinitis viruses (Sellon and Long, 2006), Brucella abortus (Hampson et al., 2009), plague (Wong et al., 2009).
Fecal–oral	Transmission by ingestion of pathogens shed in feces. May occur via either direct or indirect contact (contaminated environment, food, or fomites). Pathogens that are spread via this route are typically environmentally stable, and environmental contamination plays an important role in the spread of infection.	Enteric pathogens such as Salmonella (Dunowska et al., 2007), enteropathogenic E. coli, C. parvum (Gait et al., 2008), calf rotavirus (Foster and Smith, 2009), or canine parvovirus (Kramer et al., 2006).
Fomites	Transmission via contaminated equipment, clothing, vehicles, etc.	This route is particularly important for pathogens that survive well in the environment (e.g., enteric pathogens).
Iatrogenic	Inadvertent transmission during medical procedures (e.g., via contaminated needles or tissues).	Any pathogen introduced via inadequately sterilized equipment and contaminated tissue/blood products; e.g., inadvertent transmission of human hepatitis viruses through blood transfusions (Prati, 2006) or chicken reticuloendotheliosis virus via contaminated Marek's disease vaccine (Fadly et al., 1996).
Vector-borne	Mechanical or biological transmission via vectors such as flies, mosquitoes, ticks, etc.	Mechanical: e.g., Moraxella bovis (Postma et al., 2008). Biological: e.g., equine encephalitis viruses (Sellon and Long, 2006), Bluetongue viruses (Maclachlan et al., 2009), Rift valley fever virus (Basto et al., 2006), African swine fever virus (Basto et al., 2006), malaria (Ghosh and Jacobs-Lorena, 2009), or plague (Wimsatt and Biggins, 2009).

(Continued)

Table 3.3 (*Continued*)

Transmission pathway	Description	Examples
Water-borne	Indirect transmission via contact (e.g. drinking, swimming, rinsing, housing) with pathogen-contaminated water.	*Giardia* (Leclerc et al., 2002), Leptospirosis (Monahan et al., 2009), *C. parvum* (Xiao and Feng, 2008), avian influenza viruses (Webster et al., 1992), cholera (Ise et al., 1996), *Pseudomonas* spp. (Leclerc et al., 2002).
Sexual	Transmission via sexual contact with either an infected individual (direct transmission) or contaminated equipment used for reproductive procedures (fomites).	EAV (Holyoak et al., 2008), equine coital exanthema (Sellon and Long, 2006).
Vertical	Transmission from mother to the offspring before, during, or soon after birth, although transmission in the immediate neonatal period may also be regarded as horizontal.	BVD virus (Givens and Waldrop, 2004), equid herpesvirus type 1, and EAV (Sellon and Long, 2006), parvoviruses of many species (Terpstra et al., 2007; Lamm and Rezabek, 2008), Caprine arthritis–encephalitis virus (Weissinger et al., 2009).

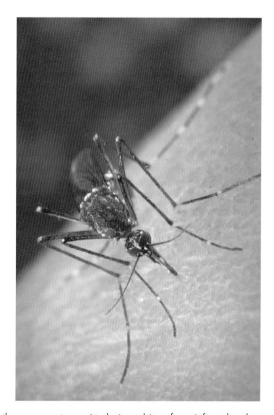

Figure 3.2 Some pathogens are transmitted via a bite of an infected arthropod, such as a mosquito. Examples include equine encephalitidies viruses, Yellow fever virus, or malaria (photo credit: CDC Public Health Image Library, James Gathany).

Respiratory Tract

The respiratory tract is protected against entry of pathogens by several mechanisms, including entrapment of pathogens in a blanket of mucous produced by Goblet cells, and their removal from the respiratory tract by coordinated movement of cilia on epithelial cells. Pathogens that evade these nonspecific mechanisms can be further removed by specific (secretory antibodies, mainly IgA) or nonspecific (phagocytyc cells, such as neutrophils and macrophages) immunological defenses (Fokkens and Scheeren, 2000; Gwinn and Vallyathan, 2006; Stannard and O'Callaghan, 2006). Despite this array of protective mechanisms, the respiratory tract is a common entry point for many pathogens (Baskerville, 1981). Examples include equine herpesviruses, feline calicivirus and herpesvirus, Newcastle disease virus, human coronavirus, equine influenza virus, as well as several bacterial and fungal species (Fennelly et al., 2004; Fischer and Dott, 2003; Hood, 2009; Li et al., 2009; Muscatello et al., 2009; Patel and Heldens, 2005; Tellier, 2006; Wong and Yuen, 2008; Wong et al., 2009; Yamanaka et al., 2008; Zicola et al., 2009).

Skin

Intact skin with a thick layer of cornified epithelium provides an effective barrier against infections with many pathogens. Typically, a break in the integrity of the skin is necessary for a pathogen to gain an entry via this route. This could be provided by skin abrasions, wounds, animal bites, insect bites, or iatrogenically via contaminated needles or contaminated surgical equipment. Although rare, some pathogens are able to penetrate intact skin as a route of entry; for example, hookworms can cause cutaneous larva migrants in humans (Haas et al., 2005; Heukelbach and Feldmeier, 2008).

Many pathogens can be transmitted either mechanically or biologically via the bites of arthropod insects. Examples include viruses (i.e., Eastern, Western, and Venezuelan equine encephalitis viruses or West Nile virus transmitted by infected mosquitoes, African swine fever virus transmitted by infected ticks or Bluetongue virus transmitted by infected midges), bacteria (i.e., *Yersinia pestis*, the causative agent of plague, most commonly transmitted by infected fleas), or parasites (e.g., *Plasmodium* spp., the causative agent of malaria in people, transmitted by infected mosquitoes) (Ghosh and Jacobs-Lorena, 2009; Maclachlan et al., 2009; Sellon and Long, 2006; Wimsatt and Biggins, 2009).

In addition, open wounds provide an easy way of entry for many infectious agents. In one study, the most common bacterial isolates from chronic wounds in horses included *Pseudomonas aeruginosa, Staphylococcus eidermidis, Serratia marcescens, Enterococcus faecalis,* and *Providencia rettgeri* (Freeman et al., 2009). Such infections may be localized and cause delayed healing of the wound itself, or they may serve as a portal of entry for further spread within the body and subsequent systemic infection. For example, cat and dog bite wounds in people, particularly those associated with *Capnocytophaga canimorsus* or *Pasteurella multocida* infections, can lead to severe systemic complications, including septic shock, meningitis, or endocarditis (Oehler et al., 2009).

Gastrointestinal Tract

Many pathogens are acquired by ingestion. Some are then transported into the various parts of the gastrointestinal tract, where they establish local infections. Examples include rotaviruses or enteric coronaviruses, which replicate in the cells at the tips of intestinal villi. Infection with coronaviruses or rotaviruses may result in development of osmotic diarrhea (Foster and Smith, 2009). Other gastrointestinal pathogens replicate in the oropharyngeal area, from where they spread systemically. For example, parvovirus-induced diarrhea is caused by infection of the intestinal crypt cells. Unlike rotaviruses and coronaviruses, parvoviruses reach the intestine via the blood stream, following systemic spread from the pharyngeal area (Meunier et al., 1985).

Local gastrointestinal infections that manifest themselves as diarrhea may, in addition, alter permeability of the gastrointestinal tract and allow commensal and pathogenic intestinal flora to gain entry into the blood stream. In a study by Johns et al. (2009), a number of bacterial species were isolated from blood collected from 9 of 31 mature horses with diarrhea within 24 hours of admission to the hospital. Horses with bacteremia were less likely to survive in comparison with horses that had negative blood cultures.

Many parasitic infections are acquired by ingestion, either through contaminated environment (e.g., pasture contaminated with nematode eggs and infectious larvae) or via a consumption of an infected host (i.e., trichinellosis through eating of raw or undercooked game or pork meat).

Other Routes

Pathogens can also establish infections in their hosts through entry via other routes, including conjunctiva (e.g., *Moraxella bovis*, a causative agent for "pink eye" conjunctivitis in cattle), urogenital track (i.e., EAV, some papillomaviruses), or placenta [e.g., equine herpesvirus type 1 (EHV-1) or feline leukemia virus (FeLV)] (Lutz et al., 2009; Postma et al., 2008; Sellon and Long, 2006).

Incubation Period

The period between infection and occurrence of clinical signs of disease is called an incubation period. The length of the incubation period can vary from hours (i.e., rotavirus, influenza virus infections), days [i.e., foot-and mouth-disease (FMD) virus], to months (i.e., rabies), or even years (i.e., acquired immunodeficiency syndrome due to the feline immunodeficiency virus infection) (Hosie et al., 2009; Lessler et al., 2009; Lutz et al., 2009; Smith et al., 1991). During the incubation period, an infected animal is clinically normal, although it is already infected with the pathogenic agent. The shedding of infectious agent can start before, around the same time, or after the end of the incubation period. The spread of pathogens that are shed before the end of the incubation period (and thus, before development of clinical signs of disease) is usually the most difficult to control. For example, feline acquired immunodeficiency syndrome develops years after primary infection with the causative feline immunodeficiency virus (FIV) (Ishida et al., 1992). Throughout this long incubation period, any infected cat can transmit FIV to other susceptible cats. Similarly, shedding of the FMD virus typically starts before infected animals develop clinical disease (Alexandersen et al., 2003). As such, FMD virus may be already widespread by the time infected animals are recognized and isolated or destroyed.

To summarize, infected animals may provide a very effective way of disseminating pathogens during the incubation period, before the infected host becomes sick itself (and can be easily identified and isolated).

The length of the incubation period for a given pathogen is important, for example, in designing effective quarantine procedures (the length of the quarantine should be longer than the length of the incubation period of the agent in question) or in back-tracking animals that had been potentially exposed to the diseased individual (all animals exposed to such individual over the time exceeding the incubation period should be back-tracked).

Mechanism of Spread in the Body

Pathogens may remain at the site of entry to cause localized infections, or they may use the initial site of entry as a portal for subsequent systemic dissemination into a variety of organs.

Local Infections

Infections with many pathogens are localized and do not result in systemic spread. Examples include scabby mouth disease in ruminants caused by a parapox virus infection, gastrointestinal infections caused by a variety of viruses, bacteria, and parasites, or localized upper respiratory tract infections (Baskerville, 1981; Buttner and Rziha, 2002; Foster and Smith, 2009).

Generalized Infections

Other pathogens spread systemically throughout the body following initial infection at the site of entry. This spread can be accomplished via the lymphatics, blood vessels, or nerves. Following dissemination of pathogens to a variety of tissues, secondary replication in those tissues may lead to generalized systemic disease. The clinical signs observed are dependent on the organ/tissue predilection of the pathogen, on the host's immune response, and on the extent of tissue damage (either directly by the pathogen or indirectly through immunopathology).

Disease

Infection with a pathogenic agent may lead to development of disease. It is important to recognize that infection is not synonymous with disease. The severity of disease following infection may vary from subclinical to death. Depending on the pathogen, clinically affected individuals may represent only the "tip of an iceberg" of all infected individuals. This is illustrated in Figure 3.3.

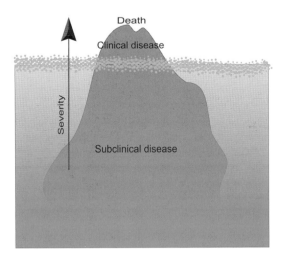

Figure 3.3 An iceberg concept of the maintenance of infections in populations. Clinical signs of disease following infection with a pathogen may vary from subclinical to death. Typically, only a small proportion of infected individuals develop disease following infection (the tip of an iceberg). The majority of infections are subclinical (submerged part of an iceberg). Subclinical infections are more difficult to recognize and therefore constitute a way of maintaining an infectious agent in populations. As with an iceberg, it is the "invisible" part that is more dangerous!

Clinical infections are reasonably easy to recognize. Diseased animals (or people) can be placed under appropriate containment conditions in order to prevent transmission of infectious agents from such individuals to other susceptible hosts. Conversely, subclinically infected individuals are difficult to recognize, as they appear clinically normal. As such, subclinically infected individuals often play an important role in the spread of infectious agents within populations. As an example, animals that are subclinically infected with FMD virus are thought to be an important risk factor for introduction of the virus into FMD-free countries (Sutmoller and Casas, 2002). Successful eradication of smallpox worldwide provides another illustration of this point (Fenner, 1993). Some of the factors that were important for success of the smallpox eradication campaign were the biological characteristics of the virus, including obvious clinical signs of infection and rare occurrence of subclinical infections. Since infected individuals were contagious (able to transmit smallpox to others) only after the development of clinical signs, it was possible to "break the chain" of smallpox transmission by a combination of vaccination and isolation of clinical cases (Fenner, 1993).

Route of Exit

Pathogens must exit their host in order to initiate infection in a new host. As such, the route of exit is inherently linked to the route of transmission of any infectious agent. Some pathogens are not able to exit their hosts, particularly if infection occurs in an accidental (or not typical) host. Such infections may still cause disease in the infected individual (sometimes severe) but typically cannot be transmitted further. For example, eastern equine encephalitis (EEE) virus normally circulates between mosquitoes and birds. Horses (and people) are considered "accidental" hosts. They become infected with EEE virus via a bite from an infected mosquito and often develop severe neurological disease following infection. However, despite the severity of clinical signs, the level of viremia in the horse is usually too low to allow infection of mosquitoes and transmission of the virus to a new host. As such, infected horses are "dead-end" hosts for EEE; the virus dies together with the infected horse (Sellon and Long, 2006).

Pathogens may use predominantly, or exclusively, one route of exit. Examples include local respiratory tract infections (exit via respiratory secretions), local gastrointestinal tract infections (exit via feces), local skin infections (exit via skin), arboviral infections (exit via ingestion of contaminated blood by an arthropod vector), or rabies virus infection (exit via saliva, which facilitates infection of a new host through biting). Other pathogens can use several different routes of exit. Agents able to cause systemic infections can often be shed through a number of routes, including respiratory secretions, feces, urine, tears, semen, or saliva. For example, EAV can be isolated from a variety of tissues and body fluids (i.e., respiratory secretions, semen, urine, placentas, aborted fetuses) following infection via a respiratory route (Holyoak et al., 2008; Sellon and Long, 2006).

Gastrointestinal Tract

The gastrointestinal tract provides a very efficient route of exit and spread for many pathogens, particularly if infection is associated with diarrhea. Voluminous, watery diarrhea is very difficult to contain, clean, and disinfect. The pathogen load in diarrhea can be extremely high. As such, watery diarrhea provides a perfect vehicle for environmental contamination, as illustrated in Figure 3.4.

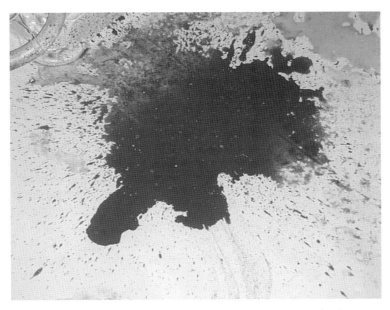

Figure 3.4   Diarrhea due to infection with canine parvovirus (CPV). Watery, diarrhea contain high viral load and provide an excellent vehicle for dissemination of CPV in the environment. CPV can remain infectious for months, particularly in areas such as grass or dirt (photo credit: Quentin Roper, with permission).

Respiratory Tract

Respiratory secretions are a common exit route for respiratory pathogens. Coughing and sneezing provide efficient ways of dispersing infectious agents via droplets and aerosols, as illustrated in Figure 3.5 (Fiegel et al., 2006; Knight, 1980; Tellier, 2006; Xie et al., 2007).

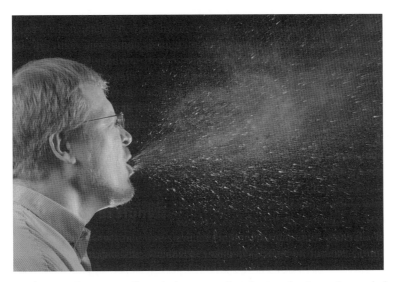

Figure 3.5   Airborne pathogens are efficiently disseminated in infectious droplets and aerosols during coughing and sneezing (photo credit: CDC Public Health Image Library, James Gathany).

Aerosols are suspensions of particles in the air and can only be formed if the particles are small enough to remain suspended. The settling time of particles depends on their size: particles larger than 100 microns settle within seconds, particles between 5 and 100 microns in diameter take minutes (up to an hour, depending on the size) to settle, and particles with a diameter <3 microns form aerosols (i.e., they do not settle and remain suspended in the atmosphere indefinitely) (Nicas et al., 2005; Tellier, 2006). Coincidently, particles of the same size as required for generation of aerosols can also gain entry to the lower respiratory tract, as they are not trapped by mucous and are not removed by the ciliary action of the respiratory epithelium (Tellier, 2006).

The length of time pathogens remain infectious in the aerosolized form depends on several factors, including the physiochemical properties of each individual pathogen (particularly its environmental stability), concentration of infectious particles, air currents, temperature, and humidity. For example, influenza viruses have been shown to remain infectious in aerosols for up to 24 hours, whereas the FMD virus can remain infectious for days (Bartley et al., 2002; Faquet et al., 2005; Tellier, 2006). As such, influenza viruses typically require direct contact between infected and susceptible individuals (or sharing the common airspace within a relatively short period of time). The FMD virus, on the other hand, can be transmitted between animals not only via direct contact or common equipment, but also indirectly by wind over large distances (Amaral Doel et al., 2009; Gloster et al., 1982, 2003, 2005).

Other Routes

Numerous other routes are used by a variety of pathogens to exit their hosts. Pathogens that cause localized skin infections enter and exit via the same route. Examples include papillomaviruses or some poxviruses, such as the orf virus. The orf virus is a parapoxvirus that causes localized proliferative lesions of the skin in ruminants and people (Haig and Mercer, 1998). The virus can be isolated from such lesions that are a source of infection to other animals either by direct contact or indirectly via contaminated fomites and environment (Buttner and Rziha, 2002; Chan et al., 2009).

Vesicular fluid in animals infected by FMD virus contains high titers of infectious virus that can be spread to in-contact animals or indirectly via fomites (Alexandersen et al., 2001). Infectious agents that cause abortions are typically present in high quantities in aborted fetuses (i.e., elephant endotheliotropic herpesvirus, porcine parvovirus, or bovine viral diarrhea virus), which may provide the source of infection for others (Leon et al., 2008; Martucciello et al., 2009; Wolf et al., 2008).

Some pathogens are shed in saliva (i.e., rabies virus, FIV, or FeLV) and transmitted by bites or grooming (Hosie et al., 2009; Lutz et al., 2009; Nagaraj et al., 2006). Hantaviruses are excreted in all body excretion of infected rodents (Terpstra et al., 2007). People become infected with hantaviruses through inhalation of dust contaminated with infected rodents' droppings, as shown in Figure 3.6.

As such, exposure to rodent-infested places increases the risk of acquiring a hantavirus infection.

Pathogens excreted via semen are efficiently spread during breeding. For example, EAV has been wildly spread in many parts of the world through contaminated semen used for artificial insemination (Balasuriya et al., 1999).

Finally, some pathogens are transmitted to a new host as part of a predator–prey cycle. For example, the parasite *Trichinella spiralis* encysts itself in the muscles of an infected animal and transmits to a new host when the infected animal (prey) gets eaten by its predator. Because people

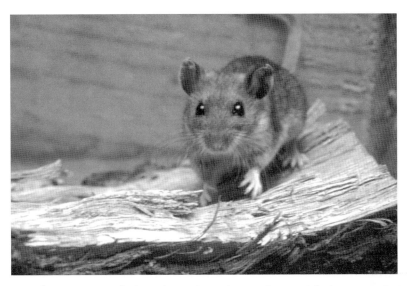

Figure 3.6   Rodents can serve as biological or mechanical vectors for many infectious agents. Rodent control should be included in any effective biosecurity program (photo credit: CDC Public Health Image Library, James Gathany).

are rarely eaten by other animals, infected humans are usually dead-end hosts for *Trichinella* transmission.

Survival in the Environment and Persistence in the Host

In order to maintain themselves in the populations, pathogenic agents had to develop strategies to survive either within their hosts or in the outside environment.

Transmission patterns and the life cycle of a pathogen often reflect its ability to survive within certain environmental conditions. Close contact between infected and susceptible individuals is a prerequisite for transmission of pathogens that do not survive well outside their hosts, whereas environmental contamination and transmission via fomites are more important in transmission of pathogens resistant to adverse environmental conditions. For example, pathogens associated with gastrointestinal infections have to survive adverse conditions encountered in the gastrointestinal tact, such as low pH of the stomach and enzymatic action of digestive enzymes. As such, these pathogens are often also resistant to adverse environmental conditions and survive well outside their hosts. Examples include rotaviruses, parvoviruses, caliciviruses, enteroviruses, *Salmonella* spp., *Cryptosporidium parvum*, and others. These pathogens can survive on inanimate surfaces for weeks to months (Kramer et al., 2006). Pathogens that show stability in diverse conditions are also typically more difficult to disinfect, increasing the likelihood of environmental contamination, particularly in the hospital setting. To further illustrate this point, the Colorado State University veterinary teaching hospital has a well-established *Salmonella* surveillance system (Dunowska et al., 2007). As part of this system, all large-animal stalls that had been used for housing *Salmonella*-shedding animals are routinely disinfected using a three-step process that consists of cleaning with a detergent and bleach solution, steaming, and a final disinfection with quarternary ammonium compound. Despite this rigorous disinfection protocol, *Salmonella* spp. were occasionally recovered from disinfected stalls (Dunowska et al., 2007).

An example of two pathogens with contrasting strategies for survival can be provided by comparing the replication cycle of herpesviruses (i.e., EHV-1) and a parvovirus (i.e., feline pan-leukopenia virus). Both pathogens are viruses, and as such they can replicate only within living cells of their hosts. Herpesviruses are fragile viruses that do not survive well outside their hosts, whereas parvoviruses are very environmentally resistant (Faquet et al., 2005). To "overcome" their environmental instability, herpesviruses have developed sophisticated strategies to evade the host immune responses, so that they are able to persist for long periods of time within their hosts (Rolle and Olweus, 2009; van der Meulen et al., 2006). One such strategy is their ability to establish latent infections (Minarovits, 2006; Reddehase et al., 2008). During latency, the viral genome undergoes very limited transcription, and infectious viral particles are not produced. In addition, many herpesviruses establish latency in immunologically privileged sites, such as neurons (Kramer et al., 2006). As such, latent herpesviruses can remain "hidden" and protected from destruction by the host immune response for years. Under certain conditions, such as during periods of immunosuppression, the latent herpesvirus may undergo reactivation and can be successfully transmitted to a new host. By contrast, parvoviruses typically do not have the ability to establish persistent infections in their hosts (Lamm and Rezabek, 2008). Since they also evoke strong, long-lasting protective immune responses in animals that survive a parvovirus infection, they require a constant supply of susceptible animals to perpetuate themselves. This apparent "difficulty" is countered by the fact that parvoviruses are environmentally stable and have been reported to survive for weeks to months outside their hosts (Gordon and Angrick, 1986).

To summarize, direct contact with an infectious individual is not a prerequisite for successful transmission of infection to a new susceptible host, particularly in a case of pathogens that survive well in the environment. Examples of diseases that can be acquired via contact with contaminated surfaces, fomites, feed or water supply, or infectious droplets carried by wind over long distances include rotaviral diarrhea in a variety of species, FMD, Salmonellosis, Cryptosporidiosis, Leptospirosis, and others (Foster and Smith, 2009; Gait et al., 2008; Gloster et al., 1982; Monahan et al., 2009). Figure 3.7 shows common items that act as fomites in the transmission of infectious agents.

In addition, most pathogens can be transmitted via more than one route. For example, large droplets are considered by many as the main route for transmission of mammalian influenza viruses. However, the importance of transmission by direct contact, aerosols, or fomites under certain conditions should also be considered (Tellier, 2006). Table 3.3 summarizes the routes of disease transmission.

SPREAD WITHIN POPULATIONS

In epidemiological terms, the likelihood of development of an epidemic is characterized by a reproductive number R_0. The R_0 denotes the number of secondary infections that would theoretically result from an introduction of one infected individual into a fully susceptible population (Lavine et al., 2008). Diseases with high R_0 have the tendency to spread fast and may be difficult to control, despite implementation of control strategies. FMD is an example of such a fast-spreading disease with high R_0, which was calculated to be 30 and 176 for nonvaccinated piglets and dairy cows under experimental conditions, respectively (Orsel et al., 2009). Conversely, diseases with low R_0 do not spread rapidly, and implementation of the appropriate control measures is likely to be successful in preventing epidemics. For example, the R_0 for canine rabies was estimated to be between 1 and 2 in various parts of the world

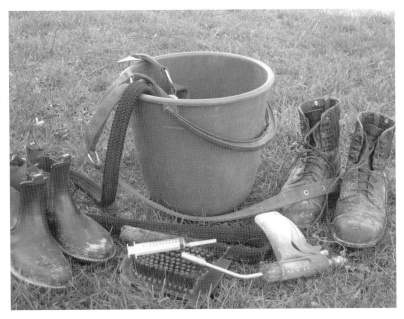

Figure 3.7 Contaminated fomites provide an efficient way of transmission of infectious agents (photo credit: Magda Dunowska).

(Hampson et al., 2009). As such, canine rabies should be amendable to effective control, and, in fact, rabies was successfully eliminated from a number of countries using a combination of strategies, including vaccination of wildlife (Niin et al., 2008). Finally, diseases with R_0 less than 1 are not capable of evolving into epidemics and would die on their own even without implementation of any control efforts.

The reproductive number R_0, or successful perpetuation of infectious agents in a population, is dependent on a variety of factors, depicted in a traditional epidemiological triangle as those related to the pathogen, the host, and the environment. This is illustrated in Figure 3.8.

The Pathogen

Species Specificity

Pathogen-related factors that play a role in disease transmission include physiochemical and biological characteristics of the agent in question. Important pathogen characteristics, such as virulence, persistence in the host, or survival in the environment, have been described in the sections above. One additional pathogen characteristic that plays an important role in disease transmission is species specificity.

Some pathogens are species specific, whereas others can easily infect a variety of species. In general, pathogens that are able to infect members of several species are more difficult to control, as there are bigger numbers of susceptible hosts available to maintain the chain of transmission. From the public health point of view, diseases caused by pathogens that are able to infect both animals and humans are particularly important. Such diseases are referred to as zoonoses. Special care is required if dealing with zoonotic infections in order to avoid inadvertent transmission of the infectious agent from infected animals to humans. As an example, *C. parvum* is a water-borne

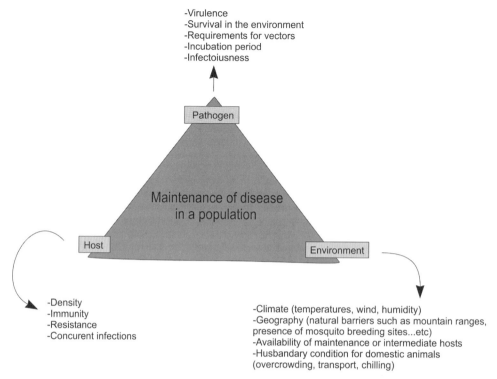

-Virulence
-Survival in the environment
-Requirements for vectors
-Incubation period
-Infectoiusness

Pathogen

Maintenance of disease
in a population

Host

Environment

-Density
-Immunity
-Resistance
-Concurent infections

-Climate (temperatures, wind, humidity)
-Geography (natural barriers such as mountain ranges,
presence of mosquito breeding sites...etc)
-Availability of maintenance or intermediate hosts
-Husbandary condition for domestic animals
(overcrowding, transport, chilling)

Figure 3.8   Classical epidemiological triangle: The outcomes of infection are dependent on several factors, which can be divided into those related to the host, the pathogen, and the environment.

protozoon parasite that is a common cause of diarrhea in many species, including calves, kids, goats, foals, alpacas, and people. Outbreaks of diarrhea due to *C. parvum* infection have been described among veterinary students, animal handlers, and other people with close contact with animals (Gait et al., 2008; Xiao and Feng, 2008). As such, a calf shedding *C. parvum* poses a risk of infection not only to other calves, but also to in-contact animals of other species, including humans. Similar to *C. parvum*, rotaviruses have been associated with gastrointestinal disease in young animals of variety of species, including humans. However, unlike *C. parvum*, rotaviruses tend to be species specific (Cook et al., 2004; Nakagomi and Nakagomi, 1991). As such, the same hypothetical calf with diarrhea due to rotavirus infection is less likely to be a source of rotaviral infection for its human handlers or in-contact animals of different species. Despite this general rule, recent studies based on comparison of rotavirus genomes from different species suggested that interspecies transmission might have occurred in the past, and it might have contributed to genetic exchange between animal and human rotaviruses (Muller and Johne, 2007). Therefore, care should be exercised in treating animals with any infectious disease, as its full zoonotic potential may not be fully realized.

Strength of the Host Immune Response

This characteristic depends not only on the pathogen, but also on the infected host, and as such constitutes both the pathogen-related and the host-related factor. Nonetheless, some pathogens tend to evoke strong, long-lasting immune responses, whereas immune responses to other pathogens tend to be short-lived. Examples of pathogens that evoke long-lasting immune protection include some poxviruses, parvoviruses, or paramyxoviruses. In contrast, immunity to reinfection with herpesviruses, influenza viruses, or many bacterial pathogens tends to be short-lived and animals may become reinfected several times in their life span.

The Host

Host factors important in transmission of infectious agents include resistance/susceptibility to infection with a given pathogen, the density of susceptible hosts, and availability of carrier/intermediate hosts.

Resistance/Susceptibility to Infection and Disease

The severity of disease observed following infection with any pathogen varies. Typically, severe disease is observed in relatively few hosts, and many infections tend to be subclinical. As mentioned earlier, susceptibility to infection and susceptibility to disease are not synonymous. For example, animals subclinically infected with the FMD virus are highly contagious and constitute a serious risk for introduction and spread of FMD disease in FMD-free areas (Sutmoller and Casas, 2002).

Animals may remain healthy following exposure to an infectious agent for several different reasons, with different consequences with relation to their role in further spread of infection. Some animals may be resistant to infection with a given pathogen. They do not become infected and do not develop disease following exposure to such pathogen. For example, horses are resistant to infection with the FMD virus. As such, horses are unlikely to play an important role in the spread and maintenance of FMD in a given geographical area.

Animals may also remain healthy following exposure to an infectious agent if they are immune to this agent. Such animals mount fast, effective immune response following infection, which controls the offending pathogen. As such, they are susceptible to infection but resistant to disease. Immune animals are thus also unlikely to constitute an important source of infection for other animals. It should be noted that vaccinated animals may still be involved in the transmission of infectious agents, for example, when vaccine failure occurs, as in several equine influenza outbreaks (Powell et al., 1995; van Maanen et al., 2003; Yamanaka et al., 2008).

Awareness of which animal species can act as reservoir hosts for certain pathogens is important in implementing effective infection control programs. As an example, healthy reptiles are a common source of *Salmonella* infection (Bertrand et al., 2008). Other examples include rodents, which can be a source of hantavirus infections in humans (Meerburg et al., 2009), or cattle, which may act as carriers for *E. coli* 0157 infection in children (Warshawsky et al., 2002).

Determinants of resistance/susceptibility to infection and disease with a particular agent are complex and include not only species, breed, or individual genetic differences, but also factors such as age, nutritional status, or the presence of stressors. The latter include extreme temperatures, overcrowding, transport, or any concurrent infections. For example, in a study by Svensson and Liberg (2006), calves kept in groups of 12–18 animals had a higher incidence of respiratory illness and grew slower than calves housed in groups of 6–9 animals. In summary, the dynamics of disease spread and presentation vary between different populations of animals.

Host Density and Availability of Carrier/Intermediate Hosts

Many pathogens need a constant supply of susceptible hosts in order to maintain themselves in populations. These include indicator hosts (those in which clinical signs of disease are apparent), as well as carrier hosts or vectors. This is particularly important for viruses and some parasites, which cannot multiply outside their hosts, and less important for free-living organisms, such as bacteria. The requirement of a constant supply of susceptible hosts is particularly important for viruses and some parasites, which cannot multiply outside their hosts, and less important for free-living organisms, such as bacteria. It is often fulfilled by a constant supply of young animals, which tend to be more susceptible to a variety of infections. For pathogens that require complex transmission cycles involving vectors, maintenance, or intermediate hosts, the availability of such hosts is an important factor in the spread of infection. Consequently, elimination of even one group of hosts/vectors aids in control of disease in a given area (e.g., elimination of mosquitoes for control of arboviral infections or elimination of rodents for control of hantaviruses).

A high level of immunity in any given population would minimize or break altogether the ability of the pathogen to be maintained in such a population. This is a basis for infection control programs based on vaccination. Examples of successful disease eradication efforts based on maintenance of high level of immunity in a population include global eradiation of smallpox, eradication of rinderpest from the majority of the world, or local eradication of rabies in several countries (Blystone, 2001; Fenner, 1993; Niin et al., 2008).

The higher the density of susceptible hosts, the easier it is for a pathogen to maintain the cycle of infections. As such, a global increase in the number of people, together with an increase in human mobility across the globe, provides an ideal situation for human pathogens to spread into new areas. Similarly, disease control in intensive animal production units provides specific challenges associated with density of susceptible animals in such units.

The Environment

Environmental conditions play an important role in maintaining or breaking the transmission cycle of an infectious agent. Any activity that changes the established balance between hosts and their pathogens (including availability of the vectors or reservoir hosts) is likely to result in altered disease transmission patterns. Examples of human activities that have been associated with altered disease patterns include deforestation or provision of mosquito breeding sites via irrigation or urbanization (Mackenzie and Williams 2009).

CONCLUSION

A number of steps are necessary for the transmission of an infectious agent from the infected individual to a susceptible host. Common steps for all infections include entry, development of disease (may be subclinical), exit, and transmission to a new host. Pathogens have developed a variety of strategies that allow them to maintain themselves in populations. The ability of any pathogen to be successfully transmitted from one host to another depends on a variety of factors, including those related to the pathogen, the host, and the environment. Each pathogen can typically be transmitted via a number of routes, even though some may be more common (and therefore more important to address in the infection control efforts). Knowledge of primary transmission routes and factors associated with these routes is important in establishing effective control strategies. Pathogens are able to adapt to changing conditions. As such, established transmission patterns may not remain static. Factors likely to influence such changes include availability of susceptible hosts, as well as climatic and geographical conditions.

REFERENCES

Alexandersen S, Oleksiewicz MB, Donaldson AI. 2001. The early pathogenesis of foot-and-mouth disease in pigs infected by contact: a quantitative time-course study using TaqMan RT-PCR. *J Gen Virol* 82(Pt 4):747–755.

Alexandersen S, et al. 2003. Studies of quantitative parameters of virus excretion and transmission in pigs and cattle experimentally infected with foot-and-mouth disease virus. *J Comp Pathol* 129(4):268–282.

Amaral Doel CM, Gloster J, Valarcher JF. 2009. Airborne transmission of foot-and-mouth disease in pigs: evaluation and optimisation of instrumentation and techniques. *Vet J* 179(2):219–224.

Balasuriya UB, et al. 1999. Genetic stability of equine arteritis virus during horizontal and vertical transmission in an outbreak of equine viral arteritis. *J Gen Virol* 80(Pt 8):1949–1958.

Bartley LM, Donnelly CA, Anderson RM. 2002. Review of foot-and-mouth disease virus survival in animal excretions and on fomites. *Vet Rec* 151(22):667–669.

Baskerville A. 1981. Mechanisms of infection in the respiratory tract. *N Z Vet J* 29(12):235–238.

Basto AP, et al. 2006. Kinetics of African swine fever virus infection in *Ornithodoros erraticus* ticks. *J Gen Virol* 87(Pt 7):1863–1871.

Beineke A, Puff C, Seehusen F, Baumgartner W. 2009. Pathogenesis and immunopathology of systemic and nervous canine distemper. *Vet Immunol Immunopathol* 127(1-2):1–18.

Bertrand S, et al. 2008. Salmonella infections associated with reptiles: the current situation in Europe. *Euro Surveill* 13(24).

Blystone M. 2001. Rinderpest: one virus's impact on veterinary history. *Vet Herit* 24(1):8–12.

Bunning ML, et al. 2002. Experimental infection of horses with West Nile virus. *Emerg Infect Dis* 8(4):380–386.

Buttner M, Rziha HJ. 2002. Parapoxviruses: from the lesion to the viral genome. *J Vet Med B Infect Dis Vet Public Health* 49(1):7–16.

Chan KW, et al. 2009. Differential diagnosis of orf viruses by a single-step PCR. *J Virol Methods* 160(1-2):85–89.

Chastel C. 2007. [Global threats from emerging viral diseases]. *Bull Acad Natl Med* 191(8):1563–1577.

Cook N, et al. 2004. The zoonotic potential of rotavirus. *J Infect* 48(4):289–302.

Dunowska M, et al. 2007. Comparison of Salmonella enterica serotype Infantis isolates from a veterinary teaching hospital. *J Appl Microbiol* 102(6):1527–1536.

Fadly AM, et al. 1996. An outbreak of lymphomas in commercial broiler breeder chickens vaccinated with a fowlpox vaccine contaminated with reticuloendotheliosis virus. *Avian Pathol* 25(1):35–47.

Fauquet CM, et al. 2005. *Virus Taxonomy: VIIIth Report of the International Committee on Taxonomy of Viruses*, Elsevier Academic Press, Burlington, MA.

Fennelly KP, et al. 2004. Airborne infection with Bacillus anthracis–from mills to mail. *Emerg Infect Dis* 10(6):996–1002.

Fenner F. 1993. Smallpox: emergence, global spread, and eradication. *Hist Philos Life Sci* 15(3):397–420.

Fiegel J, Clarke R, Edwards DA. 2006. Airborne infectious disease and the suppression of pulmonary bioaerosols. *Drug Discov Today* 11(1-2):51–57.

Fischer G, Dott W. 2003. Relevance of airborne fungi and their secondary metabolites for environmental, occupational and indoor hygiene. *Arch Microbiol* 179:75–82.

Fokkens WJ, Scheeren RA. 2000. Upper airway defence mechanisms. *Paediatr Respir Rev* 1(4):336–341.

Foster DM, Smith GW. 2009. Pathophysiology of diarrhea in calves. *Vet Clin North Am Food Anim Pract* 25(1):13–36, xi.

Freeman K, et al. 2009. Biofilm evidence and the microbial diversity of horse wounds. *Can J Microbiol* 55(2):197–202.

Gait R, et al. 2008. Outbreak of cryptosporidiosis among veterinary students. *Vet Rec* 162(26):843–845.

Ghosh AK, Jacobs-Lorena M. 2009. Plasmodium sporozoite invasion of the mosquito salivary gland. *Curr Opin Microbiol* 12:394–400.

Givens MD, Waldrop JG. 2004. Bovine viral diarrhea virus in embryo and semen production systems. *Vet Clin North Am Food Anim Pract* 20(1):21–38.

Gloster J, et al. 2003. Airborne transmission of foot-and-mouth disease virus from Burnside Farm, Heddon-on-the-Wall, Northumberland, during the 2001 epidemic in the United Kingdom. *Vet Rec* 152(17):525–533.

Gloster J, Freshwater A, Sellers RF, Alexandersen S. 2005. Re-assessing the likelihood of airborne spread of foot-and-mouth disease at the start of the 1967-1968 UK foot-and-mouth disease epidemic. *Epidemiol Infect* 133(5):767–783.

Gloster J, Sellers RF, Donaldson AI. 1982. Long distance transport of foot-and-mouth disease virus over the sea. *Vet Rec* 110(3):47–52.

Gordon JC, Angrick EJ. 1986. Canine parvovirus: environmental effects on infectivity. *Am J Vet Res* 47(7):1464–1467.

Guthrie AJ, et al. 2003. Lateral transmission of equine arteritis virus among Lipizzaner stallions in South Africa. *Equine Vet J* 35(6):596–600.

Gwinn MR, Vallyathan V. 2006. Respiratory burst: role in signal transduction in alveolar macrophages. *J Toxicol Environ Health B Crit Rev* 9(1):27–39.

Haas W, et al. 2005. Behavioural strategies used by the hookworms *Necator americanus* and *Ancylostoma duodenale* to find, recognize and invade the human host. *Parasitol Res* 95(1):30–39.

Haig DM, Mercer AA. 1998. Ovine diseases. Orf. *Vet Res* 29(3-4):311–326.

Hampson K, et al. 2009. Transmission dynamics and prospects for the elimination of canine rabies. *PLoS Biol* 7(3):e53.

Heukelbach J, Feldmeier H. 2008. Epidemiological and clinical characteristics of hookworm-related cutaneous larva migrans. *Lancet Infect Dis* 8(5):302–309.

Holyoak GR, Balasuriya UB, Broaddus CC, Timoney PJ. 2008. Equine viral arteritis: current status and prevention. *Theriogenology* 70(3):403–414.

Hood AM. 2009. The effect of open-air factors on the virulence and viability of airborne *Francisella tularensis*. *Epidemiol Infect* 137(6):753–761.

Hosie MJ, et al. 2009. Feline immunodeficiency. ABCD guidelines on prevention and management. *J Feline Med Surg* 11(7):575–584.

Ise T, et al. 1996. Outbreaks of cholera in Kathmandu Valley in Nepal. *J Trop Pediatr* 42(5):305–307.

Ishida T, et al. 1992. Long-term clinical observations on feline immunodeficiency virus infected asymptomatic carriers. *Vet Immunol Immunopathol* 35(1-2):15–22.

Johns I, et al. 2009. Blood culture status in mature horses with diarrhoea: a possible association with survival. *Equine Vet J* 41(2):160–164.

Knight V. 1980. Viruses as agents of airborne contagion. *Ann N Y Acad Sci* 353:147–156.

Kramer A, Schwebke I, Kampf G. 2006. How long do nosocomial pathogens persist on inanimate surfaces? A systematic review. *BMC Infect Dis* 6:130.

Lamm CG, Rezabek GB. 2008. Parvovirus infection in domestic companion animals. *Vet Clin North Am Small Anim Pract* 38(4):837–850, viii–ix.

Lavine JS, Poss M, Grenfell BT. 2008. Directly transmitted viral diseases: modeling the dynamics of transmission. *Trends Microbiol* 16(4):165–172.

Leclerc H, Schwartzbrod L, Dei-Cas E. 2002. Microbial agents associated with waterborne diseases. *Crit Rev Microbiol* 28(4):371–409.

Leon A, et al. 2008. Detection of equine herpesviruses in aborted foetuses by consensus PCR. *Vet Microbiol* 126(1-3):20–29.

Lessler J, et al. 2009. Incubation periods of acute respiratory viral infections: a systematic review. *Lancet Infect Dis* 9(5):291–300.

Li X, et al. 2009. Occurrence and transmission of Newcastle disease virus aerosol originating from infected chickens under experimental conditions. *Vet Microbiol* 136(3-4):226–232.

Lutz H, et al. 2009. Feline leukaemia. ABCD guidelines on prevention and management. *J Feline Med Surg* 11(7):565–574.

Mackenzie JS, Williams DT. 2009. The zoonotic flaviviruses of southern, south-eastern and eastern Asia, and Australasia: the potential for emergent viruses. *Zoonoses Public Health* 35:221–270.

Maclachlan NJ, Drew CP, Darpel KE, Worwa G. 2009. The pathology and pathogenesis of bluetongue. *J Comp Pathol* 141(1):1–16.

Martucciello A, et al. 2009. Detection of bovine viral diarrhea virus from three water buffalo fetuses (*Bubalus bubalis*) in southern Italy. *J Vet Diagn Invest* 21(1):137–140.

Meerburg BG, Singleton GR, Kijlstra A. 2009. Rodent-borne diseases and their risks for public health. *Crit Rev Microbiol* 35:221–270.

Meunier PC, et al. 1985. Pathogenesis of canine parvovirus enteritis: sequential virus distribution and passive immunization studies. *Vet Pathol* 22(6):617–624.

Minarovits J. 2006. Epigenotypes of latent herpesvirus genomes. *Curr Top Microbiol Immunol* 310:61–80.

Monahan AM, Miller IS, Nally JE. 2009. Leptospirosis: risks during recreational activities. *J Appl Microbiol* 107:707–716.

Morens DM, Folkers GK, Fauci AS. 2008. Emerging infections: a perpetual challenge. *Lancet Infect Dis* 8(11):710–719.

Muller H, Johne R. 2007. Rotaviruses: diversity and zoonotic potential–a brief review. *Berl Munch Tierarztl Wochenschr* 120(3-4):108–112.

Muscatello G, Gilkerson JR, Browning GF. 2009. Detection of virulent *Rhodococcus equi* in exhaled air samples from naturally infected foals. *J Clin Microbiol* 47(3):734–737.

Nagaraj T, et al. 2006. Ante mortem diagnosis of human rabies using saliva samples: comparison of real time and conventional RT-PCR techniques. *J Clin Virol* 36(1):17–23.

Nakagomi O, Nakagomi T. 1991. Genetic diversity and similarity among mammalian rotaviruses in relation to interspecies transmission of rotavirus. *Arch Virol* 120(1-2):43–55.

Nicas M, Nazaroff WW, Hubbard A. 2005. Toward understanding the risk of secondary airborne infection: emission of respirable pathogens. *J Occup Environ Hyg* 2(3):143–154.

Niin E, et al. 2008. Rabies in Estonia: Situation before an after the first campaigns of oral vaccination of wildlife with SAG2 vaccinne bait. doi 10.1026, 26(29–30). Available at: http://dx.doi.org.

Oehler RL, et al. 2009. Bite-related and septic syndromes caused by cats and dogs. *Lancet Infect Dis* 9(7):439–447.

Orsel K, et al. 2010. Different infection parameters between dairy cows and calves after an infection with foot-and-mouth virus. *Vet J* 18(1):116–118.

Patel JR, Heldens J. 2005. Equine herpesviruses 1 (EHV-1) and 4 (EHV-4)–epidemiology, disease and immuno-prophylaxis: a brief review. *Vet J* 170(1):14–23.

Postma GC, Carfagnini JC, Minatel L. 2008. *Moraxella bovis* pathogenicity: an update. *Comp Immunol Microbiol Infect Dis* 31(6):449–458.

Powell DG, Watkins KL, Li PH, Shortridge KF. 1995. Outbreak of equine influenza among horses in Hong Kong during 1992. *Vet Rec* 136(21):531–536.

Prati D. 2006. Transmission of hepatitis C virus by blood transfusions and other medical procedures: a global review. *J Hepatol* 45(4):607–616.

Radford AD, et al. 2009. Feline calicivirus infection. ABCD guidelines on prevention and management. *J Feline Med Surg* 11(7):556–564.

Reddehase MJ, et al. 2008. Murine model of cytomegalovirus latency and reactivation. *Curr Top Microbiol Immunol* 325:315–331.

Rolle A, Olweus J. 2009. Dendritic cells in cytomegalovirus infection: viral evasion and host countermeasures. *APMIS* 117(5-6):413–426.

Sellon DC, Long MT, eds. 2006. Section II: Viral diseases, in *Equine Infectious Diseases*, Saunders, Philadelphia, pp 116–235.

Smith JS, Fishbein DB, Rupprecht CE, Clark K. 1991. Unexplained rabies in three immigrants in the United States. A virologic investigation. *N Engl J Med* 324(4):205–211.

Stannard W, O'Callaghan C. 2006. Ciliary function and the role of cilia in clearance. *J Aerosol Med* 19(1):110–115.

Sutmoller P, Casas OR. 2002. Unapparent foot and mouth disease infection (sub-clinical infections and carriers): implications for control. *Rev Sci Tech* 21(3):519–529.

Svensson C, Liberg P. 2006. The effect of group size on health and growth rate of Swedish dairy calves housed in pens with automatic milk-feeders. *Prev Vet Med* 73(1):43–53.

Tellier R. 2006. Review of aerosol transmission of influenza A virus. *Emerg Infect Dis* 12(11):1657–1662.

Terpstra FG, et al. 2007. Viral safety of C1-inhibitor NF. *Biologicals* 35(3):173–181.

Thiry E, et al. 2009. Feline herpesvirus infection. ABCD guidelines on prevention and management. *J Feline Med Surg* 11(7):547–555.

van der Meulen KM, Favoreel HW, Pensaert MB, Nauwynck HJ. 2006. Immune escape of equine herpesvirus 1 and other herpesviruses of veterinary importance. *Vet Immunol Immunopathol* 111(1-2):31–40.

van Maanen C, et al. 2003. Diagnostic methods applied to analysis of an outbreak of equine influenza in a riding school in which vaccine failure occurred. *Vet Microbiol* 93(4):291–306.

Warshawsky B, et al. 2002. Outbreak of *Escherichia coli* 0157:H7 related to animal contact at a petting zoo. *Can J Infect Dis* 13(3):175–181.

Webster RG, et al. 1992. Evolution and ecology of influenza A viruses. *Microbiol Rev* 56(1):152–179.

Weissinger MD, Theimer TC, Bergman DL, Deliberto TJ. 2009. Nightly and seasonal movements, seasonal home range, and focal location photo-monitoring of urban striped skunks (mephitis mephitis): implications for rabies transmission. *J Wildl Dis* 45(2):388–397.

Wilson A, Mellor PS, Szmaragd C, Mertens PP. 2009. Adaptive strategies of African horse sickness virus to facilitate vector transmission. *Vet Res* 40(2):16.

Wimsatt J, Biggins DE. 2009. A review of plague persistence with special emphasis on fleas. *J Vector Borne Dis* 46(2):85–99.

Wolf VH, Menossi M, Mourao GB, Gatti MS. 2008. Molecular basis for porcine parvovirus detection in dead fetuses. *Genet Mol Res* 7(2):509–517.

Wong D, et al. 2009. Primary pneumonic plague contracted from a mountain lion carcass. *Clin Infect Dis* 49(3):e33–e38.

Wong SS, Yuen KY. 2008. The management of coronavirus infections with particular reference to SARS. *J Antimicrob Chemother* 62(3):437–441.

Xiao L, Feng Y. 2008. Zoonotic cryptosporidiosis. *FEMS Immunol Med Microbiol* 52(3):309–323.

Xie X, et al. 2007. How far droplets can move in indoor environments–revisiting the Wells evaporation-falling curve. *Indoor Air* 17(3):211–225.

Yamanaka T, et al. 2008. Epidemic of equine influenza among vaccinated racehorses in Japan in 2007. *J Vet Med Sci* 70(6):623–625.

Zicola A, et al. 2009. Feline herpesvirus 1 and feline calicivirus infections in a heterogeneous cat population of a rescue shelter. *J Feline Med Surg* 11:1023–1027.

4 Zoonotic Diseases

Leslie Hiber and Kit T. Darling

"Veterinary practices are unique environments that bring humans into close contact with many different ill animals. In the practice environment, whether in a building or 'in the field', veterinary personnel are frequently exposed to recognized and unrecognized infectious pathogens, many of which are zoonotic" **(NASPHV, 2008).**

This chapter will identify some of the most frequently seen zoonotic diseases (diseases that are transmitted between animals and humans), provide an overview of their presentations in humans and animals, and discuss the transmission mechanisms and risks associated with each disease. The chapter will also reference precautions to help prevent transmission and discuss effective disinfection and cleaning processes and chemicals. Though the focus of this text is not on treatment, general treatment information will be mentioned.

ANTHRAX

Etiology

Anthrax is a disease caused by a spore-forming, gram-positive, rod-shaped bacteria called *Bacillus anthracis*. This disease is found worldwide, particularly in warmer climates ($>60°$F, $15.5°$C) (Greene, 2006). Moist, alkaline soils with high nitrogen content are the perfect environment for the proliferation of this organism. *B. anthracis* commences its life cycle in a noninfectious vegetative form. Toward the end of the growth phase of its life cycle when the vegetative form is exposed to oxygen, it will morph into infectious spores. Anthrax spores are often found as a contaminate in soil and on vegetation in fields where farm and domestic animals can ingest them.

Transmission

Transmission of anthrax spores can occur via direct contact or aerosol transmission. Direct transmission occurs by either ingestion of the spore or through contact with a break in the skin. Farm animals can ingest the spore through contaminated feed, soil, or vegetation in the fields. Carnivores can get anthrax through the consumption of contaminated meat and carcasses. Humans that come in contact with infected animals and their products (i.e., blood, wool, or hides) can contract anthrax through breaks in the skin or by eating undercooked, infected meat.

Veterinary Infection Prevention and Control, First Edition. Edited by Linda Caveney and Barbara Jones with Kimberly Ellis.
© 2012 John Wiley & Sons, Inc. Published by John Wiley & Sons, Inc.

Anthrax spores can also be inhaled via contaminated dust from the environment or from handling animal products (wool and hair). Anthrax may also be transmitted by biting flies.

Clinical Signs in Animals

The incubation period (time from exposure to the pathogenic organism to the onset of clinical signs) of anthrax in infected animals is usually 3–7 days but can range up to about 20 days (CFSPH, 2008). Clinical signs are dependent on the affected species. Cattle, sheep, and goats are the most commonly affected species; however, any mammal is susceptible to anthrax infections.

The acute form in ruminants can include fever, disorientation, muscle tremors, excitement followed by depression, dyspnea, abortion, and bloody discharges from the mouth, nose, and anus. Clinical signs usually reveal themselves for up to 2 days prior to staggering, trembling, dyspnea followed by rapid collapse, terminal convulsions, and death (CFSPH, 2008). The chronic form includes subcutaneous edematous swelling in the ventral neck, thorax, and shoulders. Both acute and chronic forms are usually fatal, and often the only clinical sign is death.

Horses can develop fever, chills, anorexia, depression, and severe colic with bloody diarrhea. Within 3 days to a week, they can develop swellings in the neck, sternum, lower abdomen, and external genitalia, which is then often followed by death (CFSPH, 2008).

Pigs can experience sudden death; however, mortality in this species is lower compared with ruminants and horses. With mild infections, pigs will portray signs of local inflammation, including swelling, fever, and enlarged lymph nodes. Recovery from a mild infection is common, but progressive swelling of the throat can lead to dyspnea and difficulty swallowing. This can lead to suffocation or asphyxiation and death.

Dogs and cats are considered relatively resistant to anthrax infections. Exposure to the spore does not guarantee infection in these species, and often they develop asymptomatic infections. Animals that do manifest clinical signs display ones that are similar to infections in pigs. Clinical signs specific to dogs and cats include acute, often hemorrhagic, gastroenteritis, which in younger and immunocompromised animals can lead to death.

Clinical Signs in Humans

In humans, the most common form of infection is cutaneous anthrax. The organism, after entering the body via a break in the skin, produces a toxin that initially causes a papule to form, similar to a boil. This progresses to a vesicle which then can rupture, forming a black central scar due to focal necrosis. The head, forearms, and hands are common sites of infection. Fatality due to cutaneous anthrax is 5–20% if left untreated (Acha and Szyfres, 2003).

Inhalation of anthrax spores can cause very serious symptoms and can have a greater than 85% mortality rate if left untreated (Heymann, 2004). Symptoms begin very mild and can include fever, malaise, mild cough and chest pain, along with acute respiratory distress. Within 3–5 days, severe fever, cyanosis (blue coloring to the skin and mucous membranes due to a lack of oxygen), and sudden death can occur (Acha and Szyfres, 2003). Both the cutaneous and inhalation infection of anthrax have about a 1- to 7-day incubation period (Heymann, 2004).

Gastrointestinal infection of anthrax spores is rare and can portray the same symptoms as severe food poisoning. These clinical signs can include violent vomiting and bloody diarrhea followed by fever, septicemia, and sometimes death. The mortality rate if left untreated is about 50% (Heymann, 2004). The incubation period is 12 hours to 5 days (Acha and Szyfres, 2003).

Diagnosis

Diagnosis of anthrax is confirmed by searching for the causative bacteria in blood, tissue, and other discharges via stained smears. In pigs, bacteremia (presence of bacteria in the blood) is rare; therefore, lymphatic tissue is directly examined rather than a blood sample. Bacterial culture can be used to make a diagnosis if samples are fresh; however, it is important to note that prior use of antibiotics may reduce the ability to isolate the organism. If available, polymerase chain reaction (PCR) assay can be used with blood or pleural effusion to rapidly detect these bacterial nucleic acids. Immunofluorescence assay (IFA) may also be used to detect bacteria in the blood or tissues.

Necropsy of any animal with suspected or confirmed anthrax infections is unadvisable. Opening of an infected carcass will expose the vegetative form of the organism to oxygen, causing sporulation to occur and consequently releasing the resistant infectious spores into the surrounding environment.

Treatment

Antibiotics may be an effective treatment if started early. Additional supportive care dependent on the clinical signs may also be necessary.

Disinfection/Prevention

Anthrax spores are extremely resistant to heat, radiation, disinfectants, and desiccation (process of extreme drying). They can remain viable in certain soils and environments for more than 40 years if the conditions are right (CFSPH, 2008). All areas, equipment, and surfaces that may have been contaminated by infected animals or tissues need to be cleaned and disinfected properly. Due to the resistant nature of the spores, normal disinfectants are not sufficient to properly clean an area or surface. Specific disinfectants that can be used include sodium hypochlorite (bleach), phenolics, formalin, or glutaraldehyde/formaldehyde. Instruments should be autoclaved or boiled at 250°F (121°C) for 30 minutes (CFSPH, 2008).

Any known or suspected infected animals should be strictly isolated, and the infected areas or premises should be quarantined. Infected dead animals should be destroyed by incineration or buried deep (not below the water level) to prevent environmental contamination and further transmission of the disease. Vaccinations for livestock are available in the United States and should be given to livestock housed in an endemic area.

BRUCELLOSIS

Etiology

Brucellosis is an infectious disease caused by gram-negative intracellular bacteria of the genus *Brucella*. Brucellosis is also known around the world by a variety of different names, including Undulant fever, Bang's disease, and Mediterranean fever. The *Brucella* genus consists of a variety of different species, including *B. abortus* (infects cattle, horses, and dogs), *B. melitensis* (infects sheep and goats), *B. suis* (infects domestic and feral pigs, horses, and dogs), *B. ovis* (infects sheep), *B. neotomae* (infects rodents), and *B. canis* (infects dogs and wild canidae). Humans are susceptible to infection with *B. abortus, B. melitensis, B. suis, and B. canis.*

Transmission

Transmission of brucellosis can occur by direct contact and aerosol routes. The highest concentration of the bacteria in infected animals is found in vaginal discharges, semen, and urine but can also be found in milk, blood, placenta, and fetal fluids and tissues. Dogs have been known to shed this organism vaginally for up to 6 weeks postabortion and for up to 3 months in the urine (Greene, 2006). In horses with fistulous withers or poll evil, *Brucella* sp. can also be found in the bursa. *Brucella* can infect a susceptible host by entering through mucous membranes (especially those of the oral cavity, vagina, and conjunctiva), breaks in the skin, and ingestion. In cattle, the udder is often colonized due to direct contact of contaminated hands.

Fomites (inanimate objects) can also be a source of transmission. Contaminated equipment can harbor the bacteria if not properly sterilized between patient uses. *Brucella* thrives in conditions with high humidity, low temperatures, and no sunlight. It can live for several months in water, aborted fetuses, manure, hay, equipment, and clothes (CFSPH, 2008).

Humans can become infected by ingesting contaminated, unpasteurized milk and cheese products or by direct contact with or aerosolization of contaminated bodily fluids of infected animals. Airborne infection can occur in stalls and stables of infected animals and for those people working in laboratories.

Clinical Signs in Animals

The incubation period in animals and humans can be difficult to ascertain as the onset of clinical signs are not obvious. In cattle, sheep, goats, and dogs, late-term abortions are common and may be the only sign of brucellosis. Other reproductive complications include retained placenta, decreased lactation, stillbirths, and infertility. Cattle and pigs may also display signs of arthritis after chronic infections. Goats specifically may exhibit signs of mastitis and lameness.

Clinical signs in canines are generally nonspecific. Most owners report signs of lethargy, loss of libido in breeding dogs, and premature aging (dry, lusterless coats, loss of vigor, slowing down). On physical exam, there can be generalized lymph node enlargement and splenomegaly but usually no outward signs of infection (e.g., no fever). In females, brucellosis should be suspected when apparently healthy bitches abort 2 weeks before term (Greene, 2006). In infected males, infertility is common along with enlarged scrotum and scrotal dermatitis due to constant licking. Chronically infected males may have unilateral or bilateral testicular atrophy. Dogs have been shown to remain bacteremic for months to years, and males can shed *Brucella* in the semen intermittently for up to 5 years (Quinn, 1997).

Horses with brucellosis will often have an inflammation of the supraspinous or supra-atlantal bursa called fistulous withers or poll evil. The bursa sac develops a thick wall and fills with a clear, viscous, straw-colored fluid. If the sac ruptures, it can lead to secondary infections. In horses with chronic infections, the ligament and dorsal vertebral spine near the affected bursa may become necrotic. Abortions due to *Brucella* are rare in horses.

Clinical Signs in Humans

Brucellosis in humans can cause similar symptoms as the flu. It generally has an acute onset of intermittent fever, headache, weakness, malaise, fatigue, profuse sweating, depression, weight loss, generalized aching, vomiting, and diarrhea. Many people have spontaneous recovery after a period of 2–4 weeks (CFSPH, 2008). With chronic infections, an undulating fever (fever can come and go) is common along with irritability, insomnia, mental depression, and emotional instability. Chronic cases can last from 3 months to a year or more without treatment (CFSPH, 2008).

Diagnosis

Brucellosis can be diagnosed by serology (testing using blood serum), culture, or other tests dependent on the host that is being tested. Serology is most commonly used for diagnosis. Serological testing is species dependent but can include rapid slide agglutination test, IFA, and ELISA. The rapid slide agglutination test is a good in-house, rapid, sensitive, and cheap way to detect antibodies early on. It is also very specific with a 99% correlation between a negative test and lack of infection (Greene, 2006).

Brucella can also be detected by culturing blood, semen, urine, vaginal secretions, and milk. An assortment of other tissues usually taken at time of necropsy can also be cultured. In canine patients, blood is the most practical fluid or tissue for isolation of *Brucella*. Dogs can remain bacteremic for as long as 18 months postinfection, but the amount of organisms found can be intermittent (CFSPH, 2008). Therefore, if testing is being done for screening of newly acquired animals into a breeding program, it is recommended that they should be isolated until two serotest results at a 1-month interval are negative (Greene, 2006). It is important to note that antibiotic administration may interfere with successful isolation of the organism.

Direct examination of abortion products, vaginal discharges, milk, semen, and other various tissues can be used as a presumptive diagnosis. However, if small numbers of organisms are present, the detection of any characteristic bacteria by this method will not be helpful.

PCR testing, if available, has also been developed for some species and might be more sensitive than blood culture or serology.

Treatment

Treatment options for animals with brucellosis are dependent on a variety of different factors, including clinical signs, species affected, and length of infection (acute or chronic). Treatment is more likely to be successful in animals infected for less than 3 months (Quinn, 1997). In dogs, long-term appropriate antibiotic combination therapy is necessary. Therapy should be chosen based on serologic testing and the blood culture susceptibility pattern. Bacteremia may reoccur weeks or months after the antibiotic therapy is discontinued; therefore, retesting should be performed 6–9 months following the treatment regimen (Quinn, 1997). Infected, intact males should be neutered to prevent any accidental transmission to females. The organism can still persist in neutered males, but the risk for shedding is reduced.

There is no useful treatment for cattle or pigs infected with *Brucella* (CFSPH, 2008). In sheep, antibiotics can be used; however, infertility can still be a problem. Horses with infected bursa may need to have them surgically removed to help rid them of the infection.

Disinfection/Prevention

Given the right conditions (high humidity, low temperatures, no sunlight), *Brucella* can live for months in the environment. Therefore, it is important that the proper disinfectants are used to clean up after an infected animal and their contaminated fluids. This organism is susceptible to a variety of disinfectants, including sodium hypochlorite (bleach), alcohol, and most quaternary ammonium compounds. The use of moist heat at 250°F (121°C) for a minimum of 15 minutes or dry heat at 320–340°F (160–170°C) for a minimum of 1 hour can also be used to destroy the bacteria (CFSPH, 2008).

Vaccinations for *Brucella* are available for cattle, sheep, and goats. It is important that precautions are enforced to prevent transmission of this disease within herds and breeding populations and to humans. Current protocol recommended by the USDA is that infected herds should be quarantined; individual animals should be tested and, if infected, slaughtered to help eradicate the disease from the herd. Screening of new dogs for brucellosis prior to entering a breeding program is necessary to prevent transmission to the rest of the population (see *Diagnosis*).

If working with infected animals and/or carcasses, be sure to wear the proper protective clothing (boots, impermeable clothing, gloves, face masks, goggles) and to practice good hand hygiene before and after handling the animals. Ensure that proper environmental cleaning and disinfection is performed, especially after handling aborted fetuses and fluids. Laboratory workers also need to follow good lab practices and precautions to prevent accidental exposure or infection. Also, avoid consumption of raw milk and unpasteurized dairy products.

CAMPYLOBACTER

Etiology

Campylobacteriosis is an intestinal bacterial infection caused by a gram-negative bacterium called *Campylobacter*. *Campylobacter* is the most common cause of bacterial diarrheal illness in the United States. *Campylobacter* is found worldwide in the intestinal tracts of animals. There are three main strains that tend to cause disease in domestic animals and humans: *C. jejuni* and *C. coli* (domestic animals and humans), and *C. fetus* (sheep, cattle, and humans). There are other strains that exist in these populations; however, they seem to be of minor importance in causing disease in domestic animals.

Transmission

Campylobacter is usually transmitted via the fecal–oral route by direct contact or by contaminated fomites. The bacteria can be found in feces, vaginal discharges, aborted fetuses, fetal membranes, and semen, which can in turn contaminate food and water sources. Contact with infected pets and livestock along with consumption of tainted undercooked meats and poultry, raw milk, raw clams, other contaminated foodstuffs, and unchlorinated water (swimming lakes) are common sources of *Campylobacter*. Flies can also be a mechanical vector in transmitting the bacteria.

Clinical Signs in Animals

Many animals can be asymptomatic carriers of *C. jejuni* and *C. coli*. The animals that are at most risk of developing clinical signs are the young (usually younger than 6 months of age), those that are stressed or have concurrent disease, or those that are immune compromised (Greene, 2006). The incubation period is about 1–10 days, usually 2–5 days (Halvorson et al., 2004). In dogs, clinical signs can include the following: diarrhea that may be watery, bile streaked, contain mucus and sometimes blood; fever; leukocytosis; partial anorexia; and occasional vomiting.

Most cases of diarrhea last for 3–7 days; however, in chronic cases, diarrhea may be intermittent and it may persist for two or more weeks to several months (CFSPH, 2008).

In calves and other young livestock, clinical signs may include thick, mucoid diarrhea with occasional flecks of blood, and possible fever. Signs will usually last 3–7 days; however, like dogs, they may have intermittent diarrhea for weeks to months (CFSPH, 2008).

In cattle and sheep, infection may cause infertility, early embryonic death, and a prolonged calving season; this is commonly known as bovine genital campylobacteriosis (CFSPH, 2008). Late-term abortions, stillbirths, and weak lambs can occur in sheep but are uncommon in cattle and other domestic animals. Infections in sheep can be followed by metritis (inflammation of the lining of the uterus) and occasionally death. Sheep can either continue to shed the bacteria life long or can fully recover with immunity to reinfection.

Clinical Signs in Humans

The incubation period in humans is about 2–5 days (CFSPH, 2008). Clinical signs include diarrhea (frequently bloody), abdominal pain, malaise (feeling ill), fever, nausea, and occasional vomiting. Chronic cases may display cough, headache, signs of meningitis (usually in premature neonatal infants), weight loss, and possibly abortion in the later half of pregnancy. Clinical signs may persist for about a week and are usually self-limited, although many infections are asymptomatic (Heymann, 2004).

Diagnosis

Diagnosis of campylobacteriosis is achieved most commonly by fecal culture. In humans, serologic testing is available; however, there is currently no serological testing available for infected animals. Direct gram stain identification of these bacteria can be done; however, the organisms tend to look like other enteric pathogens. Therefore, diagnosis cannot be done based on morphology alone.

Treatment

Antibiotic therapy in animals is not usually warranted in the cases of *Campylobacter* infection. Efficacy of antibiotic therapy in these cases is not truly known. Antibiotics are, however, often given to animals with cases of severe diarrhea to help minimize exposure to people and other pets in the household. Therapy in exposed sheep may prevent them from aborting in cases of an outbreak. Treatment of secondary symptoms may also be necessary in severe cases.

Disinfection/Prevention

Fortunately, *Campylobacter* is susceptible to many disinfectants, including, bleach, quaternary ammonium compounds, ethanol, and phenolics. It is susceptible to moist heat at 250°F (121°C) for at least 15 minutes and dry heat at 320–340°F (160–170°C) for at least 1 hour (CFSPH, 2008).

Although this bacterium is easily killed, it is important that precautions be taken when handling infected animals. Good hand hygiene, disinfection protocols, good environmental conditions, and control of flies and rodents are important to prevent the transmission of disease. Fecal contamination into water and feed sources should be prevented.

Vaccines are not available for dogs; however, vaccines can be used to prevent abortions in sheep and for both prophylaxis and treatment of bovine genital campylobacteriosis. It is important to note that, if vaccinated, the animal may remain a life-long carrier. Humans should also avoid consuming untreated water (swimming in contaminated lakes), unpasteurized milk products, and undercooked chicken.

CRYPTOSPORIDIUM

Etiology

Cryptosporidiosis is caused by an intracellular coccidian parasite called *Cryptosporidium*. This parasite can be found worldwide and is common in reptiles, birds, and mammals, including rodents, domestic livestock, cats, dogs, people, and numerous wild mammals. *C. parvum* is primarily responsible for causing disease in most mammals (including humans), although there are other zoonotic strains that have been isolated from a variety of different animals: *C. meleagridis* (turkey), *C. felis* (cats), *C. canis* (dog), *C. muris* (mouse), and *C. hominis* (unknown host specificity).

Transmission

Cryptosporidiosis is mainly transmitted by the fecal–oral route (direct and indirect transmission) but can also occur by aerosols. Oocysts, which are the thick-walled spore phase of this parasite's life cycle, are shed in the feces of infected animals. They are highly infectious and resistant to environmental conditions. About 50% of dairy calves and about 10% of puppies in shelters shed oocysts (CFSPH, 2008). Fecal contamination of food and water sources (swimming lakes and pools) are common sources of infection.

Clinical Signs in Animals

Cats infected with either *C. parvum* or *C. felis* and dogs infected with either *C. parvum or C. canis* are often asymptomatic, and clinical illness may only occur with concurrent disease, stress, or immunosuppression. Clinical signs may include persistent diarrhea, abdominal cramps and pain, nausea, vomiting, and fever.

Cryptosporidium is common in calves, and they are generally more susceptible at 1–3 weeks of age (CFSPH, 2008). The incubation period in calves is about 3–7 days (Halvorson et al., 2004). Similar to cats and dogs, calves can be asymptomatic carriers, and clinical illness may be more severe with concurrent disease and immunosuppression. Clinical signs in calves include diarrhea of varying severity (from mild to profusely watery), dehydration (due to severe diarrhea), anorexia, tenesmus (straining, often ineffectual), and weight loss.

Clinical Signs in Humans

In humans, the incubation period is usually about 1–12 days, the average being 7 days (Heymann, 2004). Severity of disease in people, like animals, usually depends on the immunocompetence of the person. In healthy individuals, the disease is usually self-limiting and people are often asymptomatic. In immunosuppressed individuals (i.e., AIDS patients), the disease may be chronic, often lasting a month or longer, and severe. Clinical signs may include profuse, watery diarrhea with cramping, abdominal pains, nausea, anorexia, flatulence, malaise, vomiting, weight loss, fever, and muscle pain. This parasite can also affect the respiratory system (pulmonary and tracheal cryptosporidiosis), and clinical signs then may include coughing often accompanied by a low-grade fever.

Diagnosis

Cryptosporidiosis is diagnosed by fecal floatation. However, due to the small size of the oocysts, staining of a direct smear should also be completed in order to aid in the visualization of the parasites. Oocysts can readily be seen on direct smears as they do not stain. It is important to remember that the oocysts can be shed intermittently, therefore repeat sampling may be necessary.

Treatment

Conventional antibiotic drug therapy has not been proven to be effective for the elimination of *Cryptosporidium*. The disease is usually self-limiting, but if clinical signs are severe enough, treatment of secondary symptoms (i.e., dehydration) may be initiated.

Disinfection/Prevention

Cryptosporidium is extremely resistant to environmental conditions. The oocyst can live in a moist environment for 2–6 months (CFSPH, 2008). Oocysts are resistant to most disinfectants, including bleach. The only chemicals that have been proven to be effective against the parasite are a prolonged exposure to ammonia or formol saline, moist heat (steam or pasteurization), freezing and thawing, or desiccation.

In order to prevent the transmission of *Cryptosporidium*, it is important to follow good hygiene and environmental cleaning protocols. If working with infected animals and/or feces, gloves and other protective clothing should be worn. Calves should be born in a clean environment and should be housed individually for the first couple of weeks. Good hygiene should be followed between handling of the calves, and rodents and flies should be kept under control. People should avoid eating undercooked meat and unwashed veggies and fruit due to potential contamination.

GIARDIA

Etiology

Giardiasis is an infection caused by a protozoal parasite called *Giardia intestinalis* (also called *G. lamblia, G. duodenalis,* or *Lamblia intestinalis*). It is the most common intestinal parasite and is found worldwide in humans and many species of domestic and wild animals. This protozoan can be found in two forms: the cyst and the trophozite. The infective and resistant form is a cyst, which, after being ingested, releases one or two trophozites (the noninfective motile form) into the small intestines. From there, the trophozites multiply and encyst along the way through the colon and are eventually shed in the feces.

Transmission

Transmission of *Giardia* occurs by the fecal–oral route. Common paths of transmission include the following: not using good hand hygiene after handling an infected animal or its feces, contaminated fomites, and consumption of contaminated food and water.

Clinical Signs in Animals

Most infections in adult animals are asymptomatic. In younger animals, the most common clinical sign is acute diarrhea. Other common signs in both adults and young animals may include the following: acute, chronic, or intermittent diarrhea or semi-formed soft stools (light-colored, mucoid, and may contain undigested fat often with a foul odor); poor hair coat; flatulence; and weight loss or failure to gain weight. Those animals that are stressed, immunocompromised, or housed in large groups have a greater incidence of clinical disease. The incubation period is usually 5–14 days (CFSPH, 2008). It is also important to note that both asymptomatic and symptomatic animals can excrete infective cysts.

Clinical Signs in Humans

Like animals, most humans with giardiasis are asymptomatic. Common clinical signs in people may include foul-smelling diarrhea (greasy appearance), abdominal cramps, bloating, flatulence, nausea, fatigue, weight loss, and possibly dehydration (due to severe diarrhea). The incubation period in people is between 1 and 25 days (usually within a week), and illness can last anywhere from 1 to 2 weeks in the acute form or months to years in the chronic form (CFSPH, 2008). Chronic illness is usually seen in immunocompromised individuals. Similar to younger animals in a large group setting, infants and children in day care situations are also at a higher risk of infection.

Diagnosis

The most definite way to diagnosis giardiasis is by finding the cysts and/or trophozites in a direct fecal smear. Although their presence does not necessarily indicate that they are causing an illness, as patients are often asymptomatic. A negative smear does not necessarily mean a negative diagnosis, as the parasites are shed intermittently. At least three negative samples over a period of 3–5 days are needed to definitively rule out infection (Greene, 2006). ELISA testing can be used to detect *Giardia* antigens, and IFA can also be used to help visualize these organisms.

Treatment

Antiparasitic medications commonly used in humans are often used off-label in many infected companion animals. They are often treated even if asymptomatic due to the zoonotic potential of the parasite.

Disinfection/Prevention

Giardia can live for long periods of time in an ideal environment. It prefers a moist, cool environment and can survive freezing for up to 2 weeks (CFSPH, 2008). However, it is susceptible to direct sunlight and desiccation. Sodium hypochlorite (bleach) is the disinfectant of choice. More recently, quaternary ammonium compounds are also able to successfully eliminate the organism from the environment; read the label kill claims for this information. It is also important to note that *Giardia* is resistant to chlorination levels typical in pool and tap water.

Good prevention techniques include the following: keep pets and livestock away from water sources to prevent fecal contamination of the water or to prevent the animal from picking up the organism from contaminated water; prompt removal of feces from the environment; good environmental conditions and cleaning; wash all raw fruits and vegetables prior to consumption; and good hand hygiene.

LEPTOSPIROSIS

Etiology

Leptospirosis is caused by spiral-shaped bacteria (spirochetes) called leptospires, genus *Leptospira*. This bacterium has many distinct serovars, which can affect a wide variety of animal species worldwide.

Transmission

Transmission of *Leptospira* can occur by direct or indirect contact or by aerosolization. Leptospirosis can be transmitted via contaminated food, water, equipment, and surfaces; spread in aerosolized urine or water; or by direct contact with contaminated urine. The spirochetes can also be found in aborted fetuses or in normal fetuses after calving. The spirochetes can enter the host, both animals and humas, via intact mucous membranes (e.g., eyes, nose, and mouth) or through breaks in the skin. Human cases have also been known to be transmitted via sexual intercourse, rodent bites, breast feeding, and with laboratory accidental exposures. *Leptospira* spp. do not multiply outside the host; however, animals may excrete the bacteria for months after infection. The organism may live in moist soil in a humid environment or in stagnant, slow-moving warm water for months at a time.

Clinical Signs in Animals

The incubation period is usually about 7–12 days but can range anywhere from 2 to 29 days (CFSPH, 2008). Leptospirosis can affect many domestic animals, including cattle, pigs, sheep, and dogs. Leptospires can affect many tissues, including the kidneys, liver, spleen, central nervous system, eyes, and genital tract. Infections can be asymptomatic, mild or severe, and acute or chronic. The severity of disease in most animals is dependent on immunity of the host and age of the host; typically the younger animals are often more severely affected. Clinical signs in dogs are generally nonspecific and may include fever, anorexia, vomiting, dehydration, increased thirst, stiffness, abdominal and muscle pain, kidney and liver disease, hematuria, shivering, and weakness.

Infected cattle can have clinical signs that range in severity. Leptospirosis can cause decreased milk production, fever, anorexia, conjunctivitis, diarrhea, jaundice, hemogloburinuria, pneumonia, or signs of meningitis. Calves with severe disease may die within 3–5 days (CFSPH, 2008). Adult cows may have transient and mild clinical signs that may go unnoticed. Abortion may be the only clinical sign and can occur 3–10 weeks after infection (CFSPH, 2008).

In horses, infections are usually subclinical, with ocular disease being the most prominent syndrome. In severe cases, leptospirosis may be accompanied by liver, kidney, or cardiovascular disease along with abortions.

Clinical Presentation in Humans

Clinical signs in humans can vary from asymptomatic to severe. Flu-like symptoms are often the first symptoms, which can then develop into more severe life-threatening illness involving the kidneys, liver, brain, lung, and heart. The incubation period in humans is about 7–12 days, and most people who are infectious can excrete the bacteria in the urine for 60 days or less (CFSPH, 2008). In humans, leptospirosis can also be transmitted through breast milk. Mortality rate of people with leptospirosis is about 1–5% (CFSPH, 2008).

Diagnosis

Diagnosis of leptospirosis is based on an antibody test (that only proves if there was exposure at some point in time), clinical signs, and ruling out other diseases. PCR tests for leptospires have not been proven to be completely accurate, and this particular bacterium is not easily cultured due to its fastidious nature.

Treatment

Treatment of leptospirosis is most successful if caught early in the disease process. Antibiotics and other supportive care (i.e., transfusions, fluids) dependent on clinical signs are generally included in the treatment plan. Vaccinations are available for pigs, cattle, and dogs; however, vaccines are usually serovar-specific. Leptospirosis vaccines do not completely help to prevent infection or the shedding of the organism but may help in preventing disease.

Disinfection/Prevention

Good contact precautions, including use of personal protective equipment (face shields should be worn if there is a possibility of urine splashing) and hand hygiene, are critical in preventing transmission of *Leptospira* spp. If at any time the urine from an infectious or possibly infectious patient comes in contact with any mucous membranes (eyes, mouth, and nose) or open cuts on the skin, seek medical attention immediately. It is also important to promptly clean up any urine from an infectious or potentially infectious patient.

Bleach and alcohol have been proven to be effective in killing *Leptospira* spp. The spirochete is also sensitive to moist heat and pasteurization.

METHICILLIN-RESISTANT *Staphylococcus*

Contributing Author Kit T. Darling, MS, M, MT(ASCP), CIC
Staphylococcus is gram-positive cocci that appear as "grape like" clusters on gram stain and is catalase positive. Some species are coagulase positive, whereas others are coagulase negative. The genus consists of a number of opportunistic pathogens that are important in veterinary medicine. The species of most clinical importance are *S. aureus* and *S. intermedius* group, including *S. psuedintermedius*. Soon after methicillin was used to treat penicillin-resistant staphylococci in humans, methicillin-resistant *S. aureus* (MRSA) was reported in 1961. Initially,

MRSA was associated with nosocomial infections in hospitals. In the 1990s, MRSA was isolated from people who had not been associated with a hospital, thus the emergence of community-acquired MRSA. In 2003, Salgado et al. (2003) identified MRSA colonization in 1.3% of the people studied, and only 0.2% of these people did not identify any health care–associated risks. MRSA is a worldwide problem. Recently MRSA has become a concern in veterinary medicine. This section will address MRSA in animals as well as other species of methicillin-resistant *Staphylococcus*.

Methicillin-Resistant *Staphylococcus aureus*

The first report of MRSA in animals was in 1972, in the milk from a Belgian cow with mastitis (Devriese and Hommez, 1975). MRSA has been reported in a variety of animals, including dogs, cats, sheep, horses, chickens, rabbits, birds, pigs, etc. The incubation period in animals is highly variable, like that in humans. Also similar to humans, animals can be colonized with MRSA as well as developing clinical disease (CSFPH, 2006). Some epidemiological studies of the prevalence in animals have been done. The true carriage rate of MRSA in animals is difficult to determine from these studies due to sampling bias, inadequate microbiology culture methodology, and variable geographical and strain differences (Morgan, 2008). A wide variety of animals, such as dogs, cats, horses, and other animals, have been reported as asymptomatic carriers of MRSA. Colonization occurs when the bacteria are present on the skin or mucous membranes but do not invade the tissue. Colonization may be transient or long term. Infection occurs when the bacteria successfully enters the body and invades the tissue. Most frequently, MRSA has been isolated in skin and soft-tissue infections, including abscesses, dermatitis, fistulas, intravenous catheters, postsurgical wounds, and implant infections. Less frequently, MRSA may be the causative organism in pneumonia, rhinitis, septic arthritis, osteomyelitis, bacteremia, metritis, and mastitis. The organism is transmitted by direct contact through breaks in the skin or mucous membranes or indirectly from items or the environment contaminated with MRSA.

The risks factors for colonization and infection in animals are similar to those for humans. The risks include living in a household with a colonized human or animal, hospitalization or surgery, underlying disease causing immunosuppression, and recent history of antimicrobial therapy. A study in 2006 suggested transmission of MRSA between pets and humans in veterinary clinics and households (Weese et al., 2006). In this study, both animal-to-human and human-to-animal transmission appeared to occur.

MRSA strains are resistant to beta-lactam antibiotics, which include penicillin and cephalosporins. The mecA gene that is expressed as a protein in the bacterial cell wall promotes beta-lactam resistance. Beta-lactam antibiotics damage bacteria by inactivating penicillin-binding proteins, PBP2a (CFSPH, 2006). *S. aureus* may have virulence factors and produce toxins causing very serious disease processes. An example is toxic shock syndrome toxin 1 (TSST-1), which causes toxic shock syndrome. In addition, some strains of *S. aureus* carry Panton-Valentine leukocidin (PVL), which can cause necrosis, leukocyte destruction, and severe inflammation. Strains with PVL have been associated with serious infections in humans and animals (Rankins et al., 2005).

Other Methicillin-Resistant *Staphylococcus*

For a number of years, coagulase-positive staphylococci have been considered important pathogens in veterinary medicine. The coagulase-positive staphylococci include *S. aureus,*

S. intermedius, S. schleiferi, S. lutrae, S. delphini, and *S. pseudintermedius. S. schleiferi* and *S. hyicus* have some biochemical differences that make them easy to differentiate from *S. intermedius, S. delphini,* and *S. pseudintermedius.* Commercial kits are available to identify *S. schleiferi* and *S. hyicus.* The phenotypic characteristics of *S. intermedius, S. delphini,* and *S. pseudintermedius* are similar, and commercial kits are not available to differentiate these species (Sakashi et al., 2007). *S. intermedius* has been reported as a prevalent organism in dogs, cats, horses, goats, and pigeons. Previous information has documented that *S. intermedius* is more frequently isolated from dogs and *S. aureus* is more frequently isolated from humans. *S. intermedius* may be isolated from skin, hair, and mucous membranes of healthy dogs. This organism can be isolated from pyoderma, otitis externa, and other suppurative conditions (Quinn et al., 2002). Originally the bacteria that were reported as *S. intermedius* may have included *S. delphini* and *S. pseudintermedius.* In 2005, Devriese et al. (2005) described a novel species *S. pseudintermedius.* This organism was identified on the basis of 16S rRNA sequence analysis. The isolates were from a cat, dog, horse, and parrot.

S. pseudintermedius has been isolated from healthy dogs and cats. Pyoderma, otitis externa, wound infections, abscesses, and other tissues can be caused by this opportunistic pathogen. Now methicillin-resistant *Staphylococcus pseudintermedius* (MRSPI) has been isolated from dogs, cats, and humans (Weese and van Duijkeren, 2010). Studies are needed on the risk factors associated with MRSPI infections. *S. pseudintermedius* is not a common organism isolated from humans. Even though several cases of zoonotic transmission of MRSPI have been reported between dogs and humans, it is not as much of a zoonotic concern as MRSA.

Prevention and Control

The establishment of infection prevention and control policies are important to minimize the risk for transmission of methicillin-resistant *Staphylococcus.* The precautions should include isolating the animal, barrier precautions, and disinfection of patient care equipment (thermometers, stethoscope, blood pressure cuffs, scissors, gurneys, etc.) and the environmental surfaces.

The animal should be placed in an appropriate isolated area and restricted to that area unless emergency medical procedures are needed (Weese, 2005). Gloves are worn when handling the patient, blood and body fluids, and contaminated patient care equipment or environmental surfaces. After removing gloves, perform hand hygiene either by washing hands or by using alcohol-based hand sanitizer. Gowns are worn to prevent the bacteria from contaminating the clothing. Face protection is worn if a procedure is likely to generate splashes, such as wound lavage. Wounds are covered to contain drainage and prevent transmission of the bacteria. Transport the patient on a gurney. If this is not possible, disinfect the floor where the patient has walked. Clean and disinfect all patient care equipment, environmental surfaces, and other items that the patient touches. Hand hygiene is performed after removing personal protective equipment (gloves, gowns, masks, etc.) and after contact with the patient or the environment or items that the patient has touched.

When a patient with methicillin-resistant *Staphylococcus* is discharged from the veterinary hospital, it is important to give the client information and instructions to help prevent transmission of the bacteria to people and other animals in the household. The following are some suggestions:

1. Follow your veterinarian's instructions.
2. Use good hand hygiene (handwashing or use alcohol hand sanitizer) before and after contact with the infected animal.

3. Use gloves when caring for wounds or when in contact with blood or body fluids.
4. Keep open wounds covered.
5. Clean and disinfect environmental surfaces and items that had contact with the infected animal. Use an EPA product (EPA number will be listed on the label) that is effective against MRSA or a bleach solution. Follow the instructions on the label of the product. A bleach solution is made by mixing 2 teaspoons of bleach into 1 quart of water.
6. Wash any items that become soiled by the animal separately from the other laundry, using hot water and laundry detergent (and bleach if possible). Dry in a hot dryer.
7. Anyone in the household that is immunocompromised, recently had surgery, or is very young or elderly should avoid contact with the infected animal or items soiled by the animal.

RABIES

Etiology

Rabies is caused by an infection with an enveloped RNA rabies virus in the genus *Lyssavirus*, family Rhabdoviridae. Rabies can be found worldwide and can potentially infect all mammals (contact your state health department to determine which animals are at the greatest risk for transmission of the rabies virus). Worldwide, more than 30,000 people die from rabies each year and 10–12 million receive postexposure treatment (Greene, 2006).

Transmission

The rabies virus can be found, after sufficient incubation, in the salivary glands, saliva, nervous tissue, and cerebrospinal fluid of infected animals. It has also been detected in other tissues and organs, including the lungs, adrenal glands, kidneys, bladder, heart, ovaries, testes, prostate, pancreas, intestinal tract, cornea, germinal cells of hair follicles in the skin, sebaceous glands, tongue papillae, and the brown fat of bats. Despite the detection in various tissues, the virus is not transmitted via blood, urine, or feces.

It is transmitted most often in saliva via a bite from an infected animal; however, transmission can occur if infected saliva or neurological tissues come in contact with mucous membranes or a break in the skin.

Most human exposures to rabies occur through domestic animals (dogs, cats, cattle, and horses) that, in turn, have been exposed to wild animals that are infected with the virus. Most exposures exist in areas where rabies virus infections in wildlife and feral domestic animals are an endemic.

Clinical Signs in Animals

The incubation period in animals generally ranges from 10 days to 6 months (or longer) but is dependent on a variety of factors: the amount of virus transmitted, virus strain, site of inoculation (bites closer to the head or spinal cord have a shorter incubation period), host immunity, and the degree of innervation (proximity to nerve supply) of the bite site (CFSPH, 2008; Greene, 2006).

Initial clinical signs in an animal infected with the rabies virus usually last 2–3 days (Greene, 2006). A behavioral change may occur in this initial stage in which the animal can become apprehensive, restless, shy if they were outgoing, or vice versa. A slight, low-grade fever may also be found in this initial stage. The animal may then experience both or one of either the next two stages, often referred to as the furious and the paralytic (dumb) forms of rabies infection.

The furious form can last around 1–7 days and is more commonly found in the cat than the dog. Animals with this form are often restless, photophobic, easily excited, can become hyperesthetic, and appear that they are barking or snapping at nonexistent objects. As the disease progresses, they become more vicious and vocal, and they often eat unusual objects. Confined animals will often try to bite or attack their enclosures. Wild animals with this form are usually seen in the daylight alone and no longer display a fear of humans. In the terminal stages, seizures, lack of muscular coordination, disorientation, and paralysis are seen, and within about 4–8 days of the onset of clinical signs, death occurs (CFSPH, 2008).

The paralytic, or dumb, form of rabies lasts around 2–4 days, and the predominant clinical sign is progressive paralysis. Cats commonly display the paralytic form following the furious form beginning around day 5 of clinical illness (Greene, 2006). Increased salivation, a dropped lower jaw, and a change in the tone of the bark are indications that cranial nerve, masticatory muscle, and laryngeal paralysis have occurred. Paralysis of these muscles can cause an animal to look like it is choking while trying to drink water to quench extreme thirst. Ataxia and lack of coordination may occur due to ascending spinal paralysis. Respiratory failure is the final clinical sign prior to death.

A horse or mule infected with the rabies virus may seem distressed or extremely agitated. These clinical signs are often mistaken for colic signs. Cattle may seek solitude, stop ruminating, and have an abnormal bellow. Survival in all mammals is extremely rare once the clinical signs become visible.

Clinical Signs in Humans

The incubation period in humans is generally 1–3 months but can range from 2 days to several years (CFSPH, 2008). Initial signs include headache, fever, anxiety, with pain and discomfort at the bite site. As the disease progresses, hypersalivation, confusion, abnormal behavior, hypersensitivity to light and sound, and violent behavior may occur. Some individuals refuse to drink water, have excessive salivation, and may experience painful pharyngeal spasms when attempting to swallow liquids. Death occurs usually due to convulsions or respiratory arrest due to paralysis. As in other mammals, survival is rare and infection is generally considered fatal once clinical signs are evident.

Diagnosis

Identification of the rabies virus is done by direct IFA of brain tissue postmortem. There are currently no definitive or efficient diagnostic tests that can be done premortem. Make sure to investigate the proper way to collect and submit the samples per the laboratory that is being used, as mishandling of the tissue can cause false negatives to occur, or the tissue may not be able to be used for testing.

Treatment

Once clinical signs of rabies are evident, there is no treatment to stop the progression of the disease. Postexposure vaccinations in mammals (except humans) have not been proven effective (due to the lack of studies). Contact your state health department for further information regarding postexposure protocol in humans. The protocol for animals can be found on the National Association of State Public Health Veterinarians (NASPHV) website (http://www.nasphv.org).

Disinfection/Prevention

Rabies virus can remain viable in a carcass for several days at 68°F (20°C). It can survive much longer when the body is refrigerated (Greene, 2006). The virus is susceptible to a variety of disinfectants, including lipid solvents (i.e., soap), quaternary ammonium compounds, and bleach. The virus does not survive very long in the environment, except in cool dark areas, as it is readily inactivated by sunlight (CFSPH, 2008).

Prevention measures are mainly focused on pre-exposure prophylactic vaccinations. Vaccinations are available for most domesticated animals, including dogs, cats, ferrets, cattle, sheep, and horses. A vaccinated animal that bites a human and is not displaying any clinical signs associated with rabies needs to be quarantined and observed for 10 days (CFSPH, 2008). If the animal is unvaccinated and bites a human, it should be euthanized and tested. Any animal that is clinical and bites a human should be euthanized and tested immediately. Contact the state health department, where the bite occurred, for further specific information regarding where the animal must be quarantined and who must be contacted.

Wild animals should be avoided, especially those that are displaying rabid clinical signs (see *Clinical Signs in Animals* section). Wild animal and feral dog populations are sometimes vaccinated via the aid of bait to help reduce the threat of rabies transmission to domesticated animals and humans.

People who work with animals or animal tissues, or conduct recreation in environments with high risk of exposure, should also undergo pre-exposure prophylaxis. In particular, the risk of veterinary personnel being exposed to rabid animals is more than 300 times greater than that of the general population (Greene, 2006). Pre-exposure vaccination does not eliminate the need for treatment postexposure; however, it does provide a variety of benefits, including the following: some protection if exposure is unknown or if postexposure treatment is delayed, eliminates the need for rabies immunoglobulin, and decreases the number of postexposure vaccinations that need to be given. All individuals who are exposed (vaccinated or not) should seek treatment as soon as possible. Treatment includes immediate wound cleansing and disinfection, rabies postexposure vaccination, and the administration of human rabies immunoglobulin (if not previously vaccinated).

When working directly with an alive or dead rabies suspect animal, double gloves, safety glasses and face masks or respirators should be worn. Individuals who are vaccinated need to have a titer checked every 2 years to determine whether they are still adequately protected by the original vaccine.

SALMONELLA

Etiology

Salmonellosis is caused by a gram-negative, aerobic, rod-shaped bacteria. There are over 2400 different serotypes of *Salmonella* spp., but the most typical ones seen in clinics and humans are *S. enteritidis* and *S. typhimurium* (CFSPH, 2008; Greene, 2006). Salmonella is naturally found in many wild and domestic animals. It usually does not become an issue for these animals until their immune system is weakened (due to other disease) or they are stressed, possibly by transportation, crowding, food deprivations, weaning, parturition, exposure to cold, sudden change of feed, or overfeeding following a fast. It is also very common for a horse to break with *Salmonella* after a major surgery (i.e., colic surgery).

Transmission

Transmission can occur by ingesting the bacteria in contaminated food, such as undercooked meat, animals being fed a raw food diet, animal-derived animal treats, and water sources. In a clinic setting, transmission can occur by ingesting the bacteria by the fecal–oral route via contaminated hands or fomites. Both animals and humans can be carriers without being clinical for this infection. Animals shed *Salmonella* continually for the first week after infection and then intermittently for the next 3–6 weeks or longer (Greene, 2006).

Clinical Signs in Animals

The incubation period in most animals is 3–5 days, either from time of exposure to organism or, if they are carriers, from the onset of a stressful situation (Greene, 2006). Clinical signs in animals can range from asymptomatic to severe dependent on the immune status and age of the host (the very young and old tend to have more severe clinical signs) and the number of infecting organisms. Most infected patients develop gastroenteritis signs, including vomiting, diarrhea, fever, anorexia, malaise, and abdominal pain. Infections usually resolve within 2–7 days and often do not require treatment unless the patient becomes severely dehydrated (CFSPH, 2008). In horses, if the enteritis is severe and treatment is not given, death can occur as a result of dehydration and toxemia as quick as 24–48 hours (CFSPH, 2008). Infection can also cause abortions and joint problems in some ruminants and horses.

Clinical Signs in Humans

In humans, *Salmonella* is associated with a sudden onset of headache, abdominal pain, cramping, diarrhea, nausea, vomiting, and/or dehydration. The incubation period in humans is 1–3 days. Fecal shedding can last several days to weeks, and humans can become temporary carriers for several months or longer (CFSPH, 2008). Antibiotics are also known to prolong the carrier state in many adults.

Diagnosis

Isolation of the *Salmonella* by culture is the most definitive way to diagnose salmonellosis. Because animals can shed *Salmonella* intermittently, five consecutive fecal cultures or three PCR samples need to be submitted ideally over a 2- to 3-week time period (Greene, 2006). However, it is common practice to take samples in large animals (horses, cows) all from within the same day if they are clinical. Until all the samples come back negative, salmonellosis cannot be ruled out.

Treatment

Treatment is dependent on the severity of clinical signs. If it is deemed necessary to use antibiotics for salmonellosis, appropriate antibiotics should be chosen based on the susceptibility pattern of the specific type of *Salmonella* sp. It is important to note that administration of antibiotics may contribute to the patient becoming a prolonged carrier of *Salmonella*. Secondary treatment may be needed if clinical signs are severe (i.e., dehydration).

Disinfection/Prevention

Any patient that presents with diarrhea or breaks with diarrhea while staying at the clinic or hospital should be immediately isolated, and proper precautions should be instituted as *Salmonella* can be easily spread to other patients and can be hard to get rid of in the environment. Isolation precautions include disposable gloves, gowns, and boot covers; face shield; footbaths at every entrance and exit into the isolation facility; patient-specific equipment; limited foot traffic through the area; limited personnel exposure; and excellent hand hygiene. If possible, all equipment should be designated for an isolation area only. However, if the equipment must be used on other patients, it must be properly cleaned and disinfected before use.

Salmonella can survive in the environment for a long period of time, especially in wet and warm environments. Therefore, it is important to make sure that cleaning and disinfection are done properly and thoroughly to prevent transmission. There are a variety of different disinfectants on the market that can be used to kill these gram-negative bacteria. Read the label carefully to ensure that it is effective against *Salmonella*. If an outbreak of *Salmonella* occurs at your clinic, it is a good idea to get the strain serotyped to ensure that it is indeed the same strain being shared (i.e., to determine whether it is a nosocomial infection being acquired from the clinic or hospital).

TOXOPLASMOSIS

Etiology

Toxoplasmosis is a disease caused by *Toxoplasma gondii*, an obligate intracellular coccidian parasite. It is found worldwide more commonly in warm, humid climates. Cats are the definitive host for this parasite; however, it can cause infection in almost every warm-blooded animal. Cats, sheep, goats, and swine are most commonly known to be infected, followed by dogs and horses, which tend to have lower infection rates. Cattle are relatively resistant to infection (CFSPH, 2008).

There are three major infectious stages that the parasite will transition through: sporozoites in oocysts (the oocyst is a protective, thick-walled structure) that are excreted in the feces, tachyzoites (actively multiplying stage found in tissues), and bradyzoites (slowly multiplying stage) enclosed in tissue cysts (thick-walled structures often found in the muscles and central nervous system) (CFSPH, 2008; Greene, 2006).

Transmission

Transmission of *T. gondii* can occur via ingestion of infected animal tissues or contaminated water and food, via the fecal–oral route through contact with infected feces or soil, or via inhalation of aerosols. Congenital infection can occur in some species, including sheep, goats, small rodents, and humans (CFSPH, 2008). Other more uncommon routes of transmission include lactation, transfusion of body fluids, or transplantation of tissues or organs (Greene, 2006).

The most common ways for humans to become infected with *T. gondii* is by ingestion of viable cysts in undercooked meat or ingestion of oocysts shed in the feces of a recently infected cat. Transplancental infection of the human fetus can occur via tachyzoite spread when a pregnant woman is infected for the first time (no previous exposure) and is more severe if infected during the first trimester.

Clinical Signs in Animals

Clinical signs in animals are dependent on age, sex, host species, strain of *T. gondii*, number of organisms, and the stage of the parasite ingested (Greene, 2006). The majority of animals infected with the parasite are asymptomatic, whereas those that are symptomatic often have underlying disease or were infected in utero or lactationally (CFSPH, 2008; Greene, 2006).

Cats that are symptomatic are usually young or immunocompromised, and the most severely affected are those that acquire the disease transplacentally or lactationally. These kittens may be stillborn, die before weaning, or exhibit a variety of clinical signs, including inflammation of the liver, lungs, and central nervous system; lethargy, depression; hypothermia; or enlarged abdomen due to enlarged liver and ascites.

Older cats may demonstrate lethargy, anorexia, dyspnea (most often due to concurrent pneumonia), persistent or intermittent fever, weight loss, icterus caused by hepatitis, vomiting, diarrhea, abdominal effusion, stiffness of gait, shifting leg lameness, neurologic deficits, dermatitis, and death (Greene, 2006). Central nervous system signs are more common in older cats, but severity is dependent on the site of the lesion (CFSPH, 2008). Ocular clinical signs can also occur, which can include generalized retinitis or irregular reddish, dark, or pale retinal foci; glaucoma, corneal opacity, and panophthalmitis are often due to chronic low-grade infections (CFSPH, 2008).

Like cats, infected dogs are usually asymptomatic, and, if clinical, it is usually in puppies or immune-compromised older dogs. Clinical signs may include hyperexcitability, depression, seizures, head tilt, paresis, paralysis, pelvic limb muscles become rigid but nonpainful, acute hepatitis (become icteric), abdominal effusion, lethargy, fever, vomiting, diarrhea, retinitis, uveitis, and death (CFSPH, 2008).

In sheep, goats, and swine, abortions and stillbirths are common if infected during pregnancy. Infected young often are uncoordinated, weak, feverish, dyspneic, and have a high mortality rate. In the horse, fever, encephalitis, ataxia, and retinal degeneration have been reported, whereas in cattle, reported clinical signs are fever, respiratory distress, nasal discharge and conjunctival hyperemia (CFSPH, 2008).

Clinical Signs in Humans

In humans, the incubation period is about 10–23 days postingestion of contaminated meat and 5–20 days postingestion of oocysts from infected cats (Heymann, 2004). However, most infections are asymptomatic and self-limiting, usually persisting 1–12 weeks, after which immunity is readily aquired (CFSPH, 2008; Greene, 2006). Individuals that are immunocompromised or pregnant may experience fever, malaise, headache, sore throat, lymphadenopathy, and rash. Severe clinical signs may include myositis, mycoarditis, pneumonitis, and neurological signs (CFSPH, 2008).

The primary disease that develops in infected children is retinochoroiditis (Greene, 2006). The severity of disease in infants infected in utero is dependent on when the infection occurred.

If infected during the first trimester, clinical signs will be more severe and may include severe ocular disease, hydrocephalus, convulsions, and intracerebral calcification. In the worst cases, abortion or stillbirths may occur (CFSPH, 2008). The fetus/child infected in the later stages of pregnancy may display varying degrees of ocular disease, fever, rash, hepatomegaly, splenomegaly, pneumonia, or generalized infection (CFSPH, 2008).

Diagnosis

In cats, fecal flotation may be used to identify oocysts in the feces if the cat is actively shedding the oocyst (usually occurs in early infection or due to a stressful event). Unfortunately, there is no single serologic assay that exists to definitively confirm a positive toxoplasmosis patient (Greene, 2006). Serological tests used in the diagnosis of toxoplasmosis include IFA, ELISA, complement fixation, the Sabin-Feldman dye test, direct and indirect hemagglutination, latex agglutination, and modified agglutination tests. IgG and IgM titers drawn 3–4 weeks apart can be used to differentiate recent versus older infections (CFSPH, 2008).

The parasite in the trophozite form may be detected more commonly in peritoneal and thoracic fluid but may also be found in blood, cerebrospinal fluid, fine-needle aspirates, transtracheal or bronchoalveolar washings, aqueous humor in ocular disease, or postmortem in a variety of other tissues (CFSPH, 2008; Greene, 2006).

Treatment

There are currently no drugs that are effective in killing *T. gondii*. However, there are medications available to slow down the replication process. Some antibiotics are available to help with this process, and supportive care is often necessary for active infections.

Disinfection/Prevention

T. gondii is most susceptible to disinfectants in the unsporulated oocyst form. In this stage, they are susceptible to most disinfectants, including bleach, quaternary ammonium compounds, and alcohol. In the oocyst form (mature infective stage), *T. gondii* is resistant to most disinfectants but may be deactivated by iodine, formalin, and ammonia. They can withstand exposure to extreme temperatures (freezing, heat, and desiccation) for up to 18 months or longer (Greene, 2006). Scalding or boiling items in hot water, at temperatures greater than 150°F (65.5°C), will also kill any form of the parasite. Steam cleaning is useful to decontaminate hard, impervious surfaces.

Pregnant women should be especially careful when handling raw meat and should avoid contact with cat feces. Pregnant women working with cats, their feces, or any potentially infectious material should wear gloves at all times and practice meticulous hand hygiene after.

All cat feces and litter should be disposed of daily before sporocysts become infective (24 hours is necessary for oocysts to reach the infective stage). All individuals should perform good hand hygiene directly after handling cat feces and or infective material.

All meat should be thoroughly cooked prior to ingestion, and all surfaces that the raw meat may have come in contact with should be properly disinfected after use. Freezing of meat in home freezers for at least 24 hours is also an effective way to kill this parasite (Greene, 2006).

Outdoor feral cats are an excellent source of *T. gondii;* therefore, sandboxes should be kept covered at all times while not in use, and gloves should be worn when gardening or handling soil that may have been contaminated by cat feces, followed by good hand hygiene.

CONCLUSION

Zoonotic diseases are an important risk factor for veterinary personnel to be aware of, whether while working in a veterinary clinic or hospital, at shelters, on personal farms, or while interacting with personal pets. The diseases discussed in this chapter are among the more common zoonotic diseases that may be encountered; however, the information provided may not give sufficient detail for specific circumstances. Further research should be done by those consistently working with species that may contract/transmit zoonotic diseases.

REFERENCES

Acha PN, Szyfres B. 2003. *Zoonoses and Communicable Diseases Common to Man and Animals, 3rd ed.*, Pan American Health Organization, World Health Organization, Washington DC.

[CFSPH] The Center for Food Security and Public Health. 2006. *Methicillin Resistant Staphylococcus aureus*, Iowa State University, College of Veterinary Medicine, Ames, IA, pp 1–9.

CFSPH. 2008. *Handbook for Zoonotic Diseases of Companion Animals*, Iowa State University, College of Veterinary Medicine, Ames, IA.

Devriese LA, Hommez J. 1975. Epidemiology of methicillin-resistant *Staphylococcus aureus* (MRSA) in dairy herds. *Res Vet Sci* 19:23–27.

Devriese LA, et al. 2005. *Staphylococcus pseudintermedius* sp. *Nov.*, a coagulase positive species from animals. *Int J Syst Evol Microbiol* 55:1569–1573.

Greene CE. 2006. *Infectious Diseases of the Dog and Cat, 3rd ed*, Saunders Elsevier, St. Louis, MO.

Halvorson K, et al. 2004. *Infectious Disease Control Policies for the Veterinary Medical Teaching Hospital Small Animal Clinic Texas A&M University*, Texas A&M University, College of Veterinary Medicine, College Station, TX.

Heymann DL, ed. 2004. *Control of Communicable Diseases Manual, 18th ed.*, American Public Health Association, Baltimore, MD.

Morgan M. 2008. Methicillin-resistant *Staphylococcus aureus* and animals: zoonosis or humanosis? *J Antimicrob Chemother* 62:1181–1187.

[NASPHV] National Association of State Public Health Veterinarians, Veterinary Infection Control Committee. 2008. Compendium of veterinary standard precautions for zoonotic disease prevention in veterinary personnel. *J Am Vet Med Assoc* 233(3):415–433.

Quinn PJ. 1997. *Microbial and Parasitic Diseases of the Dog and Cat*. Saunders, Philadelphia, PA.

Quinn PJ, et al. 2002. *Veterinary Microbiology and Microbial Disease*, Blackwell Publishing, Ames, IA.

Rankins S, et al. 2005. Panton valentine leukocidin (PVL) toxin positive MRSA strains isolated from companion animals. *Vet Microbiol* 108(1-2):145–148.

Sakashi T, et al. 2007. Methicillin-resistant *Staphylococcus pseudintermedius* in a veterinary teaching hospital. *J Clin Microbiol* 45(4):118–125.

Salgado CD, Farr BM, Calfee DP. 2003. Community-acquired methicillin-resistant *Staphylococcus aureus*: a meta-analysis of prevalence and risk factors. *Clin Infect Dis* 36:131–139.

Weese JS. 2005. Methicillin-resistant *Staphylococcus aureus*: an emerging pathogen in small animals. *J Am Anim Hosp Assoc* 41:150–157.

Weese JS, et al. 2006. Suspected transmission of methicillin-resistant *Staphylococcus aureus* between domestic pets and humans in veterinary clinics and in the household. *Vet Microbiol* 115:148–155.

Weese JS, van Duijkeren E. 2010. Methicillin-resistant *Staphylococcus aureus* and *Staphylococcus pseudintermedius* in veterinary medicine. *Vet Microbiol* 140:418–429.

5 Disease Prevention Strategies

Nathan Slovis, Barbara Jones and Linda Caveney

"Medicine is the only profession that labors incessantly to destroy the reason for its own existence."
James Bryce, 1914

INTRODUCTION

Perpetuation of infectious disease requires three elements: an infectious agent, a suitable host, and a mode of disease transmission. With this in mind, infection control is best achieved by eliminating or isolating the source of the infectious organism, reducing host susceptibility, and preventing the transmission of disease between patients (Elchos et al., 2008). Although all three factors are necessary for successful disease transmission, two aspects of infection prevention lend themselves more easily to intervention in the acute phase of an infectious disease outbreak and in a clinical, hospital setting: isolating the agent of disease and controlling spread of disease between animals. This chapter focuses on general principles of intervention in the infectious disease process by eliminating the reservoir for the agent, controlling the route of transmission of the pathogenic organism, and protecting the animal.

CONTROLLING THE INFECTIOUS AGENT

Animal Source

Animal sources of infectious disease include both clinically healthy animal carriers of disease as well as clinically ill patients that are actively infected. The first step for disease prevention strategies should be to identify the source of infectious organisms. If patients are showing signs of clinical illness, they should immediately be isolated. If an animal has had known exposure to an infectious disease, diagnostic tests should be performed to identify the pathogen and initiate appropriate therapy.

The apparently healthy animal that is a carrier poses a problem for the general practice population. Once admitted to a facility, animals are under stress and this often suppresses the immune system and can stimulate the shedding of pathogens. Patients should be continually

Veterinary Infection Prevention and Control, First Edition. Edited by Linda Caveney and Barbara Jones with Kimberly Ellis.
© 2012 John Wiley & Sons, Inc. Published by John Wiley & Sons, Inc.

assessed for any signs of infectious diseases. Diagnostic tests should be performed to obtain a definitive diagnosis of an infectious organism.

Eliminating the Reservoirs

The source or reservoir of the infectious agent—also known as the fomite—might be found in the environment, on the equipment, or even on the hands of staff members. Virtually any object can serve as a fomite: Blood, saliva, nasal secretions, urine, or feces from an infectious patient can be carried from that patient to another on equipment, clothing, muzzles, buckets, clippers, and stethoscopes. The list is virtually endless. Traffic from animal transport carts, equipment carts, and shoes all can spread any infectious material from one area to another.

The focus for controlling the source of the infectious agent must be on all hygienic practices performed within the facility. This includes hand hygiene, environment management, facility design, and equipment cleaning and disinfection.

Hand Hygiene

Hand hygiene is the single most important way to prevent the spread of infections in any health care or animal setting. Hand antisepsis reduces the incidence of health care–associated infections (Larson, 1988, 1999). Trials have studied the effects of hand washing with plain soap and water versus some form of hand antisepsis on health care–associated infection rates (Maki, 1989; Mortimer et al., 1962). Health care–associated infection rates were lower when antiseptic hand washing was performed by personnel. In another study, antiseptic hand washing was associated with lower health care–associated infection rates in certain intensive care units, but not in others. The microbial ecology of health care pathogens may not be entirely within our control; however, interventions such as hand hygiene can be implemented to aid in the prevention of transmission.

Human skin is colonized with two categories of bacteria: transient and resident (Price, 1938). Transient flora colonize the superficial layers of the skin and are more amenable to removal by routine hand washing. These transient bacteria often are acquired by health care workers (HCW) and therefore are more frequently associated with health care–associated infections. Resident flora are attached to the deeper layers of the skin and are considered more resistant to removal. However, the resident flora are less likely to be responsible for health care–associated infections (Price, 1938).

Background Information

For generations, hand washing with soap and water has been considered a measure of personal hygiene (Rotter and Mayhall, 1999). The concept of cleansing hands with an antiseptic agent probably emerged in the early nineteenth century (Boyce et al., 2002). In 1822, a French pharmacist demonstrated that solutions containing chlorides of lime or soda could eradicate the foul odors associated with human corpses, and that such solutions could be used as disinfectants and antiseptics (Boyce et al., 2002). It was not until 1843 that Oliver Wendell Holmes concluded independently that puerperal fever was spread by the hands of health care personnel (Rotter and Mayhall, 1999). Unfortunately, it took decades until hand washing gradually became accepted as one of the most important measures for preventing transmission of pathogens in health care facilities.

Evidence of Transmission of Pathogens on Hands

Transmission of health care–associated pathogens from one patient to another via the hands of HCWs requires the following sequence of events (Boyce et al., 2002):

- Organisms present on the patient's skin, or those shed onto inanimate objects in close proximity to the patient, are transferred to the hands of HCWs.
- These organisms survive for at least several minutes on the hands of personnel.
- Handwashing or hand antisepsis by the worker is inadequate (or omitted entirely), or the agent used for hand hygiene is inappropriate.
- Finally, the contaminated hands of the caregiver come in direct contact with another patient, or with an inanimate object that will come into direct contact with the patient.

Various studies have documented that HCWs can contaminate their hands (or gloves) simply by touching inanimate objects in the patient's room (Boyce et al., 1997; Hayden et al., 2001; Ojajarvi, 1980; Samore et al., 1996). Several investigators have studied transmission of infectious agents by using different experimental models (Ehrenkranz and Alfronso, 1991; Patrick et al., 1997). Organisms were noted to be transferred to various types of surfaces in much larger numbers from wet hands than from hands that were thoroughly dried. It is therefore imperative that all HCWs have dry hands before performing a procedure on a patient.

Review of Preparations Used for Hand Hygiene

In the United States, the antiseptic handwashing products intended for use by HCWs are regulated by the Food and Drug Administration's Division of Over-the-Counter Drug Products. Requirements for in vitro and in vivo testing of HCW handwashing products and surgical hand scrubs are outlined in the FDA's document, "Tentative Final Monograph for Healthcare antiseptic Drug Products (TFM)." These requirements differ from the methods widely used in Europe (European Standard 1500-1997).

It is important to emphasize that scientific studies have not established the extent to which counts of bacteria or other microorganisms on the hands need to be reduced to minimize transmission of pathogens in health care facilities; whether the counts on the hands must be reduced by 1 $\log_{10}$ (90% reduction), 2 $\log_{10}$ (99% reduction), 3 $\log_{10}$ (99.99% reduction), or 4 $\log_{10}$ (99.999% reduction) is unknown.

Plain Soap (Non-Antimicrobial)

Soaps are detergent-based products that contain esterified fatty acids and sodium or potassium hydroxide. Their cleaning activity is associated to the detergent properties. These properties are responsible for suspending dirt, soil, and various organic substances from the hands. The CDC (2002) defines hand washing as "vigorous, brief rubbing together of all surfaces of lathered hands, followed by rinsing under a stream of water." Hand washing suspends microorganisms and mechanically removes them by rinsing with water. The principal here is *removal* of loosely adherent transient flora—not *killing*. There are several studies (that contradict each other) about the efficacy of plain soap in the removal of pathogens on hands. For example, hand washing with plain soap and water for 15 seconds reduced the bacterial counts on the skin significantly (by 0.6–1.1 $\log_{10}$), whereas another study found that hand washing with plain soap failed to remove pathogens from the hands of hospital personnel (Ehrenkranz and Alfronso, 1991; McFarland et al., 1989; Rotter and Mayhall, 1999).

Alcohol-based Hand Antiseptics

The majority of alcohol-based hand antiseptics contain isopropanol, ethanol, n-propanol, or a combination of these products. The antimicrobial activity of alcohols is due to their ability to denature proteins (Ali et al., 1991). Alcohol solutions containing 60–95% alcohol are most effective, and higher concentrations are actually less effective because proteins are not easily denatured in the absence of water (Ali et al., 1991; Harrington and Walker, 1903; Price, 1939). Alcohols have excellent in vitro germicidal activity against gram-positive and gram-negative vegetative bacteria, including multidrug-resistant strains, *Mycobacterium tuberculosis*, and various fungi.

The alcohol antiseptics are not appropriate for use when hands are visibly dirty or contaminated with organic debris. Nor are alcohol antiseptics effective against bacterial spores, *Cryptosporidium* spp., and nonenveloped viruses.

Alcohol antiseptics have been documented in the prevention of healthcare-associated pathogens (Ehrenkranz and Alfronso, 1991; Mackintosh and Hoffman, 1984; Marples and Towers, 1979). These products also have been noted to be more effective for standard hand washing or hand antisepsis by HCWs, compared with soap or antimicrobial soaps (Blech et al., 1985; Cardoso et al., 1999; Dineen et al., 1965; Leyden et al., 1991; Lilly and Lowbry, 1978; Paulson et al., 1999; Rotter et al., 1980, Rotter, 1984; Rotter and Koller, 1992; Zaragoza et al., 1999).

The ideal volume of alcohol-based hand hygiene product applied to the hands is not exactly known (and is affected by the type of alcohol used and its concentration), but some ideas can be extrapolated from several studies (Larson et al., 1987; Mackintosh and Hoffman, 1984; Marples and Towers, 1979). For example, if hands feel dry after rubbing together for 10–15 seconds, an insufficient volume of product was likely applied. Refer to the product label for manufacturers' recommended amounts.

Alcohol-impregnated towelettes contain limited amounts of alcohol, and a single towlette's effectiveness is comparable to soap and water (Butz et al., 1990; Ojajarvi, 1991). It is therefore recommended to use more towelettes for hand antisepsis.

A field trial of alcohol-based hand rubs (low-viscosity rinses, gels, and foams) found that ethanol gel was slightly more effective (compared with ethanol solution) at reducing bacterial counts on the hands of HCWs (Ojajarvi, 1991).

Chlorhexidine-Based Antiseptics

Antimicrobial activity of chlorhexidine gluconate begins when the compound attaches to—and subsequent disrupts—microorganisms' cytoplasmic membranes. This results in precipitation of cellular contents (Boyce et al., 2002; Osterholm et al., 2000). Chlorhexidine's antimicrobial activity occurs more slowly than that of alcohols. Chlorhexidine has good activity against gram-positive bacteria and slightly less activity against gram-negative bacteria and fungi.

Unlike alcohol-based products, the antimicrobial activity of chlorhexidine is only minimally affected by the presence of organic material, including blood. Chlorhexidine is a cationic molecule; its activity can be reduced by natural soaps, various inorganic anions, nonionic surfactants, and hand creams containing anionic emulsifying agents (Denton, 1991; Larson et al., 1987; Walsh et al., 1987). Antiseptic formulations usually contain 2–4% chlorhexidine gluconate. Chlorhexidine has substantial residual activity (Aly and Maibach, 1979; Larson et al., 1990; Pereira et al., 1997). The addition of low concentrations (0.5–1%) of chlorhexidine to alcohol-based preparations has resulted in greater residual activity than alcohol alone (Aly and Maibach, 1979).

Iodine and Iodophor-Based Antiseptics

Iodine has been recognized as an effective antiseptic since the 1800s. However, iodine can irritate and discolor the skin. Iodophors have replaced iodine as the active ingredients of most antiseptics. Iodine and iodophor molecules rapidly penetrate the cell wall of microorganisms and inactivate cells by forming complexes with amino acids and unsaturated fatty acids, resulting in impaired protein synthesis and alteration of cell membranes (Gottardi, 1991). Iodophors are composed of elemental iodine, iodide, or tri-iodide together with a polymer carrier. Iodine and iodophors have bactericidal activity against gram-positive, gram-negative, some spore-forming bacteria, viruses, and fungi. Povidone-iodine 5–10% and iodophor (most preparations contain 7.5–10% povidone-iodine) formulations are considered to have good antimicrobial activity.

Quaternary Ammonium Compound–Based Antiseptics

Quaternary ammonium compounds are composed of a nitrogen atom linked directly to four alkyl groups, which may vary in their structure and complexity. Alkyl benzalkonium chlorides, benzethonium chloride, cetrimide, and cetylpyridium chloride are the most widely used antiseptics in this group of compounds. The antimicrobial activity of this group of compounds likely is attributable to adsorption to the cytoplasmic membrane, with subsequent leakage of low-molecular-weight cytoplasmic constituents. Compounds within this group are primarily bacteriostatic and fungistatic; they are more active against gram-positive bacteria than against gram-negative bacilli. Their antimicrobial activity is adversely affected by the presence of organic material, and they are not compatible with anionic detergents (Merianos, 1991). A recent study of surgical intensive care unit personnel found that cleaning hands with antimicrobial wipes containing a quaternary ammonium compound was as effective as using plain soap and water for hand washing; however, both were less effective than decontaminating hands with an alcohol-based hand rub (Hayes et al., 2001).

Triclosan-Based Antiseptics

Triclosan is a nonionic, colorless substance that has been incorporated into soap products. Concentrations of 0.2–2% have been noted to have antimicrobial activity. Triclosan enters bacterial cells, affecting the cytoplasmic membrane as well as synthesis of RNA, fatty acids, and proteins. Triclosan has a broad range of antimicrobial activity, but it is often bacteriostatic. Like chlorhexidine, triclosan does have persistent activity on the skin. However, triclosan has recently been shown to have considerable health risks that might include effects on the endocrine system (EPA, 2010; FDA, 2010). Research is underway to help characterize the relevance and potential effects in humans that have been first observed in animals (FDA, 2010).

Choosing the Appropriate Hand Hygiene Product

When evaluating hand hygiene products for potential use in health care facilities, one must consider factors that can affect the overall efficacy of such products. For example, accessibility of hand hygiene facilities affects the frequency of hand washing or antiseptic washing by personnel, according to studies (Bischoff et al., 2000; Freeman, 1993; Kaplan and McGuckin, 1986; Preston et al., 1981). It is not uncommon in some facilities to have only one sink available in areas housing many patients or sinks located far away from the patient, which will discourage hand washing by personnel. In contrast, alcohol-based hand sanitizer devices can be located adjacent to patient housing and at many accessible sites in patient care areas.

Another impediment to hand hygiene could be the lack of credible information on the importance of improved hand hygiene to control health care–associated infection. Recent evidence supports the belief that improved hand hygiene can reduce health care–associated infection rates. Facility personnel should understand that failure to perform appropriate hand hygiene is now considered the leading cause of health care–associated infections and outbreaks of multiresistant organisms (Boyce et al., 2002). In nine hospital-based studies of the impact of hand hygiene on the risk of health care–associated infections, the majority demonstrated a direct relationship between improved hand hygiene practices and reduced infection rates.

Technique for Hand Washing

Hand washing using soap and running water should be performed whenever hands are visibly dirty. Bar soaps should not be used because there is a potential for indirect transmission of infectious pathogens from one person using bar soap to the next. Refillable soap dispensers (mounted on the wall) or disposable pump dispensers should be used. The procedure for hand washing is the following:

- Wet the hands with warm water (not hot water, which will lead to skin dryness).
- Dispense at least 3–5 ml of a liquid soap.
- Lather up vigorously to cover all surfaces of both hands for a minimum of 15 seconds. Be sure to address the fingertips and areas between the fingers, as well as the back of the hands and base of the thumbs.
- Rinse the hands under running water in a rubbing motion until no soap residue remains. (Residual soap can also lead to skin dryness.)
- Dry the hands thoroughly with a blotting motion.
- Turn off the water using the paper towel—not with bare hands—to avoid recontaminating the hands.

Technique for Alcohol-Based Hand Sanitizers

Alcohol-based hand sanitizers are available in foam and gel formulations. The key is to have enough product to thoroughly cover the hands and to rub hands until the alcohol in the product evaporates. The procedure for alcohol-based hand sanitizer application is the following:

- Carefully evaluate your hands to be sure they are visibly clean.
- Dispense the product (approximately 1–2 full pumps or a 2- to 3-cm diameter circle) in the palm of one hand.
- Spread the product over all surfaces of hands—paying particular attention to the fingertips, areas between the fingers, back of the hands, and the base of the thumbs.
- Continue rubbing with the product until the hands are dry. This generally takes 20–30 seconds. Hands must be fully dry before touching the patient or any environmental surface.

When Hand Hygiene Should Be Performed

Hand hygiene, whether it be through hand washing or the use of an alcohol-based hand sanitizer (if hands are not visibly dirty), should be performed in all of the following situations:

- Before and after contact with a patient.
- After touching any blood, body fluids, excretions, secretions, or items contaminated by these—even if gloves are worn.

- Before and after contact with items in the patient's environment.
- Between procedures on the same patient to prevent cross-contamination of different body sites.
- Before putting on gloves and immediately after taking gloves off.
- After handling any laboratory specimens or cultures.
- Before and after eating food or taking smoking breaks.
- After using the restroom or blowing your nose.

It is important to keep in mind that intact skin is the body's first line of defense against infectious organisms. Maintaining skin health and integrity is an essential component of hand hygiene (CCAR, 2008). Skin that is chapped, cracked, cut, or abraded can easily become a route of entry for pathogenic organisms. Water-based skin lotions should be made available so they can be applied when skin health is compromised. Petroleum-based lotions can weaken latex gloves and increase permeability.

Environmental Cleaning and Disinfection

Proper cleaning and disinfection procedures are an effective way to minimize infectious microorganisms in the environment. Cleaning must be done to remove dirt and organic materials before a disinfectant can be applied to the surface. The appropriate dilution of the disinfectant and adequate contact time are key factors when eliminating microorganisms from the environment. Chapter 6 provides necessary information to create an effective disinfection protocol.

Facilities

Ideally all animal housing facilities should have floors and walls that are constructed of nonporous materials. Porous, textured, cracked, or pitted surfaces—as well as dirt or wooden surfaces—can harbor microorganisms and are difficult to clean and disinfect. For instance, in a large-animal facility, there is no reliable method for decontamination of dirt floors. Removable rubber mats—as an alternative flooring surface—can also harbor infectious organisms beneath them. This problem occurs because mats are difficult to remove, disinfect, and replace routinely due to their weight and size.

Management practices that may predispose patients to infectious organisms include sharing of stalls or kennels among animals and excessive manure build-up in the free runs or stalls. Whenever possible, one animal should be housed in its assigned stall or kennel. If there are more animals than housing facilities, then pairs or small groups of animals should always enter the same housing unit. This type of preplanning will aid in the reduction of cross-contamination between animals.

Footbaths or footmats decrease the mechanical transfer of pathogenic microorganisms from one area of the facility to another. Footbaths are shallow containers of a disinfectant solution. Footmats are covered with a durable, easily cleaned material that is saturated with a disinfectant. Footbaths or footmats should be placed at entrances to large-animal facilities, entrances to any isolation facility, and anywhere personnel will be walking on a surface that could be more contaminated than the general floor environment (CCAR, 2008).

A few problems exist with the use of footbaths or footmats. They include inadequate removal of organic debris prior to stepping into the disinfectant, inadequate contact time of the disinfectant, and not changing the disinfectant solution routinely or with appropriate frequency. These issues should be addressed in hygiene protocols of every facility.

Particularly in a large-animal facility, failure to remove gross organic debris prior to stepping into a footbath can lead to a waste of product and false sense of security. Removing visible manure can be accomplished with the use of a brush and water or by using a bath container filled with detergent and water prior to stepping on the footbath with the disinfectant. This helps to minimize the amount of debris accumulating in the bath solution. A build-up of debris will significantly diminish the effectiveness of the disinfectant. The frequency of replacing disinfectant solution is determined by the traffic flow and the organic debris build-up. At minimum, disinfectant solution should be changed daily.

Proper contact time is just as important in a footbath as it is in environmental and equipment disinfecting. Generally, most disinfectants require a 10-minute contact time to achieve the desired outcome.

When using a footbath outside of an isolation area, the disinfectant should be effective against the specific pathogen, stable in solution, and have a short contact time (Morley et al., 2005). Chapter 7 discusses the various disinfectants available for use in footbaths.

Animal Contact Items

All items used within the animal's cage or stall should be considered potentially contaminated and must be appropriately cleaned and disinfected or discarded.

Items used for feeding or watering should be made of a material that is easily disinfected, such as stainless steel. Hay nets may be used in large-animal facilities if they can be properly cleaned and sterilized with ethylene-oxide between every use. Use of disposable bedding and litter boxes is ideal and should be used if cost allows.

Thermometers are an animal contact item of particular concern because they come in direct contact with fecal matter and are difficult to completely disinfect. At a minimum, disposable thermometer covers should be used. In cases where a patient is known or suspected to be shedding an infectious agent, it is prudent to dedicate a thermometer to that patient and dispose of the thermometer after the animal has been discharged. Another possible alternative for your facility is the use of disposable temperature strips. Temperature strips usually take longer to obtain a reading rectally (compared with digital thermometers), but their disposable nature makes them a good choice in regards to biosecurity and infection control.

Clipper blades should be properly cleaned and maintained. Dull blades or improperly cleaned blades can cause skin trauma with subsequent risk for infection or transmission of pathogenic organisms between patients. Additional clippers should be available for contaminated wounds or when the animal's fur is caked with feces, urine, blood, or other body fluids. The clipper blades should be thoroughly cleaned and disinfected after each patient. The body of the clippers should also be cleaned to remove any organic material, paying particular attention to ridges, then disinfected according to the manufacturer's recommendations.

Stethoscopes have been shown to be contaminated with potentially infectious agents in both human and veterinary care facilities. In order to avoid having a stethoscope become a source of infection, it should be cleaned regularly. Refer to the stethoscope manufacturer's recommendations for cleaning and disinfection of the tubing and bell of the stethoscope (Marinella et al., 1997).

Any items used in the housing or treatment should be taken to an area for cleaning and disinfection; it is important that contaminated items not get used on another patient or come in contact with other clean and disinfected objects. Examples of these items are vinyl-coated mats or pads, heating pads, syringe pumps, and even the hard-covered medical record or cage identification tags.

CONTROLLING THE ROUTE OF TRANSMISSION

Disrupting the routes of transmission prevents spread of infectious diseases by blocking the means by which pathogens are shared. The methods by which infectious organisms are spread can be categorized into contact (direct, indirect, fomite), respiratory (airborne, droplet), ingestion (fecal–oral), and vector. Knowledge of the specific pathogen's route of transmission—as well as its persistence in the environments, infectious dose, and incubation period—is important for development of appropriate infection control procedures. Strategies for controlling the route of transmission include the use of hand hygiene, barrier protection, isolation, contact precautions, respiratory precautions and enteric precautions, as well as vector control measures.

Use of Barrier Protection

The proper use of barrier protection or personal protective equipment (PPE) is a critical component of infectious disease control protocols. The key factor here is the "proper use." This means of protection only contains the hazardous materials; it does not eliminate them. Effective use of PPE is very dependent on education and compliance of the staff members. PPE is designed to reduce the contamination of personal clothing, reduce exposure to the skin and mucous membranes of the staff, and reduce transmission of infectious organisms between patients by the staff (CCAR, 2008). The following are items included as PPE.

∗**Gloves** should be worn when there will be contact with blood, body fluids, excretions, secretions, and mucous membranes. Gloves are a means of providing a barrier to the hands; they are not a substitute for proper hand hygiene. Gloves do not provide complete protection against hand contamination. Therefore hand hygiene—either by means of handwashing or the use of alcohol-based hand sanitizer—should be used immediately after removal of gloves. When removing gloves, care should be taken to avoid contact between the skin and outer surface of the glove. When hands are gloved, avoid touching items that will be touched by personnel with ungloved hands, such as phones, doors, equipment, pens, and other hands-on items. Gloves should not be washed and reused. Gloves should be worn while handling one patient and removed prior to handling another patient. Gloves should also be changed when going from a contaminated area to a clean area on the same patient.

Gloves come in a variety of materials; choice is dependent on the intended use of the gloves. Latex gloves are commonly used. But if sensitivities develop, alternative glove materials (such as nitrile or vinyl) are acceptable.

∗**Lab coats or smocks** are a means of protecting personal clothing from contamination. These are not fluid resistant. Therefore, they should not be used as a means of PPE when there is a possibility of splashing or exposure to a larger amount of potentially infectious fluid. Lab coats and smocks should be changed whenever they become visibly soiled. They should not be worn outside the work environment and should be laundered daily.

∗**Scrubs** are worn routinely in veterinary practices because they are durable, easily cleaned, and prevent contamination of personal clothing. They should be donned at the veterinary facility and removed at the end of each day and laundered at the facility. This recommendation is for the protection of the staff member's family and their personal pets. Scrubs should be changed whenever they become visibly soiled. Separate scrubs specifically designated for use during surgical procedures should be donned prior to surgical procedures and covered with a lab coat when the staff member is outside the operating room.

∗**Nonsterile gowns** are used when handling animals with suspected or confirmed infectious diseases. These are typically used when treating a patient in an isolation room. Gowns are also commonly used when a patient with an infectious disease is being treated elsewhere in the facility (i.e., undergoing imaging or having a bandage change). They should be used only one time; hanging or reusing contaminated gowns leads to contamination of hands, clothing, or the environment. Disposable impermeable gowns provide superior protection but should not be reused. Gloves should be worn whenever gowns are worn. Gloves and gowns should be removed and placed in the laundry bin (or appropriate trash receptable for disposable gowns) prior to leaving the patient's cage/room. Hands should be washed immediately prior to performing any other tasks. Proper gown removal is critical to keep from contaminating your clothing and the environment. The outer surface of the gown should be touched with gloved hands only. The procedure for removing the contaminated gown is as follows:

- Unfasten the ties or break the ties at the waist and shoulders.
- Remove the gown, starting at the shoulders and arms, by pulling on the front (chest) area of the gown with the gloved hands.
- Ball up the gown for disposal (or laundry) while keeping the contaminated surface on the inside.
- Peel the cuffed area of the gown and gloves off the wrist and hands and place the gown in the appropriate bin.
- Wash hands immediately.

∗**Face protection** prevents introduction of infectious organisms to the mucous membranes of the eyes, nose, and mouth. This typically includes wearing a surgical mask. A full face shield or goggles should be used whenever exposure to splashes or sprays is likely to occur. Examples of these types of procedures include dental procedures, nebulization, wound lavage, and handling a patient that is suspected to have rabies.

∗**Footwear** worn in an animal clinic or facility ideally should only be worn while working in the clinic. Requirements for designated footwear vary with the species of animals being seen. In a small-animal facility, close-toed footwear with soles of nonslip material will reduce the likelihood of injury from dropped items (i.e., scalpels), slipping on wet surfaces, and contact with potentially infectious materials.

Footwear that is appropriate for working with large animals should be designed to protect the feet from exposure to manure or other organic materials. Footwear should be washable for removal of organic materials. Treads should ensure stable footing—but not so deep that it is impossible to clean them routinely with a stiff brush.

Disposable shoe covers or a dedicated pair of waterproof boots should be worn in areas where infectious material is expected to be present on the floor (i.e., isolation rooms or facilities). Donning the shoe covers when entering this area and removing them upon leaving the area will prevent the spread of infectious materials from one area of the clinic to another. This is especially important because other patients and personnel often have very close contact with the floor.

Use of Isolation

The main use of isolation protocols is to prevent transmission of pathogens between hospitalized patients (and throughout the general hospital environment) and to prevent nosocomial infection to high-risk individuals (Weese, 2004). A proper isolation area should allow for complete separation of potentially infectious cases and have an area for performing routine treatment procedures (CCAR, 2008). The size and structural aspects of isolation facilities will vary with the clinic size, types of species treated, and the diseases that are endemic to the area.

Conditions of special concerns for nosocomial transmission include patients with acute gastrointestinal disorders, acute respiratory tract infections, or those with known bacterial infections that are resistant to multiple antimicrobial drugs. Only equipment and materials needed for the care and treatment of that individual patient should be kept in the isolation room.

Preparing premade packs of disposable items for each patient admitted to isolation facilitates both having the necessary items to treat the patient and keeping unnecessary waste to a minimum. These can include items such as leashes; a digital thermometer; a few syringes, needles, and injection caps; blood tubes, tape, and gloves; vet wrap; and pens. This pack is used on the individual patient; when the patient is discharged, the items that were not used or used up completely are discarded. Reusable equipment and supplies (i.e., muzzles, grooming supplies, stethoscopes) should be designated specifically for use on patients in the isolation area. Ideally, there should be an adjacent area to the patient housing room where reusable items and equipment can be cleaned and disinfected after a patient is discharged. The cages, floor, treatment table, sink, etc. in the housing room should be thoroughly and completely cleaned and disinfected after each patient.

Ventilation should be under negative pressure (relative to adjacent areas) so the air flows into the isolation area and subsequently is vented out of the building.

Small-animal clincs lacking a designated isolation area can sometimes convert a room that has the lowest amount of human traffic—as long as the floors, walls, and furnishings can be easily cleaned and disinfected and the room can be emptied of all but essential equipment.

For large-animal patients, building a temporary facility (i.e., canvas or plastic structure or bales of straw to enclose farm animals) at least 60–70 feet from other large-animal facilities can provide medical isolation. This alternative would be reserved generally for an outbreak situation.

Access to the isolation room should be limited to a minimum number of essential personnel providing the necessary care for that patient.

While a patient is housed in isolation, it should not be taken out to urinate or defecate (for dogs or horses) in public or shared areas with other animals. Ideally, dogs should be transported on a gurney to a dedicated area for isolation patients only.

If the patient has to be taken to other areas of the clinic for diagnostic radiographs or surgical procedures, transport should be done at the end of the day, if feasible, or at a time when there is minimal animal and personnel movement in the clinic. Appropriate PPE should be worn by all staff involved in the procedure. Other animals should be kept out of the area. After the procedure is completed, thorough cleaning and disinfection should be done immediately.

Use of Transmission-Based Precautions

Upon identification of the infectious disease state, additional precautions are taken depending on the mode of disease transmission. These are broken down into contact, respiratory, or enteric precautions.

Contact Precautions

Contact precautions focus on the diseases spread by direct contact with an infected animal or the infectious agent in the environment. Examples include *Strep equi*, *Leptospirosis*, tritrichomonas, dermatomycoses, *Brucella canis*, tularemia, and plague. Potentially, items can become contaminated with the infectious pathogen and become a fomite. Clothing, brushes, and buckets used in the care of one patient should be kept away from any other patients and thoroughly cleaned and disinfected after each patient use. The use of contact precautions include the following:

- Use of appropriate signage to indicate the infectious agent.
- Facilities that house animals should provide enough space to care for the individual animals (i.e., stables, kennels, pasture, and/or free runs) without the risk overcrowding. An overcrowded facility usually results in poor sanitation because of excessive organic debris. This organic debris is a major contributor to environmental contamination by pathogens (Petersen et al., 2008).
- Keep all other patients out of direct contact range (i.e., nose-to-nose or fur-to-fur contact).
- Prevent contact between animals of differing age and immune status.
- Use barrier protection and gloves, followed by hand hygiene. Ideally, disposable, one-use gowns, coveralls, hair caps, and boot covers should always be used during contact with isolation cases.
- Contaminated clothing should be removed before handling other patients.
- Healthy patients (those in for elective procedures) should be tended to first, before animals that show clinical signs of illness.
- Proper cleaning and disinfection of all hospital areas (including parking lots, waiting rooms, exam areas, treatment areas, and passageways to hospital wards/stalls) is a critical component in contact precautions.
- Use appropriate methods for waste disposal.

For large-animal facilities, ensure the following:

- Footbaths should be placed at the entrance to large-animal facilities to help reduce organic material from clients' boots while congregating in the waiting area.
- All trucks and trailers must be thoroughly cleaned and disinfected after transporting an animal(s) from a farm to the hospital facility.
- Ambulatory veterinarians should take extra care when going from one farm to another, noting that manure can become impacted and transported in tire treads.

Respiratory Precautions

Respiratory or aerosol precautions focus on infectious organisms that are spread by aerosolization of the pathogen. This can occur from an actively sneezing/coughing animal; reaerosolization by high-pressure washing of cages, pens, or stalls; or through dust particles floating on air currents. Temperature, humidity, and ventilation all play an important role in aerosol transmission. Examples of aerosolized infectious agents include influenza viruses, equine herpesvirus type 1, *Bordatella* species, feline herpesvirus type 1 (rhinotracheitis) and caliciviruses, *Chlamydia*, Picornaviridae virus family (foot and mouth disease), and *Coxiella burnetti* (Q-fever).

Infectious agents that are spread by aerosolization are the most difficult to control. Other animals in close proximity can breathe in the infectious organism or have contact with droplet/aerosol-contaminated surfaces. Most pathogens do not survive for extended periods within airborne droplets because sunlight and air results in the desiccation of the organism(s) (Dvorak, 2008).

Respiratory precautions include the following:

- The use of individual rooms, cages, or stalls with separate ventilation systems relative to other areas of the facility. For equine patients, if this is not possible, prepare a separate, temporary housing area away from the main facility.
- Decreasing the density of the animals within confined space.
- Increasing the distance between patients—perhaps by leaving an empty stall or cage on either side of the infectious patient.
- Avoid sweeping floors or using high-pressure washers, which foster aerosolization of pathogens.
- Dust and increased activity (excerise) will cause the patient to cough, which may increase the aerosolization of the infectious disease.
- Barrier protection, gloves, and potentially masks should be used when handling patients with respiratory pathogens.
- Ensure adequate ventilation—ideally 8–15 air exchanges per hour.
- Minimize excessive moisture, dust, and odors (i.e., ammonia).
- Use of air filters can assist in pathogen removal; filters need to be changed routinely.
- Proper cleaning and disinfection of all hospital areas.
- The potential exists for any object or device used in the care of the patient to be contaminated with the infectious pathogen, thus becoming a fomite. Clothing, medical equipment, and items used in treatment should be thoroughly cleaned and disinfected after coming in contact with the patient.

Enteric Precautions

Enteric precautions are used when the pathogen is transmitted by ingestion (oral or fecal/oral route). Examples include parvovirus, *Leptospirosis,* panleukopenia, Johne's disease, Potomac horse fever, *Salmonella, Escherichia coli,* coccidia, *Clostridium perfringens, Clostridium difficile,* and rotavirus. Enteric disease can be spread by animals eating food or water contaminated with urine or feces—as well as by licking or chewing on fecal- or urine-contaminated objects in the environment.

The potential exists for any item used in conjunction with patient treatment or husbandry to become contaminated with fecal material that contains infectious pathogens, thus becoming a fomite.

Enteric precautions include the following:

- Proper cleaning and disinfection is critical for controlling the spread of enteric pathogenic agents. Cleaning items (i.e., shovels, wheelbarrows), buckets, food and water dishes, and other medical equipment need to be thoroughly cleaned and disinfected after each use. The proper use and application of disinfectants in an animal facility is discussed in Chapter 6.
- The use of barrier protection (gowns and gloves) when handling or treating these patients.
- All staff members should follow good hand hygiene procedures during and after handling any infectious patient.
- High-pressure hoses should not be used to remove animal waste materials; this can aerosolize the infectious organism and widen the area of contamination.
- Outdoor exercise areas for patients with infectious diseases must be separated from the general population's exercise area. Prompt removal and disposal of the feces with infectious

pathogens is an effective means of controlling the spread. For equine facilities, composting of the manure is recommended. Composting kills most of the pathogenic organisms that have been examined experimentally; many have not been looked at specifically but based on times, temperatures, and pHs achieved, most would be expected to be killed. Some bacteria known for environmental persistence and resistance to degradation (i.e., Johne's disease agent) may be significantly reduced but not completely eliminated.

- The equipment used for removal of manure should not be used for any other purpose. Ideally, separate dedicated stall cleaning implements should be assigned to each stall to prevent cross contamination. In general, the risk of spreading disease in fecal material can be lowered by exposing wastes to outdoor environmental conditions (sunlight, drying, high temperature, absorption of the pathogen in the soil) (Hammer and Holzbauer, 2005).
- Ensure proper storage and handling of patient food. Provide a clean and dry closed container for commercially prepared food. Food stocks should be systematically rotated and should not be "topped off" in the same containers. Food storage rooms should be kept clean and free of insects and rodents. If food is spilled, it must be cleaned up immediately and disposed of. For large-animal feed, the storage area should provide a clean and dry environment to prevent spoilage and mold growth. Hay should be stored off the floor, free of contamination from wildlife, vermin, scavengers, birds, or other livestock that might urinate, defecate, or otherwise introduce disease. Similarly, grains should be stored in ways to prevent access by disease vectors or rodents.
- Provide a ready source of clean, fresh water. Water bowls should be cleaned and disinfected daily and not shared by patients. In large-animal facilities, never put the hose end in the bucket; this can result in the hose becoming a fomite. Waterers or other watering means should be able to be properly cleaned and must maintain a constant supply of water that is free of organic material.

Table 5.1 provides a summary of the examples of intervention tactics for contact, respiratory, and enteric precautions.

Vector Control

Vector transmission occurs when an insect acquires a pathogen from one animal and transmits it to another. This occurs either mechanically or biologically. In mechanical transmission, the disease does not replicate or develop in or on a vector, such as a fly. Biological transmission (in fleas, ticks, or mosquitoes) occurs when the infectious agent replicates and/or develops in the vector, which then regurgitates the pathogen onto or injects it into an animal. This type of transmission depends on the prevalence of the agent and its distribution, as well as the agent's abundance, life expectancy, and feeding habits (Hammer and Holzbauer, 2005). Prevention of vector transmission is based on elimination, separation of host and vector, and reduction of the insect numbers.

Fly and Mosquito Management

- Control moisture and drain sources of standing water. Remove materials where fly larvae develop.
- Fecal material should be picked up and disposed of on a daily basis.
- Garbage cans should have tight-fitting lids to prevent insects from entering.

Table 5.1   Examples of Intervention Tactics

Respiratory Precautions

Avoid overcrowding, follow recommendations on appropriate density of animals per square foot of facility for in the animal housing area, waiting room, etc.

Increase the distance between animals.

Leave a cage or pens between patients.

Optimally, isolate in separate room with separate ventilation system.

Temperature, relative humidity, and ventilation management.

Schedule patients with potentially infectious diseases at the end of the day.

Limit stress and excitement.

Ensure proper ventilation with 6–10 air exchanges per hour.

High-pressure washers should not be used on cages or stalls.

Floors should not be dry mopped or swept.

Wet mop floors or use filtered vacuums.

Allow adequate ventilation after application of disinfectant.

Enteric (Fecal/Oral) Precautions

Focus on thorough cleaning and disinfection of all animal-contact items and surfaces.

Food storage in closed containers, rotated on a first in, first out basis; not adding to or topping off of older feed.

Keep food storage area clean to avoid infestation of pests (e.g., insects, rodents).

Avoid common source water bowls.

Use of barrier protection to prevent inadvertent contamination among patients.

Provide separate areas for patient exercise; patients suspected or diagnosed with infectious disease in separate exercise area from general patient populations.

Clean outdoor patient exercise areas on a routine basis.

Promptly clean up feces, urine, or bodily fluids from any area where patient traffic may occur.

Contact Precautions

Limit the number of staff who have direct contact with infectious patients.

Congested waiting areas increase the potential for patients to have direct contact.

Proper cleaning and disinfecting of cages, stalls, pens, and carriers is critical.

Use of barrier protection to prevent inadvertent contamination among patients.

Cover all patient wounds or draining tracks.

Promptly clean up any body excretions or secretions.

Use disposable items whenever possible.

If the hospital facility boards animals, tend to the boarded animals before hospitalized patients.

Fomites Play a Large Role in Infectious Disease Transmission

Human hands are a major source of disease transmission; wash or use hand sanitizer frequently. Ideally have hands-free sinks and towel dispensers.

Routinely check dispensers of hand sanitizer, soap, and paper towels.

Avoid "topping off" of any soap dispenser.

If clothing (coveralls, exam smocks, scrubs, or other objects that are worn while caring for patients) is dirty or contaminated in any fashion, change into clean attire.

(Continued)

Table 5.1 (*Continued*)

Clean all equipment that is used on a patient before using again or placing it in an area where someone else may use the uncleaned item (e.g., thermometers, stethoscopes, water bowl).

Clean and disinfect boots and shoes routinely.

Have dedicated shoe wear for work purposes.

Specific Tactics for Large-Animal Facilities

Never use manure bucket to move hay or bedding.

Screen windows and use insect repellents.

House different age groups separately.

Minimize manure run-off from the manure storage area and paddocks into creeks or streams.

Drain any area where there is standing water.

Advise clients to isolate newly discharged patients when they arrive home.

Have a boot bath available for clients in the admission area.

Have a routine schedule for cleaning boot cleaning brush and disinfectant footbath.

- Use chemical insecticides as an adjunct to other insect-control measures. (Chemical insecticides alone are not enough.) Methods include animal sprays, spraying premises, or spraying with residual products. Always read the product label carefully and follow recommendations for application methods.
- Fly traps can be used in areas where chemicals sprays are prohibited (i.e., around animals, animal food, or water).

For Flea Control

- Preventative measures for the animals include spot-on treatments (Revolution, Frontline, etc.), topical flea baths (should be avoided if possible because certain topical flea baths can be toxic), or sprays. With the use of any flea-control product, always read the label and follow the manufactures recommendations for application and use.
- Environmental treatment measures are critical. Effective removal of fleas from the home or facility environment—once they become thoroughly infested—is difficult and may require repeated chemical treatments. Flea-control treatment should be administered to the animal. Bedding, blankets, and cloth toys should be laundered frequently. Premises should be vacuumed, and vacuum bags should be immediately disposed of in sealed containers. Apply the appropriate environmental flea-control product. Always read the label and follow the manufacturer's recommendations for application and use.

For Tick Control

- Use preventative measures for the animal. These include spot-on treatments. Always read the label and follow the manufacturer's recommendations for application and use.
- Animals should be examined regularly for the presence of ticks.
- Promptly remove the tick. This is accomplished by grasping the tick with a tweezer or hemostat where the mouthparts enter the skin. Slowly pull until the tick is removed; avoid leaving any part of the tick embedded in the skin. Clean the area with an antiseptic product.

PROTECTING THE PATIENT

Protecting the patient is key to preventing a pathogenic organism from entering and causing disease. Following current vaccine protocols, monitoring and providing treatment for enteric parasites—as well as good nutritional support for healthy skin and immune systems—all help avert clinical disease.

Characteristics of the animal (such as species, breed, age, sex, genetic composition, immune competence, and physiological status) play a role in the dynamic of whether an animal is a susceptible host for clinical or subclinical disease. In addition, characteristics of the infectious agent (such as microorganism type, ability to survive in the environment, virulence, size of the infectious dose, resistance to host defenses, and genetic variation) will determine whether an infection develops into clinical disease or a subclinical infection—or whether it is eliminated by the animal's healthy defense mechanisms. Environmental factors can also influence the health of animals. Table 5.2 provides a list of factors that can influence the health status of animals.

Patient Defenses

Animals have developed an elaborate defense mechanism to provide immediate, nonspecific immunity. Elements related to nonspecific immunity include anatomical structures and mechanical activity, inhibitory secretions, antimicrobial factors, and cells.

Anatomical structures include skin and mucous membranes, mucocillary clearance of the respiratory tract, turbinate design, flushing activity of urine and the lacrimal system, and peristalsis.

Inhibitory secretions include fatty acids in the skin, mucus, bile, and hydrochloric acid in the stomach.

Antimicrobial factors include lysozymes, complement, interferons, acute-phase proteins, properdin, lactoperoxidase, degradative enzymes, and toxic free radicals.

Cells include macrophages, dendritic cells, neutrophils, eosinophils, and natural killer cells.

Shortly after birth, the external surface of the body, alimentary tract, and regions of the respiratory tract become colonized by bacteria. The host and bacteria live in harmony. Bacteria

Table 5.2   Summary of Harmful Factors that Influence the Heath Status of Animals

Harmful Factors
Ineffective disease control measures
Inadequate vaccination program
Inappropriate antibiotic usage
Abuse or overuse of antibiotics
Nutritional imbalances
Contaminated food or water
Water deprivation
Overcrowding
Uncontrolled environmental temperatures
Inadequate ventilation

Adapted from Quinn et al., 2005.

that colonize many parts of the body (without producing disease states) are part of our normal flora. Different regions of the body have distinctive resident flora.

Patient Nutrition

Proper nutrition is essential to maintain healthy immune systems and skin. Feeding a balanced, good quality, commercially made diet for the appropriate age will aid in ensuring adequate nutritional intake that will support the integrity of the skin and immune system. While the patient is hospitalized, try to avoid drastically changing its diet.

Some small-animal clients are opposed to feeding their animal commercial diets; they prefer raw meat-based diets. Raw meat diets may contain a variety of enteropathogens (*Salmonella*, *Campylobacter*, *E.coli*, and *C. difficile*). Although there is no means of tracking these diseases in pets being fed raw food diets, evidence for risk can be inferred from studies in humans. There are numerous well-defined cases of food poisonings from raw or undercooked meat in the United States. There is one documented study of therapy dogs in Ontario and Alberta, Canada, statistically confirming that raw meat can increase a dog's risk of excreting harmful bacteria, like *Salmonella* (Lefebvre et al., 2008). This poses a risk to other hospitalized patients (as well as clinic staff) and may contaminate the hospital environments. Each facility should create a policy determining how to handle these situations. One option is to consider cooking the pet's normal diet for the duration of the hospitalization. If that is not possible, the following guidelines should be adopted:

- The animal fed the raw diet is considered "suspect" or infectious and should be housed in an area separate from the rest of the patients. It is recommended that these patients not be treated by staff whose immune systems may not be functioning optimally (Lefebvre et al., 2008). Enteric precautions should be instated for the patient.
- Raw meat should be kept frozen until the day before feeding. It should be thawed in the refrigerator in a sealed container.
- Any uneaten meat should be removed from the cage and discarded.
- Any items that come in contact with the preparing or serving of the meal should be cleaned and disinfected promptly after use.
- Hand hygiene should be performed after handling any raw meat or items that have been used in the preparation of the meal (CCAR, 2008).

Along with providing a nutritious diet, guidelines for routine monitoring and treatment of internal parasites should be a part of the overall support of the patient's health.

Patient Vaccination

Vaccination is currently the main technique to increase resistance of animals to infections. It is one of the most cost-effective measures for controlling infectious disease, both in food animal and companion animals.

Active immunization refers to administration of a vaccine that can induce a protective response and can produce long-lasting protection against an infectious agent (Quinn et al., 2005). The length of the protection is influenced by host factors of age, immune competence, and the presence of maternal antibodies in the bloodstream. The duration of protection achieved with inactivated vaccines is usually shorter than that induced by modified live vaccines.

CONCLUSION

Although the history of human medicine goes back into the mists of time, the concept of infection control is a relatively recent notion, and we continue to learn lessons in this area. The acceptance of the germ theory of infection, understanding of modes of pathogen transmission, antisepsis, and the rise of the antibiotic era have been key milestones in the development of modern infection control policy. Veterinarians, by understanding the general principles of intervention in the infectious disease process, will be able to eliminate the reservoir for the agent, control the route of transmission of the pathogenic organism, and protect the animal.

REFERENCES

Ali Y, Dolan MJ, Fendler EJ, Larson EL. 1991. Alcohols, in SS Block, ed. *Disinfection, Sterilization and Preservation, 4th ed.*, Lea and Febiger, Philadelphia, PA, pp 229–254.

Aly R, Maibach HI. 1979. Comparative study on the antimicrobial effects of 0.5% chlorhexidine gluconate and 70% isopropyl alcohol on the normal flora of hands. *Appl Environ Microbiol* 37:610–613

Bischoff WE, et al. 2000. Handwashing compliance by health care workers. The impact of introducing an accessible, alcohol-based hand antiseptic. *Arch Intern Med* 160:1017–1021.

Blech MF, Hartemann P, Paquin JL. 1985. Activity of non antiseptic soaps and ethanol for hand disinfections. *Zentralbl Bakteriol Hyg [B]* 181:496–512.

Boyce JM, Potter-Bynoe G, Chenevert C, King T. 1997. Environmental contamination due to methicillin-resistant *Staphylococcus aureus*: possible infection control implications. *Infect Control Hosp Epidemiol* 18:622–627.

Boyce JM, et al. 2002. Guideline for hand hygiene in health-care settings. *MMWR Recomm Rep* 51(RR-16):1–45.

Butz AM, Laughon BE, Gullette DL, Larson EL. 1990. Alcohol-impregnated wipes as an alternative in hand hygiene. *Am J Infect Control* 18:70–76.

[CCAR] Canadian Committee on Antibiotic Resistance. 2008. Infection prevention and control best practices for small animal veterinary clinics. Available at http://www.wormsandgermsblog.com/uploads/file/CCAR%20Guidelines%Final(2).pdf.

Cardoso CL, Pereira HH, Zequim JC, Guilhermetti M. 1999. Effectiveness of hand-cleansing agents for removing *Acinetobacter baumannii* strain form contaminated hands. *Am J Infect Control* 27:327–331.

[CDC] Centers for Disease Control and Prevention. 2002. *Guideline for Hand Hygiene in Health-Care Settings: Recommendations of the Healthcare Infection Control Practices Advisory Committee*. CDC, Atlanta, GA.

Denton GW. 1991. Chlorhexidine, in SS Block, ed. *Disinfection, Sterilization and Preservation, 4th ed.* Lea and Febiger, Philadelphia, PA.

Dineen P, Hildick-Smith G, Maibach HI, Hildick-Smith G, eds. 1965. Antiseptic care of the hands, in *Skin Bacteria and Their Role in Infection*. McGraw-Hill, New York, NY.

Dvorak G. 2008. *Disinfection 101*. Available at: http://cfsph.iastate.edu. Center for Food Security and Public Health, Ames, IA.

Ehrenkranz NJ, Alfronso BC. 1991. Failure of bland soap handwash to prevent hand transfer of patient bacteria to urethral catheters. *Infect Control Hosp Epidemiol* 12:654–662.

Elchos BL, et al. 2008. Compendium of veterinary standard precautions for zoonotic disease prevention in veterinary personnel. *J Am Vet Med Assoc* 233(3):415–432.

[EPA] Environmental Protection Agency. 2010. Factsheet: Triclosan. Available at http://www.epa.gov/oppsrrd1/REDs/factsheets/triclosan_fs.htm.

[FDA] Food and Drug Administration. 2010. Triclosan: what consumers should know. Available at http://www.fda.gov/ForConsumers/ConsumerUpdates/ucm205999.htm.

Freeman J. 1993. Prevention of nonsocomial infection by location of sinks for hand washing adjacent to the bedside [Abstract 60]. In Programs and Abstracts of the 33rd Interscience Conference of Antimicrobial Agents and Chemotherapy. American Society for Microbiology, Washington DC.

Gottardi W. 1991. Iodine and iodine compounds, in SS Block, ed. *Disinfection, Sterilization and Preservation, 4th ed.* Lea and Febiger, Philadelphia, PA.

Hammer C, Holzbauer S. 2005. *Equine biological risk management*. Available at: http://cfsph.iastate.edu. Center for Food Security and Public Health, Ames, IA.

Harrington C, Walker H. 1903. The germicidal action of alcohol. *Boston Med Surg J* 148:548–552.

Hayden, MK, Blom, DW, Lyle, EA, et al. 2001. The risk of hand and glove contamination by healthcare workers (HCWs) after contact with a VRE (+) patient (pt) or the pts environment (evn) [Abstract K-1334]. Presented at the 41st Interscience Conference on Antimicrobial Agents and Chemotherapy. American Society for Microbiology, Chicago, IL.

Hayes RA, et al. 2001. Comparison of three hand hygiene (HH) methods in a surgical intensive care unit (SICU) [Abstract K-1337]. Presented at the 41st Interscience Conference on Antimicrobial Agents and Chemotherapy. American Society for Microbiology, Chicago, IL.

Kaplan LM, McGuckin M. 1986. Increasing handwashing compliance with more accessible sinks. *Infect Control* 7:408–410.

Larson E. 1988. A causal link between handwashing and risk of infection? Examination of the evidence. *Infect Control Hosp Epidemiol* 9:28–36.

Larson E. 1999. Skin hygiene and infection prevention: more of the same or different approaches? *Clin Infect Dis* 29:1287–1294.

Larson EL, Butz AM, Gullette DL, Laughon BA. 1990. Alcohol for surgical scrubbing? *Infect Control Hosp Epidemiol* 11:139–143.

Larson EL, Eke PI, Wilder MP, Laughon BE. 1987. Quantity of soap as a variable in handwashing. *Infect Control* 8:371–375.

Lefebvre SL, Reid-Smith R, Boerlin P, Weese JS. 2008. Evaluation of the risks of shedding *Salmonellae* and other potential pathogens by therapy dogs fed raw diets in Ontario and Alberta. *Zoonoses Public Health* 55:470–480.

Leyden JJ, et al. 1991. Computerized image analysis of full-hand touch plates: a method for quantification of surface bacteria on hands and the effect of antimicrobial agents. *J Hosp Infect* 18(suppl B):13–22.

Lilly HA, Lowbry EJL. 1978. Transient skin flora: their removal by cleansing or disinfection in relation to their mode of disinfection of hands. *J Hosp Infect* 31:919–922.

Mackintosh CA, Hoffman PN. 1984. An extended model for transfer of micro-organisms via the hands: differences between organisms and the effect of alcohol disinfection. *J Hyg (Lond)* 92:345–355.

Maki DG. 1989. The use of antiseptics for handwashing by medical personnel. *J Chemother* 1(suppl 1):3–11.

Marinella MA, Pierson C, Chenoweth C. 1997. The stethoscope: a potential source of nosocomial infection? *Arch Intern Med* 157(7):786–790.

Marples RR, Towers AG. 1979. A laboratory model for the investigation of contact transfer of micro-organisms. *J Hyg (Lond)* 82:237–248.

McFarland LV, Mulligan ME, Kwok RYY, Stamm WE. 1989. Nosocomial acquisition of *Clostridium difficile* infection. *N Engl J Med* 320:204–210.

Merianos JJ. 1991. Surface-active agents, in SS Block, ed. *Disinfection, Sterilization, and Preservation, 4th ed.* Lea and Febiger, Philadelphia, PA, pp 283–320.

Miki DG, et al. 1990. An MRSA outbreak in a SICU during universal precautions: new epidemiology for nosocomial MRSA: downside for universal precautions [Abstract 473]. In: Program and Abstracts of the 30th Interscience Conference on Antimicrobial Agents and Chemotherapy, American Society for Microbiology, Washington DC.

Morley PS, Weese JS. 2008. Infection control in a large animal hospital, in BP Smith, ed. *Large Animal Internal Medicine, 4th ed.*, Elsevier, New York.

Morley PS, et al. 2005. Evaluation of the efficacy of disinfectant footbaths as used in veterinary hospitals. *J Am Vet Med Assoc* 226(12):2053–2058.

Mortimer EA Jr, et al. 1962. Transmission of staphylococci between newborns. *Am J Dis Child* 104:289–295.

Ojajarvi J. 1980. Effectiveness of hand washing and disinfection methods in removing transient bacteria after patient nursing. *J Hyg (Lond)* 85:193–123.

Ojajarvi J. 1991. Handwashing in Finland. *J Hosp Infect* 18(suppl B):35–40.

Osterholm MT, Hedberg CW and Moore KA. 2000. Epidemiology of infectious diseases, in GL Mandell, JE Bennett, R Dolin R, eds. *Principles and Practice of Infectious Diseases, 5th ed.* Churchill Livingstone, Philadelphia, PA.

Patrick DR, Findon G, Miller TE. 1997. Residual moisture determines the level of touch-contact-associated bacterial transfer following hand washing. *Epidemiol Infect* 119:319–325.

Paulson DS, Fendler EJ, Dolan MJ, Williams RA. 1999. A close look at alcohol gel as an antimicrobial sanitizing agent. *Am J Infect Control* 27:332–338.

Pereira LJ, Lee GM, Wade KJ. 1997. An evaluation of five protocols for surgical handwashing in relation to skin condition and microbial counts. *J Hosp Infect* 36:49–65.

Petersen CA, Dvorak G, Steneroden K, Spickler AR. 2008. *Maddie's Infection Control Manual for Animal Shelters for Veterinary Personnel, 1st ed.* Center for Food Security and Public Health, Ames, IA.

Preston GA, Larson EL, Stamm WE. 1981. The effects of private isolation rooms on patient care practices, colonization and infection in an intensive care unit. *Am J Med* 70:641–645.

Price PB. 1938. Bacteriology of normal skin: a new quantitative test applied to a study of the bacterial flora and the disinfectant action of mechanical cleansing. *J Infect Dis* 63:301–318.

Price PB. 1939. Ethyl alcohol as a germicide. *Arch Surg* 38:528–542.

Quinn PJ, et al. 2005. Infection and immunity, in *Veterinary Microbiology and Microbial Disease.* Blackwell Science, Ames, IA, pp 494–514.

Rotter ML. 1984. Hygenic hand disinfection. *Infect Control* 1:18–22.

Rotter ML, Koller W. 1992. Test models for hygienic handrub and hygienic handwash: the effects of two different contamination and sampling techniques. *J Hosp Infect* 20:163–171.

Rotter M, Koller W, Wewalka G. 1980. Povidone-iodine and chlorhexidine gluconate-containing detergents for disinfection of hands. *J Hosp Infect* 1:149–158.

Rotter M, Mayhall CG, eds. 1999. Hand washing and hand disinfection, in *Hospital Epidemiology and Infection Control, 2nd ed.* Lippincott Williams & Wilkins, Philadelphia, PA.

Samore MH, et al. 1996. Clinical and molecular epidemiology of sporadic and clustered cases of nosocomial *Clostridium difficile* diarrhea. *Am J Med* 100:32–40.

Scott E, Bloomfield SF. 1990. The survival and transfer of microbial contamination via cloths, hands and utensils. *J Appl Bacteriol* 68:271–278.

Walsh B, Blakemore PH, Drabu KJ. 1987. The effect of handcream on the antibacterial activity of chlorhexidine gluconate. *J Hosp Infect* 9:30–33.

Weese JS. 2004. Barrier precautions, isolation protocols, and personal hygiene in veterinary hospitals. *Vet Clin North Am Equine Pract* 20(3):543–559.

Woolfrey BF, et al. 1991. Human infections associated with *Bordetella bronchiseptica. Clin Microbiol Rev* 4:243–255.

Wright JG, et al. 2008. Infection control practices and zoonotic disease risks among veterinarians in the United States. *J Am Vet Med Assoc* 232:1863–1872.

Zaragoza M, et al. 1999. Handwashing with soap or alcoholic solutions? A randomized clinical trial of its effectiveness. *Am J Infect Control* 27:258–261.

6 Guidelines for Effective Cleaning and Disinfection

Linda Caveney

Creation of a disinfection protocol is a vital part of any infection control program. In establishing a disinfection protocol, some basic knowledge about chemical disinfectants is critical to the success of the program. There are many disinfectants available in today's marketplace. No one disinfectant is adequate for every situation. They all have one thing in common, however: disinfectants reduce the number of pathogenic organisms in the environment of a veterinary clinic (or any other animal containment facility, such as a transport trailer or pet carrier). Clear definition of terms and understanding the information on a manufacturer's label in order to determine the appropriate level of disinfection for each item are just a few of the topics reviewed in this section.

DEFINITION OF COMMON TERMS

As noted in previous chapters, the terms disinfectant, antiseptic, sterile, and sanitize are all commonly used but not always correctly so. Defining these terms will give a clearer understanding of the different chemical agents and their effects on microorganisms. Table 6.1 provides common vocabulary regarding cleaning and disinfection.

HOW TO READ A DISINFECTANT LABEL

Manufacturers are required to include important information about their product on the label. Labels give instructions regarding application, types of surfaces, effectiveness, and hazards to humans, animals, and the environment. These instructions must be followed conscientiously to get the desired outcome. A thorough understanding of the label claims will help you choose the appropriate product for your disinfectant protocols.

Manufacturers' claims of effectiveness are based on their products' ability to destroy three kinds of test organisms: *Staphylococcus aureus, Salmonella cholerasuis,* and *Pseudomonas aeruginosa.* If a product is stated to have a limited efficacy claim, it kills only one specific microorganism group, either gram-positive or gram-negative bacteria. *S. aureus* is the representative organism for gram-positive kill claims, whereas *S. cholerasuis* is for gram-negative

Veterinary Infection Prevention and Control, First Edition. Edited by Linda Caveney and Barbara Jones with Kimberly Ellis.
© 2012 John Wiley & Sons, Inc. Published by John Wiley & Sons, Inc.

Table 6.1   Common Vocabulary for Cleaning and Disinfection

Antiseptic	A substance that prevents growth or activity of microorganism and is usually applied topically to living tissue. The FDA is the governing agency over antiseptics in the United States.
Cleaning	The removal of all visible, nonvisible, and any other foreign material. This is the most important step in any disinfection or sterilization process. Cleaning is not the same as disinfecting. There is not disinfecting without cleaning first.
Decontamination	The process of rendering an object or person free of harmful or infectious material or toxins.
Detergents	Cleaning agents comprised of a wetting agent to reduce surface tension, a chelating agent to suspend particles in water, and a base that is either cationic, anionic, or nonionic (in reference to its positive, negative, or uncharged ionic characteristic, respectively). Detergents are commonly a blend of anionic and nonionic detergents.
	Cationic Detergents have positive electrical charges on a large portion of their organic molecules.
	Anionic Detergents have negative electrical charges on a large portion of their organic molecule.
	Nonionic Detergents have no charge.
Disinfectants	Chemical agents that destroy infectious microorganisms (bacteria, viruses, fungi) but may not kill bacterial spores on inanimate objects or surfaces. Note that, in the United States, the EPA registers all disinfecting agents as "antimicrobial pesticides."
Germicide	Chemical agents that kills pathogenic microorganisms but not bacterial spores. The suffix "–cide" denotes a killing action (e.g., bactericide, viricide), whereas the suffix "–stat" or "–static" refers to inhibiting or preventing the organism from multiplying (e.g., bacteriostat, fungistat). Germicide is the broad term. If a bactericide is used, it refers only to bacteria, and it may not kill fungus or viruses.
Sanitizing	Reducing the number of microbial contaminants on surfaces to levels judged as safe from a public health standpoint.
Spores or Endospores	Represents the dormant state of organisms (generally bacterial or fungus) that demonstrates resistance to heat, radiation, and chemical agents.
Sterilization	The use of a physical (i.e., high heat) or chemical (i.e., ethylene oxide gas) procedure that kills or destroys all forms of microbial life. The sterilization process will be discussed in Chapters 10 (High temperature) and 11 (Low temperature).
Vegetative cells	Actively growing and reproducing in their life cycle. In this category are gram-positive and gram-negative bacteria.
Viruses	Lipid (or enveloped) Viruses whose core is surrounded by a coat of lipoprotein. This category of viruses is easily killed by disinfectants.
	Nonlipid (or nonenveloped) Viruses whose core is not surrounded by lipoproteins. They are more resistant to chemical agents than lipid viruses.

kill claims. The terms "general purpose" or "broad spectrum" are used if a product is effective against both gram-positive and gram-negative organisms; in other words, the product has been tested against both *S. aureus* and *S. cholerasuis*. If the disinfectant is labeled "hospital" or "medical environment," that claim must be backed by testing against *S. aureus*, *S. cholerasuis*, and *P. aeruginosa*. *P. aeruginosa* is an opportunistic gram-negative bacillus bacterium that is responsible for many hospital-acquired, or "nosocomial," infections.

The EPA requires products to be tested under "hard water" conditions. This means the water can contain up to 400 parts per million hardness or calcium carbonate ions. Also, the EPA requires a product to be effective in the presence of a 5% serum contamination. This is to simulate actual conditions that a disinfectant will generally be used under (e.g., organic material).

The manufacturer is required to list active ingredients, which are the chemicals listed (in percentages) that actually kill or render the microorganism incapable of producing a disease state. Inert ingredients are listed as a total percentage of the proprietary ingredients—those that make the product unique. These include components such as soaps, dyes, and perfumes.

A product's precautionary statement tells of potential hazards to the user and how to minimize those hazards when using the product. Typically, precautionary statements might specify wearing gloves, goggles, skin protection, a respirator, or use of the product in a well-ventilated room. The hierarchy of terms from the most harmful to least harmful is as follows: danger–poison, danger, warning, and caution.

Manufacturers can include additional statements on environmental hazards, physical or chemical hazards (corrosive, flammable), and storage and disposal information (e.g., temperature for storage).

A product label's first aid information recommends actions to take if the product is swallowed, inhaled, or has come in contact with skin or eyes.

The disinfectant manufacturer puts the directions for use on the label for you to follow. Directions indicate where, how, and when to use the product; what the active ingredient will control; and the best application method. Some product labels will state that they are capable of cleaning as well as disinfecting (although there is really no one-step cleaning and disinfecting in the veterinary environment); some will have distinct actions depending on different dilutions of the product and/or contact time specifications. Obtaining the desired effect from the product is dependent on these conditions. They must be followed precisely. It is a violation of federal law to use a product in a manner other than what the label states. Figures 6.1 and 6.2 illustrate these components on a typical disinfectant label.

FACTORS THAT CAN ALTER THE EFFECTIVENESS OF CHEMICAL DISINFECTANTS

Concentration

As mentioned previously, the manufacturer's label information tells you the correct dilution for the desired outcome. Label information might recommend a higher concentration for the bactericidal claims or a lower concentration for bacteriostatic claims. Using more than the recommended dilution is a waste of the product, as well as creates a potential risk to the user, the environment, or the item or surface being disinfected. Bear in mind that, when cleaning an environmental surface, such as a floor, standing water on the floor will dilute the disinfectant you are applying. Therefore, you should apply all disinfectants to a dry surface.

Reuse life

Once a product is diluted for use, it will lose some of its effectiveness over time and exposure to contaminants. Always check the manufacturer's directions to learn the length of time a product will maintain its effectiveness when diluted, and don't exceed this time frame. For example, sodium hypochlorite or some quaternary ammonium products are effective for 24 hours after

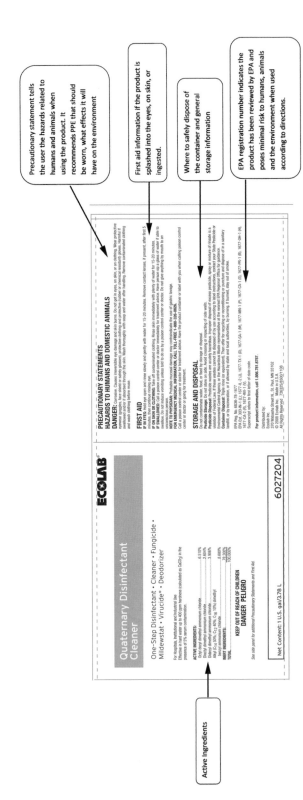

Figure 6.1 This is a diagram of a manufacturer's primary label with notations of active ingredients, safety information, and EPA registration number. Photo courtesy of Ecolab, St. Paul, MN.

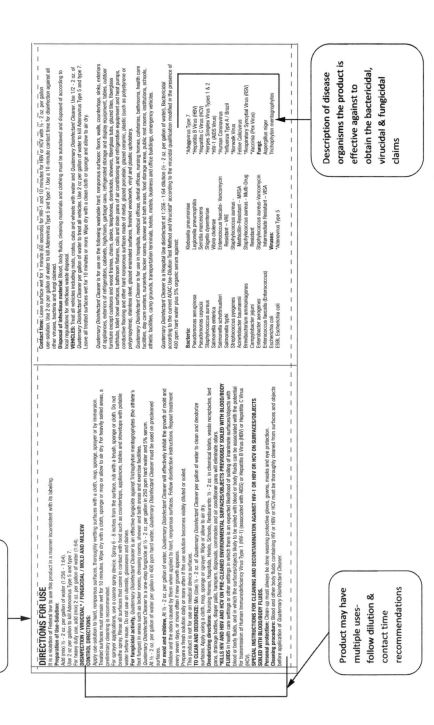

Figure 6.2 This is a diagram of a manufacturer's primary label with notations of directions for use, application, and description of diseases and organisms the product has been tested against. Photo courtesy of EcoLab, St. Paul, MN.

they are diluted if the organic load remains under 5%. Some manufacturers may recommend diluting their disinfectant with distilled water.

Stability

Disinfectants are purchased in a concentrated form and have a shelf life stated on the label by the manufacturer. They should not be used after the expiration date because the availability of the active ingredient may be decreased. Some disinfectants are sensitive to heat and light. The general recommendation is to store disinfectants in a cool, dark area to maximize their shelf life.

Organic Load

This is the amount of soil, debris, serum, blood, bedding, and/or feces/manure that is present. Removal of all organic matter is essential before the application of any disinfectant. Organic matter can prevent the disinfectant from reaching the microorganism on the surface you are trying to disinfect and/or inactivate the active ingredients in the disinfectant. Cleaning the item or surface area allows the disinfectant to come directly into contact with the microorganism, giving you the desired effect in the manufacturer claims. Using a disinfectant that is considered an effective cleaner provides added confidence that, in situations when proper cleaning has been missed or performed inadequately, the disinfectant itself will remove soil, allowing disinfection to occur. This is most commonly achieved by the addition of a surfactant. Surfactants enhance the cleaning efficacy of a product and assist in ensuring complete and even coverage of the surface by preventing beading.

Surface Features

Different surface types can greatly impact the effectiveness of disinfectants. If the surface or item is porous, uneven, pitted, or cracked, then microorganisms can hide in this irregular surface. Wooden surfaces are especially difficult to disinfect due to their grain lines and porosity.

Temperature

Manufacturers recommend a temperature range, generally 68–70°F, for their product to be effective. Too high a temperature can cause evaporation of the product or active ingredient, therefore not allowing the appropriate contact time. Conversely, too cold of a temperature can also alter the efficacy of the disinfectant.

Water Hardness

This is determined by the amount ions contained in tap water. Hardness is measured in parts per million and reflects the level of everything that is dissolved in a water supply. This includes calcium, magnesium, chloride, iron, carbonate, and any other ions. These ions form weak bonds with cleaning ingredients (soap or detergents), leading to deposits or build-up of soap scum. This, in turn, reduces the cleaning action and does not allow the disinfectant to come in direct contact with the item or surface being disinfected. Most manufacturers add chelating agents to bind with the ions. These agents tie up or hold hardness elements so they don't come out of the solution.

pH

This is the measure of acidity or alkalinity of a substance. Pure water has a pH of 7 (neutral). Lower numbers indicate acidity, and higher numbers indicate alkalinity. Some disinfectants work best at higher pH [e.g., quaternary ammonium compound (QAC) works best at a pH of 9–10], whereas others work better at a slightly lower pH (e.g., chlorhexidine gluconate or diacetate works best at a pH of 5–7). Inadequately rinsed items that contain residual soaps or anionic detergents can alter the pH of a disinfectant and reduce its effectiveness.

SPAULDING CLASSIFICATION SYSTEM

Items used in patient care and the care of environment pose a potential risk of transmitting infectious diseases to other patients or staff if they are not cleaned and disinfected or sterilized properly. Deciding which process is appropriate to use on a particular item or environment is complex. In 1968, Earle Spaulding developed a rational approach to disinfection, a classification system adopted and used today by the CDC and the health care industry. He believed that the selection of a disinfection agent should be based on the intended use of a medical item and the degree of risk of infection associated with it. The Spaulding Classification System determines the correct method for preparing instruments and other items used in patient care. There are three categories, each based on the degree of risk of infection when used on a patient. The categories are critical, semi-critical, and noncritical. These categories coincide with the different levels of disinfectant activity.

An item that enters sterile tissue or other normally sterile area of the body or the vascular system is categorized, under the Spaulding System, as a critical care item and should be sterilized. These items pose the greatest risk for transmission of infection if contaminated. A few critical care examples are surgical instruments, catheters, needles, scalpels, and biopsy forceps.

Items that come in contact with nonintact skin or mucous membranes, but do not usually penetrate normally sterile areas, are considered semi-critical. They should be processed, at a minimum, with high-level disinfection immediately before they are used. If the item is heat stable, sterilization is preferred. Examples of semi-critical items are flexible endoscopes, bronchoscopes, urinary catheters, laryngoscopes, and endotracheal tubes.

Items that come in contact with intact skin are noncritical items and require intermediate- to low-level disinfection. Examples of devices that are included in this classification are blood pressure cuffs, cardiac diagnostic electrodes, thermometers, stethoscopes, tabletops, and environmental surfaces.

Table 6.2 summarizes the classification of devices, Spaulding System, and disinfectant products.

CLASSIFICATION OF CHEMICAL DISINFECTANT ACTIVITY

There are three levels of disinfectant activity: high, intermediate, and low. Disinfectant activity is based on the resistance of microorganisms to chemical agents.

- **High-level disinfection** will destroy all vegetative microorganisms, mycobacteria, most fungi, nonlipid (small, nonenveloped) viruses, and lipid (medium, enveloped) viruses, but not necessarily a high number of spores.

Table 6.2 Classification of Devices, Spaulding Process, and Disinfectant Products*

Device classification	Device (examples)	Spaulding process classification	EPA product classification
Critical (enters sterile tissue or vascular system	Implants, scalpels, needles, other surgical instruments, etc.	Sterilization; sporicidal chemical with prolonged contact	Sterilant
Semicritical (touches mucous membranes, except dental)	Flexible endoscopes, laryngoscopes, endotracheal tubes, and other similar instruments	High-level disinfection; sporicidal chemical; short contact	Sterilant/disinfectant
Noncritical (touches intact skin)	Thermometers, hydrotherapy tanks	Intermediate-level disinfection	Hospital disinfectant with label claim for tuberculocidal activity
	Stethoscopes, tabletops, bedpans, etc.	Low-level disinfection	Hospital disinfectant without label claim for tuberculocidal activity

*Modified from Rutala (1996).

- **Intermediate-level disinfection** will kill vegetative microorganisms, mycobacteria, fungi, lipid (medium, enveloped) and nonlipid (small, nonenveloped) viruses, but not bacterial spores. Some intermediate level disinfectants may have limited activity against nonlipid viruses.
- **Low-level disinfection** will kill most vegetative bacteria and some lipid (medium, enveloped) viruses. Some low-level disinfectants have limited activity against fungi, and they are not effective against mycobacteria, spores, or nonlipid (small, nonenveloped) viruses.

Table 6.3 summarizes the microbial resistance to disinfectants.

Table 6.3 Spaulding Classification of Resistance (Descending Order)

	Category	Typical organisms or disease	Sterilant	High-level disinfectant	Intermediate disinfectant	Hospital disinfectant	Food contact surface sanitizer
Difficult	Prions	Creutzfeldt-Jakob disease					
	Bacterial spores	*Bacillus, Clostridium*	X	Sporicide			
	Mycobacterium	*Mycobacterium tuberculosis*	X	X	X		
	Nonlipid or small viruses	Poliovirus, Norovirus, HAV	X	X	X	X	
	Fungi	*Aspergillus, Candida*	X	X	X	X	X
	Vegetative bacteria	*Staphylococcus Pseudomonas Acinetobacter E. coli* MRSA, VRE	X	X	X	X	X
Easy	Lipid or medium-sized viruses	*Herpes simplex* HIV, HBV, HCV	X	X	X	X	

ADDITIONAL CONCERNS WHEN USING DISINFECTANTS

Along with the previously discussed features of disinfectant concentration, stability, and storage, there are a few other factors to consider.

Contact Time

Disinfectants applied to a clean surface need time to kill or render the microorganism inactive. The manufacturer states the minimum contact time for the product on the label. Contact time is essential to get the desired effect from the active ingredient in the disinfectant. Some may require 5 minutes to kill certain organisms, whereas it may take 10 minutes for other disinfectants to kill the same organism. Always check the manufacturer's recommendation. The area or item to disinfect needs to remain wet with the disinfectant solution for the recommended time. Some chemicals evaporate quickly (e.g., alcohol), whereas others have residual activity (e.g., some QAC). Products that dry before contact time has been achieved will not achieve complete disinfection. The ideal disinfectant will offer rapid and realistic contact times. Some manufacturers state that the product does not need to be rinsed after application; others will recommend rinsing. Misuse of the product can potentially put people or animals at risk.

Safety Precautions

The manufacturer will specify on the product label the personal protective equipment (PPE) that is required for mixing and/or applying the disinfectant. Gloves and eye protection are the most common PPE that should be worn when using disinfectants. Other types of precautions include instructions to rinse with water before allowing people or animals to return to the area and having good air ventilation in the area. Further information on safe use of the product is found on its material safety data sheet (MSDS). As required by OSHA, each facility should keep a book of all MSDSs for each chemical agent used. The MSDS contains each product's chemical identification and composition; hazard identification; first aid information, fire fighting and accidental release measures; exposure control/personal protection; handling, storage, and disposal information; stability and reactivity; toxicological and ecological information; as well as federal, state, and international regulations for storage, use, and disposal of the materials. The MSDS section on exposure control/personal protection and potential health effects can contain detailed information on effects of the product from ingestion, inhalation, skin and eye contact, and chronic exposure. Close attention to this section should be considered when choosing a disinfectant. Familiarize yourself with the kinds of information found on an MSDS (see http://osha.gov.SLTC/hazardcommunications/index.html) before an emergency arises. OSHA also has established occupational exposure limits on several chemical sterilants and disinfectants. Employers are mandated by law to ensure compliance within these limits. Training of staff should be included in you disinfection policy.

Expense

Cost of the product is also an important consideration in selecting the proper disinfectant to use. To accurately figure the cost of one product versus another, consider their relative dilution rates. For example, if a QAC is $56.00 per gallon of concentrate, with a use dilution of 0.5 ounce per gallon, it will cost $0.22 per use dilution of 1 gallon ($56.00 divided by 128 ounces per gallon, multiplied by 0.5 use dilution = $0.22). One gallon of diluted disinfectant can cover about 100–150 square feet. Therefore, if your room is about 500 square feet, it will cost about $1.10 to disinfect that room (500 times $0.22) (Dvorak, 2008).

Environmental Considerations

Most disinfectants have a certain level of health hazard associated with their use. Some disinfectants have ecological hazards. Products like hypochlorites and phenolics are hazardous to plant and aquatic life. Care should be taken not to have run-off of these products into ponds and creeks.

CRITERIA FOR ESTABLISHING A DISINFECTION PROTOCOL

No single disinfection protocol will fit all settings. A careful assessment of you facility is the first step in creating a disinfection protocol. What actually needs to be disinfected? How often will it need to be cleaned and disinfected? Who is responsible for doing the disinfecting? Remember that any medical equipment, or the environment itself, can serve as a reservoir for pathogenic microorganisms. Because animals and staff members come into contact with all areas of the environment and equipment, this has to be addressed in your protocol for cleaning and disinfection. Knowledge of the route of transmission of a particular causative agent is helpful in evaluating the scope of the area to disinfect (e.g., airborne vs. contact). Choosing a disinfectant for the job requires considerable attention. There is no ideal disinfectant that is all of the following: 1) broad spectrum, 2) able to kill every pathogenic microorganism, 3) in any environment, and 4) nontoxic, noncorrosive, and inexpensive. Table 6.4 is a summary of points of concern when choosing which disinfectant will be best suited for a particular area or equipment.

Chapter 7 will look at the different characteristics of the chemical disinfectants available for medical applications.

After assessment, the next step in any disinfection protocol is cleaning. This is perhaps the most indispensable component. If the area is not cleaned thoroughly and completely, the disinfectant will not be able to reach the targeted microorganisms. Organic materials on surfaces

Table 6.4 Selection of the Ideal Disinfectant

Speed of disinfection	Offers rapid and realistic contact time to ensure compliance and guarantee disinfection will be achieved
Spectrum of microbiocidal efficacy	One that demonstrates a broad antimicrobial effectiveness, ultimately preventing environmental contamination of a variety of microorganisms
Cleaning ability	One that contains a surfactant to enhance cleaning ability, assists in ensuring complete and even coverage of the surface being disinfected
Personnel health and safety	Should be free of volatile organic compounds, safe for the user and the occupants of the environment
Material compatibility	One with good material compatibility profiles for the task; not one disinfectant can be used on all surfaces
Environmental concerns	Offers "green" claim

can inactivate the action of most disinfectants. Cleaning will remove more than 90% of infectious organisms from a surface. Cleaning can first be accomplished "dry" with brushing or sweeping to remove bedding, kitty litter, and debris from the area. Presoak the area by applying water and detergent to the surface by spraying or wiping. Follow this with scrubbing to render a surface 99% free of bacteria. Friction is key, because the action of scrubbing will loosen and remove the visible dirt, organic material, and debris. This is a very important component of the cleaning protocol. High-pressure washers should be used with caution because they can aerosolize microorganisms and further spread contamination.

A layer of biofilm can form on a surface if thorough scrubbing is not accomplished every time an area is contaminated. Biofilm is an especially persistent medium that contains living and dead cells among a polysaccharide matrix that microorganisms secrete when they grow in water or water solutions. The presence of biofilm prevents disinfectants from reaching microorganisms.

The sequence of the cleaning process should be from the cleanest area to the dirtiest area, and from top (ceiling) to bottom (floor). If your application is in a barn-like structure, start farthest from any drains and work toward them or to a point where water exits the facility. Any equipment in the area to be cleaned and disinfected should be removed and then undergo a similar cleaning and disinfection process.

After the area is cleaned, it should be rinsed and allowed to dry completely before a disinfectant is applied. This is important because the disinfectant can be diluted by additional water; it will not be effective in that lower concentration.

The next step is application of the selected disinfectant. Previously reviewed were the considerations for selection based on the active ingredient, environment to be disinfected, temperature, pH, safety concerns, etc. One reminder: Completely read any manufacturer's product label and follow the directions as listed.

APPLICATION OF DISINFECTANTS

Application of the disinfectant can be accomplished by spraying, mopping, rags-and-bucket wiping, or low-pressure foam sprayers. Manufacturers recommend application methods on their labels. Veterinary facilities that treat companion animals will have a much different application method compared with facilities that treat farm animals and horses. For each disinfectant, choose the best application method for the area or equipment, following the manufacturer's directions for use (dilution, contact time, PPE, etc.). In this section, different methods of disinfectant application are discussed.

Spraying

Spraying with a hand pump bottle is acceptable to clean and disinfect tabletops and vertical surfaces. The area should first be cleaned of organic material, as previously described. Apply the diluted disinfectant solution to the surface, liberally covering all surface areas for the recommended contact time. Follow the manufacturer's instructions for rinsing with water after the contact time, or allow the product to dry on the surface. Some disinfectants contain detergents and claim that they are one-step cleaning/disinfectant products. They can be sprayed on the surface after the removal of gross organic material. The surface area is then wiped with a nonlinting rag or paper towel to further remove any debris. Then the surface is sprayed a second time, allowing the disinfectant to remain on the surface for the recommended contact time. Follow the manufacturer's instructions regarding rinsing with water or allowing the product to dry.

Spraying of the disinfectant does aerosolize the disinfectant; therefore, sprays should be used in a well-ventilated area. Placing the disinfectant solution in a secondary container (spray bottle) requires application of a label that states the contents of the container as well as the first aid measures. See Figure 6.3 for an example of a secondary label with notations for product contents and first aid measures.

If multiple types of disinfectants are used, dedicated bottles should be provided and labeled for each disinfectant solution. For ease of mixing a larger volume, a disinfectant can be diluted in a known-volume container (e.g., 1 gallon) then transferred to the spray bottle. This gallon container also needs to have a secondary label. The spray bottle and the gallon container should be labeled with the date of mixing. Dating the container will let everyone who uses the container know when it was mixed. Alternatively, products can be labeled with an expiration date that indicates when the product will no longer be effective. Whichever method is chosen, indicate the information in your infection control protocols and communicate to all staff members. Never top-off containers. When the spray bottle or gallon container is empty or past its efficacy date, the container should be emptied, rinsed with water, and allowed to dry before refilling.

Mopping

Mopping is used to apply a disinfectant to a larger environmental surface, such as a floor without a drain. A major risk of using a single mop and bucket is the increased potential for getting large amounts of organic material in the bucket with the disinfectant solution. The active ingredient can be rendered ineffective quite quickly, and contamination can be spread over a greater surface area. The two-bucket method of mopping overcomes this problem. One bucket is filled with clean water and equipped with a means of squeezing out excess water (e.g., mop wringer). The other bucket is filled with the disinfectant solution and also equipped with a means of squeezing excess liquid from the mop. In the case of the second bucket, the mop-squeezing procedure regulates the amount of solution being applied to the surface. When the mop is first used, place it in the disinfectant solution bucket, wring out excess solution, and apply to the surface area. The application rate is ordinarily approximately 13.5 ounces per 10.76 square feet (0.4 liter per square meter) surface area. The mop should then be rinsed in the clean tap water bucket, leaving any residual soil or debris in the tap water. Remove excess water, then place the mop in the bucket with the disinfectant solution and continue mopping the surface area. Allow the entire surface to remain wet for the appropriate contact time for the disinfectant being applied. Follow the manufacturer's instructions for rinsing the area or allowing it to dry completely after application. The tap water should be changed frequently when it appears visibly dirty; the same applies for the disinfectant solution. When moving from one ward or area to another, fresh buckets of tap water and disinfectant solution should be used. Ideally, a dedicated bucket and mop should be used for each separate area of the facility. Mop heads should be laundered daily and allowed to dry. The bucket used for the clean water should be disinfected in between areas and at the end of the day, then allowed to dry. The bucket used for the disinfectant should be rinsed thoroughly and allowed to dry at the end of each day.

Human health care facilities have adopted another method of application for floor surfaces using a disposable microfiber mop system. Microfibers are densely constructed polyester and

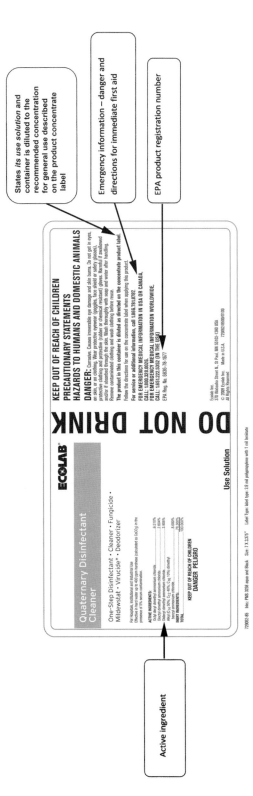

States *its use solution* and container is diluted to the recommended concentration for general use described on the product concentrate label

Emergency information – danger and directions for immediate first aid

EPA product registration number

Active ingredient

Figure 6.3 This photo illustrates a secondary label provided by a manufacturer with notations of safety information. Photo courtesy of EcoLab, St. Paul, MN.

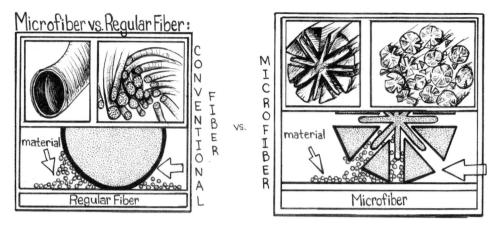

Figure 6.4 This illustration shows how microfiber works to engage particles. Illustration by Kayla Kohlenberg, Ithaca, NY.

polyamide (nylon) fibers that are 1/16th the thickness of a human hair. During the manufacturing process, the bonds between these materials are chemically and mechanically split, creating a web of ultrafine filaments and microscopic pores. This fiber has a positive charge and can absorb six to eight times its weight in liquid (EPA, 2002). Figure 6.4 illustrates a comparison between a microfiber and conventional fiber.

With this system, a special microfiber mop head is immersed in a bucket of diluted disinfectant solution. The handle is designed to attach to the mop head when it is dipped into the solution. The mop is used in the same method as traditional mops, covering the surface area of one room or ward. The mop head is removed and discarded or laundered, and another mop head is attached to continue cleaning and disinfecting another area. One advantage of using this system is that disinfectant solution does not become contaminated with organic material, and the mop is less likely to spread surface contamination further. Another advantage found in clinical and laboratory testing is that microfiber can remove up to 98% of bacteria and 93% of viruses from surfaces, using only water (Hoyle and Slezak, 2008). However, microfiber mops have some limitations. They do not clean grooved surfaces, such as grout between tiles, or rough cement surfaces well (Chou, 2009). Microfiber mops are not effective on greasy floors or those that have a high-gloss surface. If the area is extremely soiled or flooded, more than one mop may be needed. Another potential disadvantage is the cost of the system, although analysis for use in veterinary facilities should be considered.

Low-Pressure Spray/Foam Application Systems

Low-pressure spray/foam application systems are used to apply disinfect to larger areas with drains or openings to the outdoors. A low-pressure spray/foam application system allows you to cover a large area effectively and efficiently. The systems connect to garden hose–type fittings and incorporate a container that can be set to automatically mix water and disinfectant in the appropriate dilution. Figure 6.5 shows an example of a low-volume spray/foam application system.

The surface is cleaned (as previously described), and the disinfectant is applied by the sprayer/foamer for the contact time specified by the manufacturer. Alternately, hand-held spray

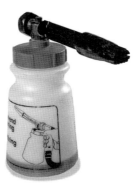

Figure 6.5 An example of a low-volume foam sprayer that is available for application of disinfectants. Photographed by Dewey Neild of Dewey Neild Photography, Ithaca, NY.

applicators (sold in garden supply stores to apply weed killer or insecticides) can be used. The container's chamber is filled with the diluted disinfectant and applied to the cleaned surface. For an illustration of a pump sprayer, see Figure 6.6.

Follow the manufacturer's instructions for rinsing the area or allow it to dry completely after application. The container is rinsed and allowed to dry after daily use.

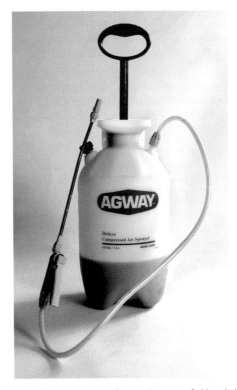

Figure 6.6 An example of a hand pump sprayer for application of diluted disinfectant. Photographed by Dewey Neild of Dewey Neild Photography, Ithaca, NY.

Rag-and-Bucket Wiping

The rag-and-bucket wiping method of disinfection can be used to clean cages and surface areas. This entails the use of a bucket of disinfectant solution and a nonlinting rag that is immersed in the solution and wrung out. The bucket's contents need to be identified with a secondary label and date. This is best accomplished with a laminated tag marked with the necessary information attached to the handle of the bucket. The area is cleaned initially (as previously described) to remove any visible dirt or debris. The moistened rag is then applied to the cage or surface area, covering the entire area with disinfectant solution. Ample solution should be applied to keep surfaces saturated for the period of contact time described by the manufacturer. If directed by the manufacturer to rinse before animals are returned to the area, wipe with a separate water-saturated, nonlinting rag or a paper towel moistened with water. The area should then be allowed to dry completely in accordance with the manufacturer's recommendations. Separate nonlinting rags should be used for each cage or surface area to be disinfected. These should be laundered and dried daily. Rags should not be allowed to sit in the bucket of diluted disinfectant solution. With the use of QAC, which is the disinfectant of choice for most environmental disinfection, the cotton in the rags can absorb the active ingredient. This is also the case with gauze sponges (Rutala, 2007).

A closed-container system with disposable nonwoven wipes is finding its place in the health care system. A roll of commercially prepared nonwoven wipes is placed in a container, and a stabilized, appropriately diluted disinfectant is added to saturate the wipes. The container is closed with a lid that has an opening at the top, allowing one saturated wipe to be dispensed at a time. Figure 6.7 shows a variety of this type of manufactured disinfecting wipes available for the health care market.

A clinical study conducted by one manufacturer compared the use of the nonwoven wipe in a closed-container system with the open-bucket method and cotton or cellulose-based wipes. The nonwoven wipe in a closed-container system delivered an optimal concentration of disinfectant to the surface, minimizing disinfectant solution contamination, changes in pH, and exposure to light and air (MacDougall and Williamson, 2007). These ready-to-use wipes are typically saturated with a QAC, alcohol, or bleach as its active ingredient. Because the wipes are stabilized, they can be used for an extended period of time in contrast to the open-bucket, in which solution has to be replaced when visibly dirty or generally every 24 hours. Closed containers can be placed in multiple areas for convenient use to encourage the cleaning and disinfection of medical equipment. One word of caution: One wipe should be used to clean and disinfect only one specific area or item; they are not to be used repeatedly over multiple areas. The disadvantage is that the cost is more than the bucket and disinfectant method. One should always check with the manufacturer of the medical equipment as to their recommended method of cleaning and choice of disinfectant. Some disinfectant wipes are not compatible with certain medical devices.

CREATING A DISINFECTION PROTOCOL

Items that need to be cleaned and disinfected in an animal care or housing area are numerous. The following are just a sample of what needs to be considered in a disinfection protocol.

- Cages, runs, stalls, including gates, doors, central walkways, floors, and walls
- Outdoor animal areas or exercise yards
- Indoor common areas, such as grooming or bathing areas

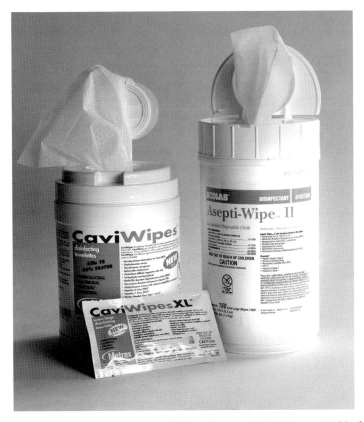

Figure 6.7 Examples of disinfecting wipes available. Photographed by Dewey Neild of Dewey Neild Photography, Ithaca, NY.

- Carriers and transport cages (for companion animals) or trailers (for large animals)
- Bedding or blankets
- Toys
- Food and water bowls
- Implements used in feces or manure pick-up (poop scoopers, shovels, picks)
- Storage or tack areas
- Food-holding or storage areas
- The entire building—entrance area and hallways, doors, and door knobs
- Office areas (if applicable), including phones, keyboards, and other commonly touched surfaces
- Vehicles used for transporting animals

For some facilities, there are specialty areas that might include the following:

- Treatment rooms, examination rooms, other visitation rooms
- Isolation areas
- Quarantine areas
- Medical or surgical areas

Some areas or items are commonly thought of as requiring cleaning, but others may not be as obvious. Areas where there are foot traffic and commonly touched surfaces can potentially act as reservoirs for infectious agents that can be transmitted to animals or humans.

Creation of a cleaning and disinfection protocol is a critical part of an infection prevention program. There is not one protocol that fits every facility. Each is unique in its design and use. The following are steps to use as guidelines in the creation of a protocol.

1. Determine what needs to be cleaned. Once you know what needs to be cleaned, then specify in detail how often it needs to be addressed. Daily? Weekly? After each animal? Also decide who will be responsible for each cleaning task.
2. Detailed cleaning. This is broken down into the physical removal of organic material and the mechanical scrubbing with a detergent. The physical removal protocol specifies how this will be accomplished. The of use shovels, poop scoops, brooms for sweeping, and/or hoses for rinsing (or a combination of these) will aid in the physical removal of gross contamination. What will be left behind is the caked-on feces or blood. Mechanical scrubbing with a detergent and water will remove the visual debris. This is accomplished with brushes, rags, scrapers, mops, or paper towels. The protocol should include the name of the detergent to be used and at what dilution. Cleaning of the shovels, poop scoops, and scrapers should also be included in the protocol.
3. Disinfecting of the item/area. This includes the selection of the proper disinfectant for a specific organism and/or a broad-spectrum disinfection for general use. Careful consideration of the disinfectant is also based on environmental features, surface composition, and safety issues (as described previously). Read the entire product label for detailed instructions. There is no ideal disinfectant for all circumstances. Whichever disinfectant you choose, be sure to include in your protocol the manufacturer's name of the product, dilution, application method, contact time, rinsing (if necessary), and drying. Different areas may require special disinfectants due to surface types or exposure to infectious organisms (e.g., parvo or feline upper respiratory virus in an isolation area). This information should all be included in your protocol. Do not overlook the disinfection of the cleaning equipment.
4. Appraisal. This is your verification that the cleaning and disinfection process actually has been accomplished. Appraisal is done most commonly by visual inspection. Although the human eye cannot see microorganisms, visual inspection will assess whether or not the cleaning process has actually occurred. Is the area free of dirt or organic material? Has attention been paid to cracks, corners, and difficult-to-reach areas? Be sure to specify who will do this. Although not routinely done by many facilities, the option of bacteriological sampling is available to determine the effectiveness of your protocol. This area is described more fully in Chapter 5.

Creating a cleaning and disinfection protocol is a very time-consuming project that has to be reviewed and updated continually. It is a critical component of an infection prevention plan. It is equally important to train all personnel on the proper procedures and safety concerns involving the use of disinfectants. A written protocol serves as a reference for everyone. Table 6.5 is an example of a cleaning and disinfection protocol for an exam room.

Table 6.5   Example of a Protocol for Cleaning of an Examination Room

This protocol provides a step-by-step description of the cleaning and disinfection of the exam room between patients, at the end of the day, and extensive cleaning and disinfection performed monthly or after a patient with known zoonotic or contagious disease state.

Items needed for cleaning:

Rubber gloves
Dust mop or vacuum cleaner
Roccal-D Plus disinfectant in flush bottle diluted with water in a 1 oz/gal ratio
Roll of paper towels
Stack of blue cloth towels (old huck towel); one towel is to be used on one surface. Multiple towels are necessary to clean and disinfect one examination room.

Microfiber mop and bucket filled with Aurora QAC disinfectant diluted with water in a 2 oz/gal ratio

Cleaning and disinfection is to be performed by technicians, animal handlers, or kennel staff.

Procedure for cleaning and disinfecting between patients:

Remove any gross debris from patient examination table with a paper towel. Place in garbage bag in the room. Using flush bottle, squirt a generous amount of Roccal-D Plus on the examination table. Wipe with a paper towel, using some friction, to remove any organic material from the table. Throw the paper towel in the garbage. Squirt the examination table with another application of Roccal-D Plus. Wipe the entire surface of table, leaving a thin film of disinfectant, allowing the surface to remain wet for the 10-minute contact time. Let the surface dry completely.

Move items on the exam room counter to one side, squirt a generous amount of Roccal-D Plus on the counter. Wipe with a paper towel, using some friction, to remove any organic material. Throw the paper towel in the garbage. Squirt the counter with another application of Roccal-D Plus. Using the blue cloth, wipe the entire surface of the counter leaving a thin film of disinfectant, allowing the surface to remain wet for the 10-minute contact time. Let the surface dry completely. Once dry, move items to cleaned area and repeat procedure on the remaining counter surface.

Clean/disinfect the high-touch areas of the room by squirting enough of the Roccal-D Plus onto a blue cloth to saturate thoroughly. Wipe the door handles, light switches, chairs, stools, and radiograph view boxes. Allow to dry.

Clean sink in the examination room by removing any gross debris from the sink with a paper towel. Place in garbage bag in the room. Using flush bottle, squirt a generous amount of Roccal-D Plus in and on the sides of the sink. Wipe with a paper towel, using some friction, to remove any organic material from the sink. Throw the paper towel in the garbage. Squirt the sink with another application of Roccal-D Plus. Using the blue cloth, wipe the entire surface and faucet handles, enough to allow the surface to remain wet for the 10-minute contact time. Allow surface to dry completely.

Vacuum or use dust mop to remove hair, toe nails, dirt, etc. from the floor of the examination room. Assess the area to determine whether mopping is necessary.

Conditions in which mopping is necessary:

Any patient has urinated or defecated in the room
Any patient suspected of having a zoonotic or contagious disease and diagnosed by the attending doctor
Any reptile patients having been examined in a room

Mopping procedure:

Use the bucket containing the microfiber mop heads that has been prepared in the morning with a dilution of 2 oz/gal of Aurora. Attach the handle to the mop head, allow excess disinfectant to drain off. Apply the disinfectant to entire floor area, including under the client chairs, stool, and garbage container. The surface of the floor should remain wet for 10-minute contact time. Remove the mop head and place it in a dirty laundry bag in dirty laundry area workroom.

(Continued)

Table 6.5 (Continued)

Remove the garbage bag and replace with another bag to line the container. Place bag in large garbage receptacle.

Collect the blue clothes used in cleaning and place in dirty laundry bag in dirty laundry area of workroom.

To be performed by animal handlers or kennel assistants.

At the end of each day:

Repeat the procedure as described above for between patients; pay particular attention to corners where debris may have collected.

Using a blue cloth thoroughly saturated with the Roccal-D Plus, wipe the exterior of all containers on the counter in each examination room.

Using a blue cloth saturated thoroughly with the Roccal-D Plus, wipe all the vertical surfaces: cabinet doors, sides of the examination table, and exam room door.

To be performed by animal handlers or kennel assistants with the help of a technician.

Monthly cleaning and disinfection of examination room

Remove contents of overhead cabinets. Using a blue cloth moistened with Roccal-D Plus, wipe the interior wall, sides, and shelves of all cabinets in each examination room. Using a blue cloth thoroughly saturated with the Roccal-D Plus, wipe exterior surface of items that cannot be immersed before placing back on shelf. Plug the sink and fill with Aurora in a 2 oz/gal dilution. Place bins and items that may be immersed in the sink; allow to remain for 10-minute contact time. Remove items, place on a blue towel that has been placed on the counter surface. Repeat procedure with all cabinets and drawers in the examination room.

The technician should be checking the expiration dates on any drugs or sterile disposable items contained in each examination room. At this time, items that are not commonly used may be reassessed as to their placement in the room.

The walls in the examination room are to be wiped down using a blue cloth thoroughly saturated with Roccal-D Plus.

The ceiling vents are to be wiped down using a blue cloth thoroughly saturated with Roccal-D Plus.

Clocks in each examination room are to be wiped down using a blue cloth thoroughly saturated with Roccal-D Plus.

Garbage container is to be filled with Aurora in the dilution of 2 oz/gal and allowed to remain for 10-minute contact time. Garbage container is taken to the wash closet where the used disinfectant can be dumped. The exterior surface of the garbage container is wiped down using a blue cloth thoroughly saturated with Roccal-D Plus. The container is allowed to air dry before placing a bag in it.

Wipe all surfaces of the client chairs using a blue cloth thoroughly saturated with Roccal-D Plus. Wipe all surfaces of the stool using a blue cloth thoroughly saturated with Roccal-D Plus. Wheels of the stool are squired with Roccal-D Plus and allowed to soak for 10-minute contact time. Excess Roccal-D Plus is wiped up using a blue towel.

At the end of each day when cleaning and disinfection is deemed complete by animal handler or kennel assistant, the office manager will verify that the cleaning and disinfection have been effectively completed through visual inspection.

CONCLUSION

The first and most critical step in any disinfection procedure is cleaning. The disinfecting agent of choice can be made following the Spaulding Classification System and product information provided by the manufacturer. Reading the entire product label, and following the dilution instructions and contact time recommendations, will provide the guidelines for rendering the environment or item free of pathogenic microorganisms. Chapter 7 will discuss the properties, advantages, and disadvantages of the various chemical disinfecting agents.

REFERENCES

Chou T. 2009. Environmental services: regulatory requirements and guidelines, in *APIC TEXT of Infection Control and Epidemiology, 3rd ed.*, APIC, Washington, DC.

Dvorak G. 2008. Center for Food Security and Public Health, Ames IA. *Disinfection 101*. Available at http://cfsph.iastate.edu.

[EPA] Environmental Protection Agency. 2002. Using Microfiber Mops in Hospitals. *Environmental Best Practices for Health Care Facilities*. Available at: http://www.epa.gov/region9/waste/p2/projects/hospital/mops.pdf.

Hoyle M, Slezak B. 2008. Understanding microfiber's role in infection prevention. *Infection Control Today* 12(11):42–44.

International Association of Healthcare Central Service Material Management. 2007. Chapter 10: Disinfection, in *Central Service Technical Manual, 7th ed.* IAHCSMM, Chicago, pp 155–174.

MacDougall KD, Williamson V. 2007. *CleanRooms*, Kimberly-Clark Professional, Roswell, GA.

OSHA Watch Special Focus-Surface Disinfection. 2005. Wipe Away Your Worries 1(1):1–7.

Rotter D. 2009. The Chemistries of Cleaning. Presented at the 7th Annual New York State Association of Central Service Professionals Educational Seminar, June 12, 2009 at Niagara Falls Conference Center, Niagara Falls, NY.

Rutala WA. 1996. APIC guidelines for selection and use of disinfectants. *Am J Infect Control* 24:315.

Rutala WA, ed. 2007. *Disinfection, Sterilization and Antisepsis: Principles, Practices, Current Issues, and New Research*, Association for Professional in Infection Control and Epidemiology, Washington, DC.

7 Chemical Disinfectants

Kristina Perry and Linda Caveney

There are various classes of chemical disinfectants. Each class is defined by its chemical nature, and each possesses unique characteristics, hazards, toxicities, and efficacy against a range of microorganisms. Commercially prepared chemical formulations are considered unique products and must be registered with the Environmental Protection Agency (EPA) or cleared by the Food and Drug Administration (FDA). A particular disinfectant is designed for a specific purpose and is to be used as indicated on the product label. The choice of which disinfectant to use is based on the targeted organism, environmental conditions (e.g., organic load, pH, temperature), and the risk it poses to the staff and animals. This chapter will give an overview of each class of disinfectant, its mechanism of action, some common trade names, the organisms it is effective against, as well as a rundown of advantages and disadvantages of using particular chemical compounds, common application methods, and special precautions or contraindications.

ACIDS

Acidic disinfectants' antimicrobial activity destroys the bonds of nucleic acids and precipitates proteins. This action is highly dependent on pH. Acidic conditions change the pH of the environment, inhibiting the growth of microorganisms. Acidic disinfectants have limited applications in the veterinary field because they are corrosive, toxic, and hazardous to handle in their concentrated form. Examples of acidic chemical compounds are acetic acid and citric acid. Household vinegar is a 4–5% solution of acetic acid (by volume) (Dvorak, 2008). Acetic acid has poor activity in the presence of organic materials.

ALKALIS

Alkaline compounds work by reacting with the lipids within the membranes of microorganisms. These compounds are very caustic and tend to emit intense and pungent fumes. Protective clothing, rubber gloves, and safety glasses must be worn whenever alkaline chemicals are used. Some examples are sodium hydroxide (e.g., lye, caustic soda), ammonium hydroxide, sodium carbonate (e.g., soda ash, washing soda), and calcium oxide (e.g., quicklime). Both sodium hydroxide and sodium carbonate (at 4% solution) have been used to disinfect areas

Veterinary Infection Prevention and Control, First Edition. Edited by Linda Caveney and Barbara Jones with Kimberly Ellis.
© 2012 John Wiley & Sons, Inc. Published by John Wiley & Sons, Inc.

where animals with foot-and-mouth virus were housed. These compounds are very corrosive to metals, especially aluminum.

Ammonium hydroxide is effective in eliminating coccidal oocysts that are resistant to a majority of common disinfectants. Sodium hydroxide in 1M concentration (40 g sodium hydroxide in 1 liter of water) at room temperature will assist in the destruction of prions. A section in Chapter 12 addresses the processing of surgical equipment contaminated with prions.

ALCOHOL

Alcohol in the health care setting generally refers to two particular water-soluble compounds: 60–70% ethyl alcohol or 90% isopropyl alcohol. They inactivate microorganisms by denaturing proteins, causing membrane damage that allows cell contents to escape. These alcohols are bactericidal against vegetative forms of gram-positive and gram-negative bacteria. They are also effective against mycoplasma, mycobacteria, pseudomonas, fungi, and enveloped viruses, but not against nonenveloped viruses or bacterial spores. Alcohol is classified as an intermediate-level disinfectant used to disinfect noncritical items, such as thermometers, stethoscopes, blood pressure cuffs, and rubber stoppers of multiple-dose medication vials. Today, 62% ethyl alcohol is the active ingredient in most alcohol-based hand sanitizers on the market. Figure 7.1 illustrates the variety of alcohol-based hand sanitizers available in the health care industry.

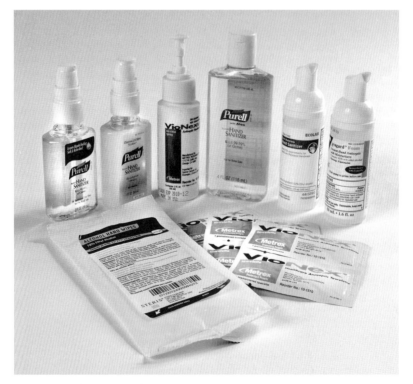

Figure 7.1   Examples of the variety of alcohol hand-sanitizing products available. Photographed by Dewey Neild of Dewey Neild Photography, Ithaca, NY.

Alcohol is fast acting, leaves no residue, and is relatively nontoxic, inexpensive, and nonstaining. Some of the disadvantages of using alcohol are that it evaporates rapidly, leaves no residual activity on the surface, is inactivated by organic material, and is extremely flammable. Some common diseases that alcohols are effective against are influenzas, *Staphylococcus aureus*, *Streptococcus*, *Salmonella*, and *Leptospira*.

ALDEHYDES

As a chemical group, aldehydes are highly reactive compounds that act to denature proteins and disrupt nucleic acids. Formaldehyde and glutaraldehyde are the most commonly found aldehydes. Formaldehyde is a monoaldehyde that exits as a gas that is freely soluble in water. Glutaraldehyde is a saturated dialdehyde. Both compounds are highly effective, broad-spectrum disinfectants that are effective against vegetative bacteria, fungi, enveloped and nonenveloped viruses, mycobacteria, protozoal oocysts, and bacterial spores.

Aldehydes are highly irritating and toxic to humans and animals via contact or inhalation. They can cause some individuals to develop allergic dermatitis, asthma, nosebleeds, and rhinitis. Persons using formaldehyde or glutaraldehyde should wear nitrile gloves, fluid-resistant gowns, and eye protection. These chemicals are also potentially carcinogenic.

Formaldehyde

Formaldehyde has limited use as an aqueous solution for surface disinfection (due to its toxicity), but is used more commonly as a gas fumigant for buildings and equipment. The efficacy of formaldehyde fumigation depends on maintaining a temperature of 57°F (14°C) and a relative humidity of 70%. Following fumigation, the building should remain closed for a minimum of 24 hours before being reoccupied.

Glutaraldehyde

Glutaraldehyde is used primarily as a high-level disinfectant for endoscopes or other medical equipment. Aqueous solutions of glutaraldehyde are acidic (these are not sporicidal), but when activated by the use of an alkalinizing agent to a pH of 7.5–8.5, the solution becomes sporicidal. Once activated, the glutaraldehyde solution has a shelf life of 14 days; some newer formulations (e.g., glutaraldehyde-phenol-sodium phenate, potentiated acid glutaraldehyde, stabilized alkaline glutaraldehyde) have a use life of 28–30 days. The antimicrobial activity is not just dependent on age of the solution but also on use conditions such as dilution and organic load. One advantage of glutaraldehyde in any formulation is its excellent biocidal properties in the presence of up to 20% organic matter.

Dilution of the solution occurs when items placed in the solution are not thoroughly dried. The addition of the water increases with each occurrence, and this dilutes the effective concentration. Chemical test strips or liquid chemical monitors are available for determining whether the effective concentration of glutaraldehyde is present despite repeated use. The minimum effective concentration (MEC) for ≥2% glutaraldehyde solutions used for high-level disinfection is 1–1.5% of glutaraldehyde (Rutala et al., 2008). The frequency of testing is determined by frequency of use: if it is used daily, it should be tested daily; if it is used weekly, test it before use. Test strips should not be used past their expiration date.

Glutaraldehyde is compatible with rubber, plastics, and metals. It is noncorrosive to endoscopic equipment. Glutaraldehyde has FDA clearance for high-level disinfection with ≥2% glutaraldehyde at 77°F (25°C) for 20–90 minutes, depending on the particular product. Increasing the temperature to 95°F (35°C) can reduce the exposure time; this is achieved by the use of an automated endoscope processor. The use of glutaraldehyde for endoscope processing is further discussed in Chapter 12.

As mentioned previously, glutaraldehyde is extremely toxic. A closed-container system in a well-ventilated room should be used for soaking equipment. OSHA has set a maximum ceiling exposure limit of 0.05 parts per million (ppm). Following the exposure time, the item must be rinsed with large volumes of sterile water or potable water that has been filtered with a bacterial retentive (0.2 micron) filter to remove any residual chemical. This rinse water cannot be reused. There is no method available to monitor sterility. An eye wash station must be available within 10 seconds travel time.

Ortho-phthalaldehyde

An alternate product to glutaraldehyde for high-level disinfection of endoscopes and medical equipment is ortho-phthalaldehyde (OPA), which contains 0.55% 1,2-benzenedicarboxaldehyde. It is bactericidal, viricidal, and fungicidal, and it kills mycobacteria and bacterial spores. OPA requires no activation, has no significant odor (as compared with glutaraldehyde), and has been tested and found to be compatible with most metals, plastics, and latex rubber. It also has excellent stability over a wide pH range (pH 3–9) and has efficacy in the presence of organic material. OPA requires no exposure monitoring, and it can be used in manual processing of endoscopes or with an automatic endoscope reprocessor. The exposure time for manual processing is 12 minutes at 68°F (20°C). The MEC must be monitored with specially formulated strips made by the same manufacturer to maintain a level of at least 0.3% OPA. It has a 14-day reuse claim. Staining of skin, mucous membranes, clothing, and environmental surfaces has been observed. Equipment processed with OPA must be rinsed thoroughly with large volumes of sterile water or potable water that has been filtered with a bacterial retentive (0.2 micron) filter. Flushing of lumens with a minimum of 100 ml of rinse water should be repeated three times. This rinse water is not to be reused. OPA is more expensive than glutaraldehyde and shows slower sporicidal activity. OPA should not be used as a sterilant because it has not been FDA-approved for that application.

BIGUANIDES

The most familiar product from this category of cationic (positively charged) compounds is chlorhexidine. This agent reacts with the negatively charged groups on cell membranes, which alters the permeability. Available forms include diacetate, acetate, and gluconate. Chlorhexidine gluconate is the most water-soluble preparation. Common trade names are Nolvasan and Virosan. Chlorhexidine is effective against vegetative bacteria (gram-positive organisms more than gram-negative), and it has limited fungicidal activity. It is not effective against all viruses, mycobacteria, or spores. The activity of chlorhexidine is greatly reduced by the presence of organic material. It is easily inactivated by anionic (negatively charged) detergents and inorganic anionic compounds. Chlorhexidine functions best in a limited pH range (5–7); it is more active at alkaline rather than acidic pH. Alcoholic chlorhexidine solutions are superior to aqueous solutions. The most common use of chlorhexidine products, found in either 2% or 4% formulation, is for surgical scrub and preoperative skin preparation. Follow the product manufacturer's recommendations for use.

Chlorhexidine diacetate (active ingredient in the trade name Nolvasan Solution) is labeled for use in disinfection of inanimate objects. Nolvasan Solution's label states the following: "it is a violation of federal law to use this product in a manner inconsistent with its labeling" (Fort Dodge Animal Health, 2003). The only animal-use claim is for dipping of the teats of cows for aid in controlling bacteria that cause mastitis. There are chlorhexidine-based solutions specifically formulated for certain animal-use applications. The label information for Nolvasan Solution recommends a dilution of 3 ounces per gallon of clean water as an effective viricidal agent (Fort Dodge Animal Health, 2003). For general cleaning of farm or veterinary premises, 1 ounce per gallon of clean water is their recommendation. Always follow the manufacturer's recommended dilution.

A major disadvantage of chlorhexidine-based products is that these products are toxic to fish; thus, the products should not be released into the environment, including creeks or streams. Also, when chlorhexidine-based products are diluted with hard water, precipitates may appear. This does not affect the antimicrobial activity.

Common application methods for use of chlorhexidine solution include mopping, spraying, soaking, and fogging of inanimate surfaces that have been precleaned with soap or detergent and rinsed with water. After proper application and appropriate contact time of 10 minutes, all surfaces must be thoroughly rinsed with clean water. When chlorhexidine solutions are applied by mopping or spraying, the room should be well ventilated, and individuals must wear long-sleeved shirts and long pants, as well as socks, shoes, and rubber gloves. When fogging, individuals must wear a full-face respirator with a canister approved for pesticides.

A commonly accepted practice within the veterinary field is the use of chlorhexidine solution for soaking of anesthetic equipment and endotracheal tubes. This equipment must be cleaned of all debris, rinsed, and allowed to dry before placing in the disinfectant solution. Following the contact time of 10 minutes, equipment must be rinsed thoroughly with tap water and allowed to dry. The disinfectant soak solution should not be in a sink where it can be diluted by water, soap, or organic materials.

HALOGENS

There are two types of halogen compounds used commonly as disinfectants and antiseptics: chlorine compounds and iodine/iodophors.

Chlorine Compounds

Sodium hypochlorite (NaOCl) is the most widely used chlorine-containing compound and is generally sold as household bleach. It is an aqueous solution of 5.25–6.15% sodium hypochlorite that denatures proteins through their electronegative nature. Sodium hypochlorite is considered a broad-spectrum disinfectant, being effective against vegetative bacteria, enveloped and nonenveloped viruses, mycobacteria, and fungi. The concentration and amount of available chlorine determines the biocidal activity.

Overall, sodium hypochlorite is inexpensive, does not leave toxic residues, and is unaffected by water hardness. It is considered to have low toxicity potential at standard dilutions and is easy

Table 7.1 Common Use Dilutions of Sodium Hypochlorite

Bleach solution ratio	Bleach dilution	Comments
1:64	2 oz [30 ml] to 1 gal [3.8 L] water	Commonly used
1:32	4 oz [120 ml] to 1 gal [3.8 L] water	Commonly used
1:10	12 oz [360 ml] to 1 gal [3.8 ml] water	Limited use, very strong

to use. Sodium hypochlorite may be irritating to eyes, mucous membranes, and skin, depending on the concentration used and the ventilation in the area. Other disadvantages of sodium hypochlorite include being corrosive to metals, and it is inactivated by organic materials, cationic soaps/detergents, and sunlight. Discoloration or "bleaching" of fabric may occur. There is reduced activity with increasing pH and lower temperatures. Toxic chlorine gas can be produced when sodium hypochlorite is mixed with ammonia or other chemicals. Sodium hypochlorite, when combined with tap water and stored in a closed, opaque container, may lose us to 50% of its free available chlorine level over a period of 1 month. The recommendation is to make a fresh solution for each application.

Some common use dilutions of sodium hypochlorite are shown in Table 7.1.

Application methods for sodium hypochlorite are by sponge, cloth, or sprayer. The areas should be cleaned thoroughly and dried prior to application of the sodium hypochlorite solution; the solution should remain for a minimum of 10 minutes and then rinsed with tap water.

Iodine Compounds

Iodine compounds are considered broad spectrum because they, like chlorine compounds, are effective against a variety of vegetative bacteria, mycobacteria, fungi, and viruses. Iodine's lethal effects are the result of penetrating cell walls and disrupting of protein and nucleic acid structures and synthesis.

Iodine solutions or tinctures have long been used by health care professionals as skin antiseptics. Iodine agents are inactivated by quaternary ammonium compounds and organic debris. Other disadvantages of iodine solutions include instability, damage to rubber and some metals, staining of fabric and skin, toxicity, and skin irritation. This inorganic form of iodine has largely been replaced by iodophors. An iodophor is a combination of iodine and a solubilizing agent or carrier. The formulation allows for both increased solubility and sustained release of free iodine. The best-known iodophor is povidone–iodine. A commonly known trade name is Betadine, which is an iodophor that combines iodine with polyvinylpyrrolidone. This formulation is relatively free of toxicity and irritancy. The amount of free iodine in an iodophor solution depends on the concentration used; the more concentrated solutions have less antimicrobial activity than the diluted solutions. Follow the manufacturer's recommendations for dilution. The appropriately diluted solutions are suitable for use on tissues or on materials that come in contact with skin or mucous membranes. Povidone–iodine solutions require frequent application and are inactivated by organic debris. Antiseptic iodophors are not suitable for use as hard-surface disinfectants because of the concentration differences. Antiseptic formulations contain less free iodine than those formulated as disinfectants (Rutala et al., 2008).

QUATERNARY AMMONIUM COMPOUNDS

Quaternary ammonium compounds (QACs) have long been used as surface disinfectants. They are categorized as low-level disinfects appropriate for cleaning floors, walls, and furnishings. Some common trade names include Roccal D-Plus, DiQuat, D-256, A456N, and Parvasol. Most have detergent properties and therefore have good cleaning ability. Some of the chemical names are alkyl dimethyl benzyl ammonium chloride, alkyl didecyl dimethyl ammonium chloride, and dialkyl dimethyl ammonium chloride. Newer chemical formulations of QAC (referred to as fourth generation) are didecyl dimethyl ammonium bromide and dioctyl dimethyl ammonium bromide. The fourth generation QACs are reported to remain active in hard water and are tolerant of anionic residue.

The bactericidal action of cationic QACs has been attributed to the inactivation of enzymes, denaturing of proteins, and disruption of cell membranes. QACs are effective against gram-positive bacteria, fungi, and enveloped viruses, and are less effective against gram-negative bacteria. They are not effective against nonenveloped viruses, mycobacteria, and bacterial spores. There is more reported activity at neutral to slight alkaline pH, and QACs are stable in storage.

QACs are generally nonirritating and have low toxicity at typical use dilutions. They have some residual activity, keeping a surface bacteriostatic for a brief time after drying. Some disadvantages to using QACs include the fact that they are easily inactivated by organic matter, hard water, anionic detergents and soaps, and also that they are less effective in cold temperatures. Furthermore, materials such as cotton and gauze pads (sponges) can absorb the active ingredient. Follow the particular QAC manufacturer's recommendation for the appropriate use dilution of the product. Once diluted with water according to the manufacturer's recommendations, the solution will generally only remain effective for about 24 hours. This is also dependent on the organic load, material used to apply the product, and temperature of the environment. Check with the manufacturer for the actual length of time a solution will remain effective.

Application methods for QAC include mopping or spraying, cloth-and-bucket method, and use of a spray foamer. The area or surface should be cleaned of organic material, using soap and water, then rinsed and dried. Next, the QAC disinfectant can be applied for the appropriate contact time of 10–15 minutes. Follow the manufacturer's recommendation for contact time and whether the product should be rinsed from the surface before the area is used by animals.

PHENOLS

Phenol or carbolic acid is one of the oldest germicidal agents used in the hospital environment. Original phenolic compounds used for the manufacture of disinfectants were obtained by distillation of coal; today, most of the phenolic compounds are synthesized. There are numerous synthetic formulations; some phenol derivatives found in hospital disinfectants are ortho-phenylphenol and ortho-benzyl-para-chlorophenol. Commonly found trade names are EnvironLph, One Stroke Environ, Pheno-Tek II, and TekTrol. Generally, phenols function by denaturing proteins and inactivating membrane-bound enzymes to alter the cell wall permeability. Phenols are typically formulated in soap solutions (to increase their penetrating powers) and at a 5% concentration. They are effective against vegetative bacteria, mycoplasmas, mycobacteria, enveloped viruses, and fungi. They are not effective against nonenveloped viruses or bacterial spores. There are numerous formulations of phenolics; the manufacturer's label should be consulted for specific recommendations before using a product.

Phenolics are categorized as low- to intermediate-level disinfectants. Usually when water is added to them, they have a milky or cloudy appearance and a strong pine odor (Pine-Sol is an example of a phenol found in the home). Phenols retain activity in hard water and in the presence of organic material. Phenolics are absorbed by porous materials. They can leave a residual film on environmental surfaces, thus maintaining its residual activity.

Phenolics are generally noncorrosive and are stable in storage. Residual films can cause skin and mucous membrane irritation. Concentrations greater than 2% are toxic to all animals, with cats and pigs being particularly sensitive. Another disadvantage of phenolic disinfectants is that some synthetic flooring may become sticky with repetitive use. Phenolic disinfectants are not recommended for use on food-contact surfaces.

Phenolics may be applied by mopping or cloth-and-bucket method. Spraying is not recommended because phenolics are toxic if inhaled. Follow the specific manufacturer's dilution, contact time, and rinsing directions.

OXIDIZING AGENTS

Oxidizing agents include a broad range of compounds that can be broken down into three general categories: hydrogen peroxide–based, peroxygen compounds, and ozone. Each form has documented activity against bacteria, viruses, fungi, and spores. They all function by denaturing the proteins and lipids of microorganisms.

Peroxide Compounds

The over-the-counter hydrogen peroxide is a 3% solution. This formulation is generally used as an antiseptic.

A stabilized 7.5% liquid form of hydrogen peroxide is used for high-level disinfection of heat-sensitive medical equipment, such as flexible endoscopes.

A new EPA-approved 0.5% accelerated hydrogen peroxide (AHP) has become available in the United States for disinfection of environmental surfaces. AHP is a formulation of hydrogen peroxide, surfactants (surface-acting agents), wetting agents (substance that reduces the surface tension of a liquid causing the liquid to spread across the surface of a solid), and chelating (to help bind metal or water hardness minerals). It can be purchased in a ready-to-use form, as wipes or as a concentrate. Benefits to using AHP disinfectants include their bactericidal and virucidal (including calicivirus and canine parvovirus) claims in a 1:16 dilution ratio with a 5-minute contact time, as well as providing fungicidal claims with 10-minute contact time. It provides exceptional cleaning properties in the presence of dried organic and inorganic material due to the strong oxidizing effect of hydrogen peroxide and the synergic effect of the ingredients in the formula. AHP is free of volatile organic compounds (VOCs), such as fragrances. AHP's noncorrosive formula is safe for most nonporous environmental hard surfaces; brass, copper, or other nonferrous metals may show signs of discoloration or pitting with use. There is a test kit available to test for the 0.5% hydrogen peroxide available in a use dilution solution. Once diluted, shelf life of AHP is 30 days. AHP breaks down into oxygen and water, doesn't leave residual chemicals on surfaces (once it has dried), has no toxic ingredients, and is nonirritating to eyes and skin. Application methods include bucket and mop, pouring the solution on a table or counter surface and wiping, or placing a small amount of solution on a towel for wiping of vertical surfaces. Spraying of the solution is not recommended as it can cause overspray onto areas you don't want the solution to be on, and aerosolization can cause discomfort for sensitive individuals breathing in chemicals all day.

Some trade names of the AHP products are Oxivir (Johnson Diversity) and Peroxigard (manufactured by Virox Technologies for Bayer, Inc. Canada). As with using any disinfectants, read and follow the manufacturer's use dilution and application recommendations to obtain the stated label claims.

Peroxygen Compounds

This group of oxidizing agents includes stabilized chlorine dioxide and peroxymonosulfate. Potassium peroxymonosulfate formulation combines a peroxygen molecule, organic acid, surfactant, and inorganic buffers to provide synergistic activity. In formulation, peroxymonosulfate is listed as having low toxic potentials, especially as powder or in concentrated solutions. Nevertheless, the manufacturer recommends wearing a mask and rubber gloves when preparing a solution and adding powder to water, to aid in mixing and avoiding irritation. It is biodegradable and does not require special disposal of prepared solutions.

Peroxymonosulfate formulation is corrosive to plain steel, iron, copper, brass, bronze, vinyl, and rubber. It has a broad microbial spectrum of activity, including bacteriocidal, virucidal (enveloped as well as nonenveloped), and fungicidal (molds and yeasts) claims. It is effective in the presence of organic material and in 200 ppm hard water. It is marketed as cleaning and disinfecting surfaces in one step, although it is recommended that heavily soiled surfaces are cleaned prior to the application of the disinfectant. In solution, it will remain stable up to 7 days in a closed-container system. It can be used in footbaths and as a surface disinfectant. One study performed at a veterinary teaching hospital at a university demonstrated that just 2 seconds of treatment time with Virkon S in either a footbath or a footmat, followed by 10 minutes of contact time, led to a 95.4–99.8% reduction in bacterial contamination. This study simulated conditions representative of those throughout large-animal hospitals (Dunowska et al., 2006). Follow the manufacturer's recommendation for appropriate use dilution. Application methods include spraying (either by hand or automatic system), mopping, cloth and bucket, soaking, and fogging (wet misting). Animals should not be housed in areas where the disinfectant is being used. Feed racks, mangers, troughs, fountains, and waterers need to be thoroughly scrubbed with soap or detergent and rinsed with water before use.

Chlorine Dioxide

Another peroxygen compound is stabilized chlorine dioxide. It is the only biocide that is a molecular free radical. It affects the cell membrane by changing membrane proteins and fats and reacts directly with amino acids in the cell. Chlorine dioxide remains gaseous in solution. In addition to being effective against bacteria and viruses, chlorine dioxide is one disinfectant that is effective against giardia cysts, oocytes of cryptosporidium, and spore-forming bacteria (such as anthrax). Chlorine dioxide has long been used to disinfect drinking water. Chlorine dioxide also has the ability to oxidize the polysaccharide matrix that keeps biofilm together. Chlorine dioxide product sold under the trade name of Clidox-S (Pharmacal Research Labs) is registered with the EPA as a high-level disinfectant in its 1:5:1 dilution (base solution + water + activator). To be used as a disinfectant, it is mixed at a 1:18:1 dilution. Clidox-S manufacturer recommends the use of a mixing station to prepare the dilution on site, at the correct dilution ratio and in the proper sequence. Once diluted, it must sit for 15 minutes prior to use, and it will remain stable for 14 days in a closed-container system. Anthium Dioxcide (manufactured by International Dioxcide, a DuPont Company) is another chlorine dioxide disinfectant that is EPA-approved for use in hospitals, food processing, agricultural, and animal-handling facilities. Follow the manufacturer's use dilution recommendations to achieve the desired bacteriocidal, virucidal, or mycobacteriocidal kill claims.

Chlorine dioxide is used in the gaseous form as a fumigant for decontamination of laboratories, clean rooms, and buildings. Special chlorine dioxide–generating units are used in this process. The area to be fumigated is sealed off, and the gas is generated and monitored continually throughout the process and records the information. The area is then opened and aerated for 3 or more hours.

Aside from all the benefits of chlorine dioxide, it is very toxic. It is a very unstable substance when it comes into contact with other materials, such as acids, chlorine, organic chemicals. It may cause a chemical reaction resulting in releasing chlorine dioxide gas, and heat explosion or fire could result. Chlorine dioxide gas can escape from a watery solution containing chlorine dioxide. When used in a confined (sealed) area, chlorine dioxide concentrations reaching 10% or more in the air become explosive. Chlorine dioxide solution exposure to the skin causes irritation and burns; moderate eye irritation resulting in watering eyes and blurry sight; inhalation of chlorine dioxide gas causes coughing, sore throat, lung edema, bronchiospasms, and headache. The OSHA limit for chlorine dioxide exposure is 0.1 ppm. Chlorine dioxide is toxic to fish and aquatic organisms.

Peracetic Acid

This strong oxidizing agent is considered a chemical sterilant in its use dilution of 0.2% peracetic acid. It can inactivate vegetative bacteria, viruses, fungi, and spores when used in automated sterilizer systems for 30–45 minutes at 50–56°C. The use of peracetic acid as a sterilant is discussed further in Chapter 11.

Oxy-Sept 333 is an example of a surface disinfectant based on a stabilized peroxyacetic acid, which is formed by a reaction between hydrogen peroxide and acetic acid. The manufacturer of Oxy-Sept 333 states that it possesses high tolerance to a wide range of water conditions (hardness, cold temperatures, and pH) and has the ability to remain effective in heavy organic loads (manure, urine, mud). The manufacturer states that it has rapid soil penetration due to the action of its surfactant with the oxidation. It has vegetative bactericidal, virucidal, and mycobactericidal kill claims. It can be applied by mopping, with a low-volume foamer, and by spraying.

Ozone

Ozone (O_3) is a variant form of oxygen that possesses strong oxidizing properties in this gaseous form. It is bactericidal, viricidal, and sporicidal. Chapter 11 discusses the use of ozone as a low-temperature sterilant.

CONCLUSION

There are many choices when selecting a disinfectant that works best for your environment. There is no one chemical that fits all situations; a combination of products should be selectively deployed. Table 7.2 is a summary of all the chemical disinfectants previously discussed to help in your selection process.

Table 7.2 Summary and Comparison of Disinfectants

Class	How they work	Advantages	Disadvantages	Hazards	Comments	Examples
Acids	Destroy bonds of nucleic acids and precipitate proteins	Effective against bacteria, enveloped viruses; limited activity against fungal spores, other viruses, and bacterial spores	Corrosive, toxic, hazardous to handle	Caustic; causes chemical burns; toxic at high concentration in the air	Changes the pH of the environment	Hydrochloric acid, acetic acid, citric acid
Alkalis	React with lipids within the membranes of microorganisms	Ammonium hydroxide effective against coccidial oocysts; sodium hydroxide assists in the destructioin of prions.	Very caustic; very corrosive to metals; ammonium hydroxide emits intense and pungent fumes; inactived by organic material	Toxic to aquatic life	Not recommended for general use	Lye, caustic soda, soda ash, washing soda, quicklime
Alcohol	Denature cell protein, causes membrane damage and cell lysis	Fast acting, leaves no residue; broad spectrum; low toxicity; no residual activity on surface; evaporates rapidly	Rapidly inactivated by organic material	Extremely flammable	Not generally appropriate as environmental disinfectant, mainly as an antiseptic	Ethyl alcohol, isopropyl alcohol
Aldehydes	Denature proteins and disrupt nucleic acids	Broad spectrum; relatively noncorrosive; sporicidal in alkali solution,	Highly toxic; inactivated by organic material	Highly irritating to eyes, skin, and respiratory tissue; carcinogenic; toxic	Requires ventilation and proper PPE; test strips required to monitor MEC	Glutaraldehyde; formaldehyde (as a fumigant); OPA as a high-level disinfectant
Biguanides	Negatively charged groups on cell membranes alters permeability	Broad spectrum against bacteria; limited against viruses; low toxicity; alcoholic solution superior to aqueous solutions; has residual effect on skin	Inactivated by organic material and soaps; function in limited pH range	Toxic to fish	Used mainly as antiseptic	Chlorhexidine diacetate, chlorhexidine gluconate

(Continued)

Table 7.2 (Continued)

Class	How they work	Advantages	Disadvantages	Hazards	Comments	Examples
Halogen chlorine compounds	Denature proteins through electronegative nature	Broad spectrum against bacteria, viruses, mycobacteria, and fungi; inexpensive; not affected by water hardness; sporicidal at higher concentrations	Inactivated by organic material; inactivated by cationic soaps and some metals; loose potency over time; discoloration of fabric; reduced activity with higher pH, lower temperatures, and presence of ammonia and nitrogen	Irritant to mucous membranes, eyes, and skin at higher concentration; corrosive; mixing with other chemicals may produce toxic gases	Must be applied to thoroughly cleaned and dry surface for disinfection; frequent application may be necessary; used to disinfect environmental surfaces	Sodium hypochlorite 5.25%
Halogen iodine compounds (iodophors)	Penetrates cell wall and disrupts protein and nucleic acid structures and synthesis	Broad spectrum against bacteria, enveloped viruses, mycobacteria and fungi, spores (some, with extended contact time); low tissue toxicity; kills immediately	Staining of tissues and plastics; inactivated by organic debris and QACs; requires frequent application	People can become sensitized to skin contact	Dilution is critical, follow manufacturer's directions; don't use skin antiseptic iodophors for surface disinfectants, use only EPA-registered hard; surface iodophors for disinfectant	Bactergent; Povidone iodine/betadine; Providone; Wescodyne

140

Agent	Mechanism of action	Properties	Precautions	Toxicity	Comments	Trade names
Quaternary ammonium compounds (QACs)	Denaturing proteins; disruption of cell membranes and inactivation of enzymes	Highly effective against gram-positive bacteria, effective against gram-negative bacteria, fungi, enveloped viruses and mycoplasmas; not effective against nonenveloped viruses or spores; stable in storage; nonirritating to skin; low toxicity at typical dilutions; some residual activity for a brief period; active at neutral to slightly alkaline pH	Inactivated by anionic detergents and soap, hard water, and organic material; loose activity at pH <3.5; less effective in cold temperatures	Toxic to fish	Different chemistries of the newer generations are more germicidal, less foaming and more tolerant to organic material.	Roccal D-Plus; Zepharin; D-256; Parvasol
Phenol	Denaturing proteins and inactivating membrane-bound enzymes to alter cell wall permeability	Broad-spectrum bactericidal, fungicidal, virucidal, and mycobactericidal; stable in storage; noncorrosive; retain activity in hard water and in the presence of organic material; leaves a film maintaining residual activity	Incompatible with cationic and nonionic detergents; unpleasant odor; some have disposal restrictions; can cause skin and mucous membrane irritations	Gross protoplasmic poison; toxic to cats and pigs	Not generally recommended for food surfaces	EnvironLph; Pheno-Tek II; TekTrol; One Stroke Environ; Pine Sol; Sporicidin; Parachlorometazylenol (PCMX)
Oxidizing agents: hydrogen peroxide based	Denaturing of proteins and lipids of microorganisms	No activation; may enhance removal of organic material; considered environmentally friendly; active against bacteria, viruses, and yeasts at lower levels; inactivates bacterial spores and cryptosporidium at higher levels	Material compatibility concerns both cosmetic and functional (brass, aluminum, zinc, copper, and nickel/silver plating); concentration of the solution needs to be monitored	Strong oxidant		Oxivir; Peroxigard

(Continued)

Table 7.2 (Continued)

Class	How they work	Advantages	Disadvantages	Hazards	Comments	Examples
Oxidizing agents: peroxygen compounds: peroxymonosulfate	Denaturing of proteins and lipids of microorganisms	Low toxicity potential; broad spectrum of activity; effective in the presence of organic material; remains stable once diluted for 7 days	Corrosive to plain steel, iron, copper, brass, bronze, and rubber	Wear gloves and face shield when preparing solution	Contains oxidizing agent, organic acid, and surfactant	Virkon-S; Trifectant
Oxidizing agents: peroxygen compound: stabilized chlorine dioxide	Denatures proteins and disrupts cell wall permeability	Broad spectrum of activity against mycobacteria, bacteria, viruses, and fungi; effective against protozoan parasites	Very unstable; needs to be prepared on site with correct dilution rates and in proper sequence (base and activator)	Very toxic	Used in water disinfection	Clidox-S; Anthium Dioxcide
Oxidizing agents: peracetic acid	Denatures proteins and disrupts cell wall permeability	Rapid action against all microorganisms; lacks harmful decomposition products; enhances removal of organic material; effective at lower temperatures	Can be corrosive; unstable when diluted	Strong oxidizing agent	Composed of acetic acid, water, oxygen, and hydrogen peroxide	Oxy-Sept 333
Oxidizing agent: ozone (gas)	Denatures proteins and disrupts cell wall permeability			No application as surface disinfectant in this gas state		

Once the choice has been made, developing appropriate written protocols and training staff members on the proper procedures are essential to achieve the desired outcome.

REFERENCES

Block SS. 2001. *Disinfection, Sterilization, and Preservation, 5th ed.* Lippincott Williams & Wilkins, Philadelphia, pp 135–361.

Dunowska M, et al. 2006. Evaluation of the efficacy of a peroxygen disinfectant-filled footmat for reduction of bacterial load on footwear in a large animal hospital setting. *J Am Vet Med Assoc* 228(12):1935–1939.

Dvork G. 2008. *Disinfection 101.* The Center for Food Security & Public Health, Iowa State University, Ames, IA. Available at: http://www.cfsph.iastate.edu.

Fort Dodge Animal Health. 2003. Subsidiary American Home Products Corporation, revised container label.

Petersen CA. 2008. *Maddie's Infection Control Manual for Animal Shelters for Veterinary Personnel, 1st ed.* Center for Food Security and Public Health, Ames, IA.

Quinn PJ, et al. 2005. Disinfection and other aspects of disease control, in *Veterinary Microbiology and Microbial Disease.* Blackwell Science, Ames, IA, pp 481–493.

Rutala WA, Weber DJ, Healthcare Infection Control Practices Advisory Committee (HICPAC). 2008. *Guideline for Disinfection and Sterilization in Healthcare Facilities.* Centers for Disease Control, Atlanta, GA, pp 38–53.

8 "Best Practice" Procedures Prior to Sterilization of Medical Equipment

Linda Caveney

Several basic factors have a direct impact on the cleaning and decontamination procedures that must precede the actual sterilization of an instrument or piece of equipment. The use of "best practice" guidelines assures that the correct procedures are followed to obtain the optimal outcome. Factors affecting sterilization include the design and location of the work area, water and cleaning agents, methods of cleaning, and cleaning protocols. Inspection for proper functioning of the surgical instruments must also be performed prior to sterilization. The purpose of this chapter is to review each of these items.

CLEANING AREA DESIGN AND LOCATION

The area that is used in the cleaning and decontamination process should be close to the point-of-use (operating room or special procedures room) so transporting of instruments can be done in an efficient manner. The cleaning and decontamination of all instruments should be done in one central area under controlled environment factors and done uniformly and consistently, following written procedures.

The walls and floor of the area should be constructed of material that allows frequent cleaning. Ideally, ventilation in the area should be under negative pressure with respect to adjacent areas, having 10 air exchanges per hour. The temperature should be maintained between 64°F and 72°F with a relative humidity between 30% and 70%. Lighting in the area should be adequate for detailed cleaning and inspection of instruments (average of 750 lux to 1500 lux according to the Illuminating Engineering Society of North America for minimum levels of illuminance for various categories of work environments; AAMI, 2009). The lighting fixtures should be selected and mounted in positions that focus the light in front of the staff member so there is no shadow effect. Traffic through the area should be restricted to those who are cleaning the equipment.

Gloves should be worn when handling the contaminated equipment throughout the cleaning and decontamination process. Hands need to be washed after the removal of gloves.

Flat work surfaces should be cleaned and disinfected after the daily equipment decontamination activities are completed. Floors should also be cleaned and disinfected daily.

Veterinary Infection Prevention and Control, First Edition. Edited by Linda Caveney and Barbara Jones with Kimberly Ellis. © 2012 John Wiley & Sons, Inc. Published by John Wiley & Sons, Inc.

WATER AND CLEANING AGENTS USED IN THE CLEANING PROCESS

Water, detergents, enzymes, and enzymatic detergents are used to clean and decontaminate surgical instruments and medical devices. Written recommendations by the original equipment manufacturer should be obtained and followed. Use of the wrong cleaning agent can damage the device and potentially harm a patient.

Water Quality and Characteristics

Water is the primary medium used as a wetting agent in the cleaning process. Important water characteristics for the cleaning process include pH level, hardness, temperature, and purity. The pH is the measure of acidity or alkalinity of a substance. The pH level influences the effectiveness of enzymes and detergents used in the cleaning process. Water hardness is a measure of the minerals, such as calcium and magnesium, found in water. Minerals can cause deposits or scale formation on instruments. The use of chelating agents (chemical agents that "tie-up" calcium and magnesium elements so that they do not come out of solution) added to water helps to minimize the formation of these deposits. Sheeting agents (chemical agents that break surface tension) can be added to the final rinse to eliminate the possibility of spots forming during the drying cycle. Softened water can also help reduce the formation of scale.

Pure water is water considered to be free of particulates, total dissolved solids, and microbes. This water has been put through a process to remove these elements. There are three main processes to obtain pure water: distillation, deionization, and reverse osmosis. A final rinse with pure water will prevent mineral or other particulates from being deposited on the instruments.

Detergents

Detergents are substances that work to free and disperse solid and liquid matter from a surface being cleaned. They have several functions:

- Lowering surface tension (as a surfactant) so the water/detergent solution can penetrate the soil of the item being cleaned
- Breaking up and dispersing (deflocculating) soil, separating clumps of dirt, and dissolving or suspending small particles in the water/detergent solution
- Keeping the soil and dirt suspended in the solution so it can be rinsed away, rather than redeposited on the item being cleaned

Detergents are formulated for specialized applications. See Table 8.1 for choosing the ideal detergent for cleaning.

Examples of specialized detergents are those formulated to work in hard water or in ultrasonic cleaners. Detergents should be compatible with the equipment being cleaned and the cleaning equipment (e.g., ultrasonic cleaner or instrument washer). The manufacturer of the instrument and the ultrasonic cleaner will provide recommendations on the types of cleaning agents that are to be used. The pH of detergents used in cleaning is neutral or mildly alkaline.

Enzymes can be added to the detergent to help "digest" large organic molecules. Enzymes are specific to their action. Protease, for example, breaks down blood, feces, mucous and albumin, whereas lipase breaks down fatty deposits, and amylase works to change the starches.

Table 8.1 Characteristics of the Ideal Cleaning Agent

Nonabrasive
Low-foaming
Free-rinsing
Biodegradable
Allows rapid disperse soil
Nontoxic
Effective on all types of clinical soil
Long shelf life
Cost-effective

Adapted from IAHCSMM, 2007 and AAMI, 2008:45.

Enzyme action is very temperature dependent; always follow the manufacturer's recommended temperature for use as well as the dilution ratio.

Lubricants

Lubricants, otherwise known as "instrument milk," are water-soluble agents designed to keep instruments in good working order. The term "milk" comes from the white, milky appearance of the solution. They help maintain the integrity of the stainless steel and prevent abrasion on blades moving against each other. Lubrication is done after cleaning. It can be applied using a spray bottle, as part of a mechanical wash process, or instrument baths. Use the proper dilution recommended by the manufacturer as well as the proper soak time. Be sure the lubricant is compatible with both the instrument and the sterilization process that will be used.

CLEANING METHODS

Cleaning is the most critical step in the sterilization process. You can clean without sterilizing, but you cannot sterilize without cleaning first. The sterilization process is dependent on direct contact of the sterilant with the surface of the item. Cleaning involves removing the visible and invisible materials from the surfaces, crevices, serrations, and lumens of instruments. Cleaning does not kill microorganisms. Decontamination involves chemical or physical means of reducing or removing contamination by infectious organisms. Dead organisms in organic debris, if left on the instrument, can cause pyrogenic or foreign body reactions. Biofilm, a cluster of living and dead bacteria encased by a slime layer (composed of polysaccharides), can form on any surface, particularly in crevices and lumens. This film provides a layer of protection for the bacteria. Biofilm also prevents the sterilant from coming into direct contact with the surface of the item. Debris left on an instrument can also cause it to malfunction.

Manual Cleaning

Manual cleaning involves the use of friction to remove the organic materials that were softened during a presoak with enzymatic detergents. Brushes specifically made to clean medical instruments should be used, rather than an over-the-counter toothbrush. See Figure 8.1 for an example of general medical instrument cleaning brushes.

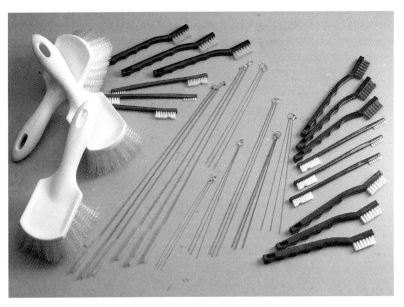

Figure 8.1 Examples of the variety of shapes and sizes of general instrument cleaning brushes available. Photograph is provided courtesy of Spectrum Surgical Instrument Corp., Stow, OH.

Specialized cleaning brushes are available in different diameters and lengths to accommodate unique cleaning needs of varying sizes of baron, frazier, and yankauer suction tubes. See Figure 8.2 for the type of brush available for cleaning frazier suction tubes.

Most brushes are made of nylon, although cotton and cloth varieties are available. Any brushes used in the cleaning process must be cleaned and disinfected to prevent the risk of cross-contamination. This should be done when the brush is heavily soiled or at the end of each day, and should be clearly stated in your cleaning protocol.

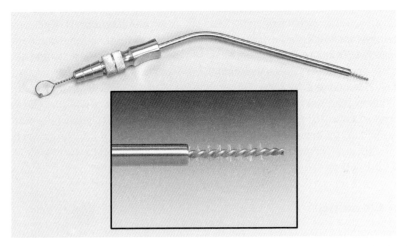

Figure 8.2 Examples of a brush available for cleaning lumens of frazier suction tips. The brush should extend past the tip of the instrument as illustrated. Photograph is provided courtesy of Spectrum Surgical Instrument Corp., Stow, OH.

Abrasive brushes should not be used because they can scratch the surface of an instrument and hasten corrosion. Rough surfaces also can cause biofilm and microorganisms to be retained. Cloths that are low-lint or lint-free can be used to clean equipment that cannot be immersed in liquids. This type of cloth should be changed regularly or when visibly soiled. Sponges can be used to clean basins, containers, or trays. They need to be replaced daily or when they become visibly soiled or stained. The structure of sponges makes them virtually impossible to clean and disinfect.

Delicate instruments, complex instruments, or instruments with lumens are all manually cleaned. Power equipment is also cleaned manually as it cannot be immersed in water.

When manually cleaning instruments or equipment, the water temperature should be between 80°F and 110°F (27°C and 44°C) and never exceed 140°F (60°C). Higher temperatures can cause proteins to coagulate (just as the white protein portion of a poached egg becomes a thickened, clotted mass). Coagulation on an instrument makes protein difficult to remove. Instruments should be scrubbed with a solution of water and a diluted detergent.

To avoid a build-up of organic materials inside the lumen of an instrument (e.g., laparoscopic forceps), a vertical soaking cylinder should be used to ensure that all internal surfaces come in contact with the cleaning solution. See Figure 8.3 for a diagram of vertical soaking.

If they are soaked horizontally, air bubbles in the lumen can keep the solution from contacting all internal surfaces. The use of brushes of the appropriate size should be used to scrub the internal channels of instruments with lumens. The brush needs to extend through the entire length of the lumen.

Mechanical Cleaning

Mechanical cleaning involves the use of an ultrasonic cleaner or automated washer. Ultrasonic cleaning is superior to manual scrubbing, reaching small areas that brushes cannot get to. Although ultrasonic cleaners assist in cleaning, they do not disinfect or sterilize.

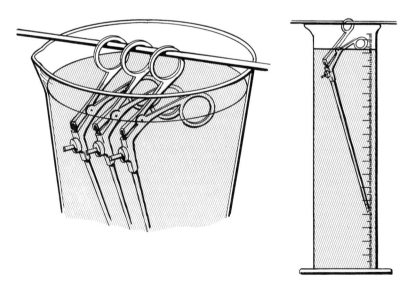

Figure 8.3   This illustrates the vertical soak method for cleaning of an instrument with long lumens. Photograph is provided courtesy of Spectrum Surgical Instrument Corp., Stow, OH.

Ultrasonic cleaners work by passing ultrasonic waves (vibrations) through a cleaning solution, causing small air bubbles to develop and become larger until they implode (collapse). The implosions draw bits of organic materials from the instruments surfaces, including the serrations, cracks, and hinges. This process is called cavitation. Following cavitation, instruments are rinsed to remove sediment and detergent from the instrument surface.

Because the ultrasonic cleaning process removes fats and lipids from the instruments, sediments remain in the ultrasonic cleaner and produce something like the ring in a bathtub. Cleaning of the tank should be done whenever the tank is emptied in accordance with the manufacturer's recommendations. When a tank is first filled, it must be "de-gassed." Excess bubbles in the water during filling reduce the energy released by the cavitation bubbles during implosion. Simply running the unit for 5–10 minutes will de-gas the water.

General guidelines for use of the ultrasonic cleaner include the following:

- Instruments placed in the cleaner should be unlocked or in the open position.
- All lumens must be completely filled with fluid so cavitation can be effective inside lumens.
- All instruments must be completely submerged in the solution.
- Unit should have a cover to contain aerosols when it is running.
- Do not overload the tray or stack instruments over the height of the tray.
- Do not mix metals within a single tray; separate unlike metals (e.g., stainless steel with nonanodized aluminum, brass, copper, chrome plating).
- Consult the instrument manufacturer's recommendations for specific information on the use of your ultrasonic cleaner.

A commercially made product is available to test the effectiveness of the ultrasonic cleaning action. A simple way to test the efficacy of the ultrasonic action is performed by using a piece of heavy-duty household aluminum foil. The size of the foil should be equal to the length and width of the chamber. Place the piece of foil in the metal basket and run through a cycle. At the end of the cycle, remove and inspect the foil. There should be large holes and numerous creases in it. The ultrasonic cleaner should be calibrated according to the manufacturer's recommendations. A preventative maintenance schedule should be adhered to for proper performance.

The use of automated mechanical washers is another method of cleaning instruments and is generally used by practices with a large number of instruments. Automated mechanical washers work on the principle of impingement, with pressurized water spraying against instruments to physically remove organic materials. They are similar to, but more powerful than, a regular household dishwasher, relying on temperature, detergents, and the spray action to clean instrument. Washers can be effective only when they are loaded properly so the force of the water comes in direct contact with all surfaces of the instruments. Delicate instruments can be displaced from a tray by the force of the spray; specially designed trays should be used for these instruments. These trays have lids or hold-downs to confine the instruments but still allow proper cleaning. Figure 8.4 shows one style of automated mechanical instrument washer available.

Consult with the washer's manufacturer for information on the preset factory cycles. The cycles vary because of the number of rinse, wash, lubricant, and drying times. Instrument cycles take longer than a cycle for trays and containers due to the decreased cleaning challenge.

CLEANING PROTOCOLS

Each instrument or medical device that has been used in patient care needs to undergo some sort of cleaning process. This deserves careful consideration because each item can affect

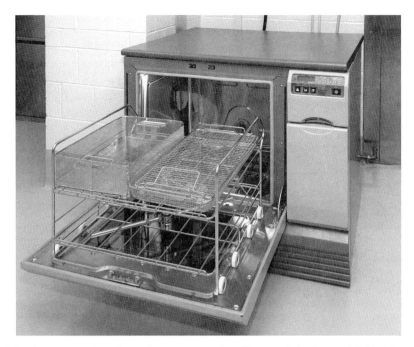

Figure 8.4 An automated mechanical instrument washer. Photograph by Dewey Neild of Dewey Neild Photography, Ithaca, NY.

subsequent patients that need use of same instrument or device. Cleaning procedures must be done consistently, efficiently, and effectively. Establishing a protocol for all items to render them "clean" and "decontaminated" is critical for infection control and patient safety. This starts within 15–30 minutes after a procedure. See Table 8.2 for point-of-use guidelines for cleaning.

Delaying the start of the cleaning process can have harmful effects on the instruments; they can begin to stain, pit, rust, and become dull. Dried blood is very difficult to remove from serrations and other areas of complex instruments. Specially designed, multienzymatic, precleaning sprays or solutions, when used with water in a soak basin at the point-of-use, help keep instruments moist so that blood and organic material will not be allowed to dry on their surfaces. Instruments taken from the surgery or procedure table should be opened or taken apart before placing them in the solution or spraying them with the enzymatic spray.

The solutions manufacturers' recommendations should be followed for the proper dilution, water temperature, and time for effective presoak procedure. Using solutions other than those specifically designed for surgical instruments can damage them and should not be used. See Table 8.3 for chemicals that can damage instruments.

Caution should be taken to ensure that sharps will not be accidentally encountered in the cleaning process.

Delicate instruments should be separated from large or heavy ones. Instruments used in laparoscopic or thorascopic procedures need to be carefully inspected for nicks or breaks in the insulation. Check the equipment manufacturer's recommendations on cleaning and processing of these and other specialty equipment. Specially designed instrument trays may require a different cleaning process than instruments or stainless steel trays. Certain trays are made of aluminum or some composite materials that can be damaged by acidic or alkaline pH detergents. The manufacturers can recommend a neutral pH detergent to use for cleaning of their trays.

Table 8.2 Point-of-use Guidelines

Action	Explanation	Example
Remove gross soil	Remove large pieces of organic material, blood, or other body fluids to allow presoak to reach the body of the instrument. Blood and saline can break down the devices protective finish if left to dry on for an extended period.	Remove fat, tissue, and blood from lumens and hard to reach crevices
Follow manufacturer's instructions for precleaning	This helps prevent the build-up of organic material or bioburden.	Flexible endoscopes should have water suctioned through the suction channel.
Keep soiled instruments moist	Spray with a premixed enzymatic product; soak in basin with enzymatic solution and water; place moist towel over instruments.	Box locks in open position in an orderly fashion to allow enzymatic product to come into contact with all areas of a device
Remove disposable components	Remove blades properly and dispose in sharps container; watch closely to ensure reusable items are not discarded.	Check for towel clamps that are attached to disposable drapes.
Separate reusable sharps from other instruments	Place sharp-pointed instruments or edges in a separate container so they can be handled safely to reduce the risk of injury.	Osteotomes, towel clamps, or skin hooks are examples of items to separate out.
Keep multipart items or sets together	This facilitates the efficiency in reprocessing an instrument set; keeping parts of items together decreases the risk of loss of instrument components.	Frasier suction tips and stylets should be kept together.
Identify items that need repair	Use an instrument repair tag system to identify a dull or malfunctioning instrument or device.	Tag is placed around the ring handle of an instrument.

Source adapted from IAHCSMM, 2007.

Following the cleaning process, verification that cleaning has been accomplished should be done. Meticulous visual inspection is the most common method used to assure the device or instrument is cleaned. If dried blood or other organic material is found on an instrument, the instrument needs to be returned to the "dirty" or decontamination area to be processed again. Do not scrape off the blood or use a brush to remove the material in the "clean" prep area.

INSPECTION OF SURGICAL INSTRUMENTS

Once an instrument or medical device has been thoroughly cleaned and decontaminated, it should be examined before it is placed back into a tray or storage. Inspection includes checking for the following:

- Proper function and alignment: For ring handled instruments, open and close while checking for stiffness; the distal tips should meet and be in alignment. Ratchet-style instruments can be tested to see whether the ratchet is sprung by closing to the first click, holding on to the

Table 8.3   Chemicals that are Harmful to Surgical Instruments

Harmful Chemicals for Surgical Instruments		
bleach	saline Solution	laundry soap
betadine	Comet	dish detergent
peroxide	iodine	Lysol
	normal hand soap	

READ INGREDIENT LABEL ON ALL SOLUTIONS
If it is NOT designed for use on surgical instruments and
sterilization, it is advisable to choose another product.

Chemical Compounds to Avoid		
aluminum chloride	barium chloride	phenol
calcium chloride	carbolic acid	sodium hypochlorite
Dakins solution	ferrous chloride	agya regina
mercury chloride	mercury salts	hydrochloric acid
potassium permanganate	tartaric acid	sulfuric acid
potassium thiocyanate	chlorinated lime	stannous chloride

Adapted from Spectrum Surgical Instruments, 1993.

distal end of the instrument, and tapping the ring end lightly on a flat surface. If the latch opens, the instrument ratchet is sprung and it needs repair. For forceps, the tips and/or teeth should meet exactly.

• Corrosion, pitting, burrs, nicks, and cracks: For ring-handled instruments, examine the box lock for cracks. See Figure 8.5 for an example of a cracked box lock.

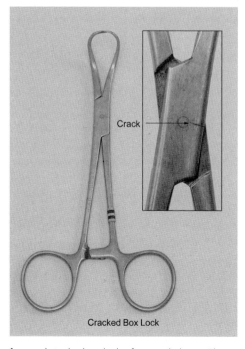

Crack

Cracked Box Lock

Figure 8.5   An example of a crack in the box lock of a towel clamp. Photograph is provided courtesy of Spectrum Surgical Instrument Corp., Stow, OH.

Table 8.4 Stain Guide for Surgical Instruments

Stain Guide for Surgical Instruments

Stain color: Brown/Orange
Cause: A result of high levels of pH in instrument cleaning detergent or laundry soap from the cleaning towels or instrument wrap.

Stain color: Dark Brown
Cause: Acidic reaction to stainless by low pH (<6) in soap or laundry detergent. If black stain cannot be rubbed off with a pencil eraser, it may be a stain resulting from an instrument coming in contact with a steam indicator strip inside the sterilization tray or peel pouch.

Stain color: Blue–Black
Cause: This is a result of plating being removed from an old instrument. This defective instrument, when put in the ultrasonic cleaner or sterilizer with other stainless instruments, will cause this stain.

Stain color: Multicolor
Cause: Excessive heat caused by a localized hot spot in the sterilizer. This rainbow-colored stain can normally be removed. If multicolor stain is on a scissor blade, resharpening is recommended.

Stain color: Light- and dark-colored round spots
Cause: Slow evaporating of water spots and the water mineral content. To reduce this problem, sterilizer door should not be opened until the steam has been completely vented.

Stain color: Blue–Gray
Cause: Liquid high-level disinfectant/sterilant solutions being used beyond recommended time limitations. This will cause the solution to become corrosive.

Stain color: Brown–Black
Cause: Dried, baked on blood.

Adapted from Spectrum Surgical Instruments, 1993.

The box lock is a common place prone to damage, and if it is not clean and dry, it will stain. Check all instruments by feeling for burrs or chips. Check to see if an instrument is stained or rusting by using a pencil eraser on the "rust" spot to remove the discoloration. Check the metal below to see if there is a pitted mark. If there is, this is corrosion and the cause of the rusting. If the metal is smooth, the source is a stain, and there is no rust. See Table 8.4 for a common stain guide.

- Sharpness of the cutting edge: Scissor cutting action should be smooth and not bind; check to see that the distal tips meet exactly. To test the cutting edge of various instruments, see Table 8.5.
- Loose set pins: Check to see that the pins are securely holding the two pieces of the ring instrument together; pins should not wobble or could become disengaged during use.
- Wear and chipping of inserts and plated surfaces: Gold-colored handles on needle holders indicate that the jaws of the instrument contain tungsten carbide inserts that can be replaced if they wear out. See Figure 8.6 for an example of a worn carbide jaw on a needle holder.
    Retractors can have areas of chipping or flaking of the surface finish; these should be replaced because chips and flakes can come off while in use during a surgical procedure.
- Concerns regarding surgical instrument identification: Marking surgical instruments to identify sets or trays is a common practice. This can be done by several methods.

Instrument marking tape is a fairly inexpensive way of doing this. The technique for applying the tape is critical. The taped site should be on the shank of the instrument (tape on a rounded surface will not allow the tape to lie flat against the instrument and can allow biofilm and debris to build up in this area). Wipe the tape site on the instrument with alcohol to remove any moisture

Table 8.5   *Sharpness Testing Standards*

General Scissors, larger than 4.5 inches
   Common Scissors: Metzenbaum, Mayo
Testing material: red test material
Procedure: Three-fourths of the scissor blade should be able to cut completely through the red test material 3 times without snagging, especially at the distal tip.

Micro-Scissors, smaller than 4.5 inches
   Common Micro-Scissors: Iris, Tenotomy
Testing material: yellow test material
Procedure: Three-fourths of the scissor blade should be able to cut completely (and smoothly) through the yellow test material 3 times without snagging, especially at the distal tip.

Laparoscopic Scissor
Testing material: Facial tissue paper
Procedure: Blades should open and close smoothly. Blades should cut through a single layer of the facial tissue paper without snagging.

Lister Bandage Scissors
Testing material: "Huck" cotton or absorbent surgical towel
Procedure: Three-fourths of the blades' length should cut through the towel once without pinching or snagging the towel.

Osteotomes
Testing material: plastic dowel rod
Procedure: Using the plastic dowel rod at a 45° angle, and the osteotome should bite into the rod. A sharpened osteotome should be 90° at the corners and look like a church steeple from the side.

Curette
Testing material: plastic dowel rod
Procedure: A curette's edge should stick into the plastic rod and remove a sample.

Single- and Double-Action Rongeurs
Testing material: 3×5-inch index card
Procedure: Jaws should cut cleanly through a single layer of an index card without tearing. The rongeurs should open and close smoothly.

Kerrison Rongeurs
Testing material: 3×5-inch index card
Procedure: Jaws should cut cleanly through a single layer of an index card without tearing. The rongeurs should open and close smoothly.

Arthroscopy Punches
Testing material: thin piece of leather
Procedure: Jaws of the punch should cleanly cut through a thin piece of leather without tearing or snagging; this testing procedure must be approved by the original equipment manufacturer. The jaws should open and close smoothly.

Cervical Biopsy Punches
Testing material: facial tissue paper
Procedure: Punch should cut cleanly through two layers of facial tissue paper without snagging or tearing.

Bone Cutters, Pin Cutters, Nail Nippers
Testing material: 3×5-inch index card
Procedure: Three-fourths of the blade's length should cut completely through an index card.

Clipper Blades
Testing material: testing twine
Procedure: Place testing twine into the blades on the far left, middle, and far right. Blades should cut cleanly through the material without snagging or tearing. There should be no broken teeth on either the cutter blade or the comb blade.

Source adapted from Schultz, 2005.

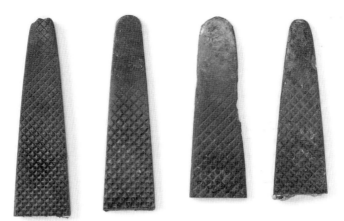

Figure 8.6 This illustrates the wear pattern of carbide inserts on needle holders. Photograph is provided courtesy of Spectrum Surgical Instrument Corp., Stow, OH.

or lubricant from the area. Wrap the tape 1.5 times around the shank, with firm, pulling tension. Do not apply excessive tape as this can interfere with the function of the instrument (e.g. not allowing the tips of a scissor to come together completely). Cut the tape at an angle, allowing the edge to lie flat. See Figure 8.7 for the result of incorrect placement of instrument tape on a pair of scissors.

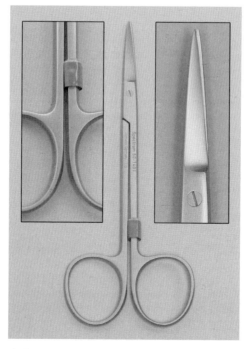

Figure 8.7 This photograph demonstrates incorrect placement of instrument tape on the shaft of a scissor, not allowing the scissor tips to meet properly. Photograph is provided courtesy of Spectrum Surgical Instrument Corp., Stow, OH.

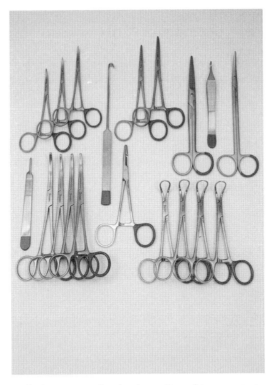

Figure 8.8 This photograph shows specialized color coding of instruments in a surgical pack. Photo is provided courtesy of Spectrum Surgical Instrument Corp., Stow, OH.

When the instrument is sterilized; the heat will help bond the tape to the instrument. Instrument tape should be replaced regularly; it should not be allowed to become dry, brittle, or discolored. Old tape can be a hazard if pieces come off during a surgical procedure.

Acid base etching is done by instrument manufacturers or repair vendors. This marks stainless steel instrument by using a stencil, solutions, and electricity. Etching is semipermanent; it can be removed by buffing during repair procedures.

Color-coding (also called "dipping") is typically done by a repair vendor. This can last for years, but once it starts chipping, it must be completely removed. See Figure 8.8 for an example of color-coding of an instrument set.

Laser etching is done by companies that offer this service. A laser is used to permanently mark an instrument.

A word about engraving: This should not be done because it damages the surface of the instrument.

Setting up a schedule for regular repair of surgical instruments with a repair vendor keeps instruments in good condition and can prolong the life of the instruments.

CONCLUSION

Cleaning is complex and contains many steps. If cleaning is not performed properly, disinfection or sterilization cannot be achieved. Manufacturers' recommendations for cleaning should be checked before establishing a cleaning procedure for an instrument or device. Cleaning detergents and processes should be reviewed periodically to assure that they are being used correctly and they are consistent with the instrument or medical device manufacturer's recommendations.

It cannot be stressed enough that cleaning is the most important step in processing any piece of medical equipment or device; if it's not clean, it cannot be sterile or disinfected.

REFERENCES

[AAMI] Association for the Advancement of Medical Instrumentation. 2009. ANSI/AAMI ST79:2006. Amendments A1 & A2, 2009. Cleaning and other decontamination processes. In: *Comprehensive Guide to Steam Sterilization and Sterility Assurance in Health Care Facilities*. American National Standards Institute, Arlington, VA, pp 43–53.

Association of periOperative Registered Nurses (AORN). 2009. *Perioperative Standards and Recommended Practices*. RP: Care of Instruments, Recommended Practice I–XII. AORN, Denver, CO, pp 611–622.

Chobin N. 2008. Providing safe surgical instruments: factors to consider. *Infect Control Today* 12(4):26–32.

[IAHCSMM] International Association of Healthcare Central Service Material Management. 2007. Cleaning and decontamination. In: *Central Service Technical Manual, 7th ed*. pp 131–154. IAHCSMM, Chicago, IL, pp 131–154.

Schultz R. 2005. *Inspecting Surgical Instruments: An Illustrated Guide*. Spectrum Surgical Instruments, Stow, OH.

Spectrum Surgical Instruments. 1993. *Surgical Instrument Cleaning Manual, 3rd ed*. Spectrum Surgical Instruments, Stow, OH.

Spectrum Surgical Instruments. 2004. *Instrument Processing Essentials, 7th ed*. Spectrum Surgical Instruments, Stow, OH.

Detergents are chemical agents that can dislodge, remove and disperse solid and liquid soils from the surface of the item being cleaned. They do this by:

9 Packaging, Preparation for Sterilization, and Sterile Storage of Medical Equipment

Linda Caveney

Preparation, packaging, and storage of sterilized items need to be done in a controlled environment by personnel who have knowledge in proper procedures. Important considerations are selection of packaging material, package configuration and preparation, the ability to present the item onto a sterile field, and where the sterile items are stored. This chapter will provide an overview of the key points in each of these steps.

PERSONNEL FACTORS

Policies should be written to ensure uniformity and consistency within the preparation and packaging area. All staff members should be familiar with the policy. Included in this policy are requirements for personal hygiene and attire, in order to minimize the introduction of microorganisms or transmission of disease. They include the following:

- Knowledge of hand-washing procedures and availability of a sink.
- Neither nail polish nor artificial nails should be worn. Nail polish that has not been freshly applied can flake off, and the flakes can contaminate items being prepared. Artificial nails can promote the growth of fungus under the nails.
- Clean uniforms should be worn in the preparation and sterilization areas. This attire should be brought into the facility and donned once in the facility (not worn to work) so as to minimize the transport of potentially infectious organisms. Attire should be changed daily, or more often if it gets wet or grossly soiled. When leaving the facility for the day, uniforms should be removed and placed in a plastic bag, then carried home to be laundered.
- Jewelry should not be worn because it can harbor microorganisms and is not easily or routinely cleaned. Furthermore, parts of the jewelry can catch, dislodge, and fall into processed items.

SELECTION OF PACKAGING MATERIALS

The choice of appropriate packaging material is determined, in part, by the sterilization process. Packaging materials suitable for steam sterilization are not the same as those for hydrogen peroxide gas plasma sterilization. Researching and obtaining test documentation from

Veterinary Infection Prevention and Control, First Edition. Edited by Linda Caveney and Barbara Jones with Kimberly Ellis. © 2012 John Wiley & Sons, Inc. Published by John Wiley & Sons, Inc.

manufacturers assures that the packaging system meets the criteria of the specific sterilization process. Perioperative Standards and Recommended Practices by the Association of periOperative Registered Nurses (AORN) recommend that, for steam sterilization, a packaging material should do the following:

- Allow steam penetration and direct contact with the items and surfaces of the package contents, and allow adequate air removal
- Provide an adequate barrier to microorganisms or their vehicles (e.g., dust or fluids).
- Resist tearing, puncture, or abrasion and prevent transfer of microorganisms
- Allow a method of sealing that results in a complete seal, is tamper-evident, and provides seal integrity
- Allow for aseptic presentation (minimal wrap memory, removal of lids from rigid containers)
- Be free of toxic ingredients and nonfast dyes
- Be nonlinting
- Permit identification of the contents
- Allow ease of use by personnel preparing and/or opening the package or rigid container
- Be large enough to evenly distribute the content mass
- Protect the package contents from physical damage
- Be shown to be cost effective
- Include manufacturer's instructions for use

For ethylene oxide (EO) sterilization, a packaging material should additionally do the following:

- Be permeable to EO, moisture, and air
- Permit aeration
- Be made of materials recommended by the sterilizer manufacturer and the sterilant manufacturer
- Maintain material compatibility with the sterilization process

In general, woven and nonwoven packaging, peel pouches, and some rigid containers are compatible with EO sterilization. However, woven materials can absorb a large amount of relative humidity; this may prevent adequate hydration of microorganisms for penetration of EO gas to all surfaces of the package contents.

For low-temperature gas plasma sterilization, a packaging material should do the following:

- Allow sterilizing plasmas to penetrate packaging material
- Be compatible with the sterilization process (nonabsorbable)
- Be constructed of material recommended by the sterilizer manufacturer and used in accordance to the packaging manufacturer's written instructions

Low-temperature gas plasma sterilization is negatively affected by absorbable packaging materials (cellulose-based packaging, textile wrappers, paper–plastic pouches, or porous wrap). More appropriate packaging for low-temperature hydrogen peroxide gas plasma sterilization is generally nonwoven polypropylene wraps and all-plastic (polypropylene) pouches with a standard heat seal.

After choosing the packing material, develop and implement policies and procedures that are consistent with both the sterilizer manufacturer's recommendations and the sterilant manufacturer's recommendations as well as the packaging manufacturer's recommendations. Choices for sterile packaging material are reusable fabric material, disposable packaging material, and rigid container systems.

Reusable Fabric Material

Historically, woven textile reusable packaging material was the standard choice. Muslin (type 140 cotton cloth) in two layers of thickness fastened together as one wrap allows sterilant (typically steam) to penetrate and provides a microbial barrier. Reusable packaging selection is a more labor-intensive packing system, because it must be collected, sorted by like fabrics, laundered appropriately, sorted, inspected, folded, and stored. (See Chapter 13 for more details on handling reusable materials.)

Disposable Packaging Material

Disposable or nonwoven materials have become a popular choice for sterilization packaging because of their effective barrier properties; they are discarded after one use. Reuse of the one-time-use product is against the manufacturers' recommendations for use and therefore will not guarantee that the product inside will be sterile or will remain sterile. There are three types of disposable packaging materials: paper, polyolefin plastic, and nonwoven flat wraps. Paper used as sterilization packaging is medical-grade, Kraft-type paper. It has been FDA approved for use as sterile packaging material; not just any paper can be use for this purpose. Paper packaging material is commonly found in various pouch sizes to accommodate instruments or soft goods. Polyolefin plastic is commonly combined with paper to form peel pouches. The paper–plastic pouches are used to package small instruments and lightweight items. They allow the user to see the contents of the pouch. Spunbound polyolefin–plastic combinations (one side is polyolefin plastic, the other spunbound polyolefin–plastic) are the packaging of choice for low-temperature hydrogen peroxide gas plasma sterilization; it does not contain any cellulose materials. This packaging is sometimes referred to as "Tyvek" pouches. Popular nonwoven packaging material is spunbond–meltblown–spunbond (SMS) flat wrap. It is made by a process in which polyolefin layers (synthetic materials that are softened by heat and hardened by cooling) are exposed to high heat and are pressure-bonded together to form sheets. These are designed for single use; they should never be reused. They come as a single sheet or double sheets that are bonded together, in various weights and sizes to accommodate the variety of tray and pack sizes commonly used.

Rigid Container Systems

Rigid container systems are box-like structures with sealable and removable lids. See Figure 9.1 for an illustration of an aluminum-style rigid container system.

They are composed of aluminum, stainless steel, plastic, or a combination of these materials. These containers have filters in the lids to allow sterilant penetration and provide a microbial barrier. The filters can be reusable or disposable, depending on specifications by the manufacturer of the container. The rigid container has an inner basket to hold the instruments. Each of these

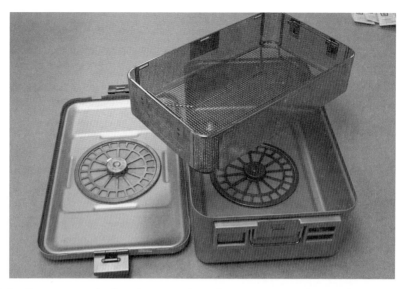

Figure 9.1   This is an example of an aluminum-style rigid container system. Photograph is provided courtesy of SPSmedical, Rush, NY.

has handles for ease in transporting and delivery of contents in an aseptic fashion. See Table 9.1 for the advantages and disadvantages in using rigid container systems.

There are specialized trays available for microsurgical instruments. Most contain silicone mats that are placed on the bottom of a shallow tray; these prevent the instruments from moving around during sterilization and handling during transport for storage or use. The lid of the

Table 9.1   Advantages and Disadvantages of Rigid Container System

Advantages	Disadvantages
	Initial cost
Provides an excellent barrier against microorganisms	Weight of the container (23 × 23 × 6 inches) empty is 8–9 pounds; staff need to be able to carry the container with instruments safely at waist height
Relatively easy to use	Sterilization and drying concerns; may require additional sterilization and drying cycle times; wet packs occur
Eliminates torn, cut, or punctured wraps	Plastic-type containers may require longer drying time
Protects instruments from damage	Additional space may be necessary as the containers are larger than traditional trays
	Additional staff may be needed; containers must be cleaned and thoroughly inspected between uses; it takes up more space in mechanical washers
	Latching mechanisms and welds can break and cannot be used until repaired
	Filter retention plates on some models can dislodge and contaminate instruments
	Verification testing within the facility using biologic indicators to ensure proper sterilant penetration and drying

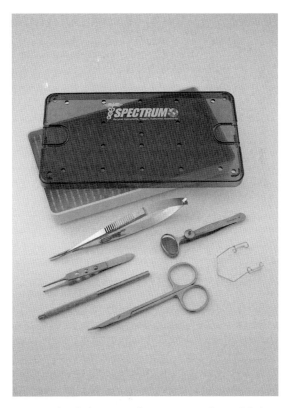

Figure 9.2 This shows a specialized plastic case for microsurgical or ophthalmic instruments. Photograph is provided courtesy of Spectrum Surgical Instrument Corp., Stow, OH.

container is secured by clips or fasteners to hold the instruments snuggly in the tray and ensures the bottom of the tray does not come off unintentionally. The cost of these specialized trays varies; but they are worth the investment in preventing damage to the expensive microsurgical instruments. See Figure 9.2 for an example of a tray for microsurgical instruments.

All packaging materials should be stored at room temperature (68–73°F; 20–23°C) and at a relative humidity range of 30–60% for a minimum of 2 hours before use. This allows adequate preconditioning for sterilization. Tests show that certain dry packaging materials—those that have been subjected to over-drying, heat-pressed woven textiles, textiles that have not been relaundered, and textiles stored in low-humidity conditions—can hinder steam penetration and cause superheating. Any reusable woven textiles (e.g., gowns, drapes, wrappers) should be laundered between every use for rehydaration (AORN, 2009). Resterilization without laundering of textiles causes the fabric to be overdry. When exposed to repeat sterilization attempts, the textiles absorb the available moisture present in the steam, thereby creating a dry or "superheated" steam effect. This is a condition that causes the steam to be unsaturated, essentially making it no more effective than hot, dry air. Saturated steam is a much better "carrier" of thermal energy than dry air (IAHCSMM, 2007). Compare this to cooking something in an oven versus a pressure cooker; the items in the pressure cooker will cook faster (due to steam and pressure) than in a dry-heat oven.

PACKAGE CONFIGURATION AND PREPARATION

Instruments or medical devices that have undergone the cleaning, decontamination, and inspection procedures are now ready to be assembled into trays or packaged as individual instruments. Instruments that have been sent out for repair and are now being returned to use need to undergo the cleaning, decontamination, and inspection (for power equipment, this includes testing to assure it works properly) before being wrapped.

Groupings of multiple instruments that are prepared for a certain specific purpose are referred to as trays or sets (e.g., orthopedic trays, screw sets). There should be documentation from the manufacturer of each instrument as to their recommended sterilization instructions. Each medical facility creates its own trays or sets for its particular needs. A list of the contents of each basic tray or set should be created in order to ensure uniformity and consistency of the packs. Lists should include the name and quantity of each instrument. Lists can also display a picture of each instrument and a picture of what the tray looks like when completely and correctly assembled. This helps train new employees and reacquaints others who need to assist in the preparation procedures.

For assembling trays, items are generally placed in stainless steel, heat-tolerant plastic or anodized aluminum trays with perforated or mesh bottoms to facilitate sterilant penetration and allow adequate drying (IAHCSMM, 2007). An absorbent sheet, generally referred to as a tray liner, can be used to absorb moisture, facilitate drying, and provide cushioning for instrument movement within a tray. See Figure 9.3 for an example of one type of tray liner.

Sharp instruments should have protective tip covers placed on them, or be placed in a special paper holder. See Figure 9.4 for examples of protective tip covers.

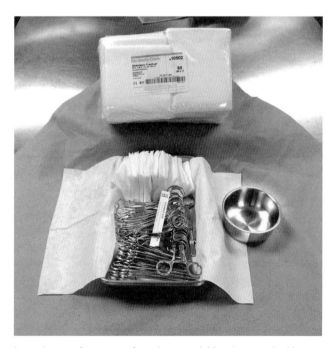

Figure 9.3 This shows the use of one type of tray liner available. Photographed by Dewey Neild of Dewey Neild Photography, Ithaca, NY.

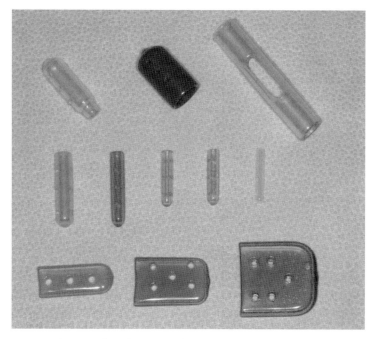

Figure 9.4   A variety of sizes and configurations of tip protectors available.

The supplier of the tip protectors should provide documentation that the coverings are compatible with the sterilization process being used. Latex tubing should not be used because it prevents steam and EO penetration to the instrument it is protecting.

If an instrument has multiple parts, it should be disassembled to allow the sterilant to come in contact with all its surfaces. Instruments that open (e.g., hemostats, scissors) with ratchets need to be kept in the open, unlocked position to allow the sterilant to contact with all surfaces. Use of specialized pins, stringers, or racks can help facilitate this. Heavy instruments are placed so that they will not damage more delicate ones.

For complex instruments, like power drills and scopes, the device manufacturer should be consulted for packaging requirements. This information includes the sterilization method (type of cycle, temperature, exposure time, and dry time) required because of the complexity of the device. Refer to Chapter 12, the section on "Processing of Powered Surgical Instruments," for further details.

All wrapped items should have chemical indicators placed in them to verify that they have been exposed to a sterilization process. The use of chemical indicators is further discussed in Chapter 10.

Peel pouches should not be placed inside wrapped or containerized instrument trays. These pouches cannot be positioned to ensure adequate steam contact, air removal, or drying. Validation for this use has not been done by any wrap manufacturer, containment device manufacturer, or paper–plastic pouch manufacturer (AAMI, 2009).

When considering the number and types of instruments to place in a tray, keep in mind the density of all the metals. A maximum weight limit of 25 pounds for containerized instruments has been set for one manufacturer's standard set with specific sterilization cycle parameters

(IAHCSMM, 2007). There is no magic weight limitation agreed upon for a wrapped tray. It should be based on the ability of staff to easily handle and transport the tray.

Too much metal mass can interfere with sterilization and/or drying in a typical preset cycle. If the metal mass in a pack is excessive, it can cause condensation, resulting in excessive moisture and a wet interior of the tray. This happens because, as steam enters the tray containing metal instruments, steam is immediately cooled when heat is transferred to the metal instrument. Over the course of the exposure cycle, all the condensate may not return to a vapor; it remains trapped in the tray or package in the form of water droplets. Tray liners can help absorb the moisture and facilitate drying. Another option is to divide the one dense tray into two smaller trays.

When wet packs do occur, the pack is considered contaminated and must be completely reprocessed. A new outer wrap (or if textiles were used, a freshly laundered wrap), a new chemical indicator, and a new tray liner (if used) should be used. Disposable products like gauze or cotton balls should be discarded. See Chapter 10, Table 10.4, for further details on procedures to follow when a wet pack is found.

Instruments ready to be assembled in a tray should be arranged in like types (e.g., all hemostats together, all towel clamps together). When possible, instruments should be presented in their order of use (e.g., towel clamps at the top of the tray). Figure 9.5 shows instruments arranged in like types and towel clamps placed at the top of the tray so they are available once the tray is opened.

All jointed instruments should be placed in with locks in the open position.

Heavier instruments should be placed at the bottom or end of a tray. The instrument arrangement in a tray should have a balance of metal density.

The tray is now ready to be wrapped. Wrapping involves the use of either reusable woven textiles or disposable nonwoven wrap. There are two methods of using flat wrappers for trays: sequential and simultaneous. Sequential wrap means the contents have been wrapped in

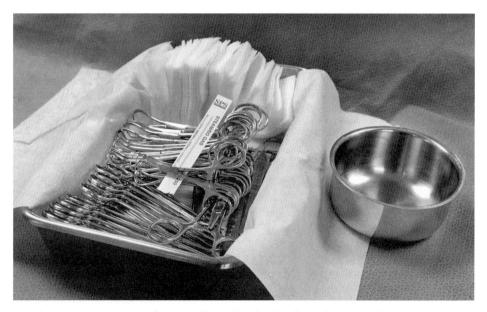

Figure 9.5 Tray arrangement illustrating like-kind and order-of-use placement. Photographed by Dewey Neild of Dewey Neild Photography, Ithaca, NY.

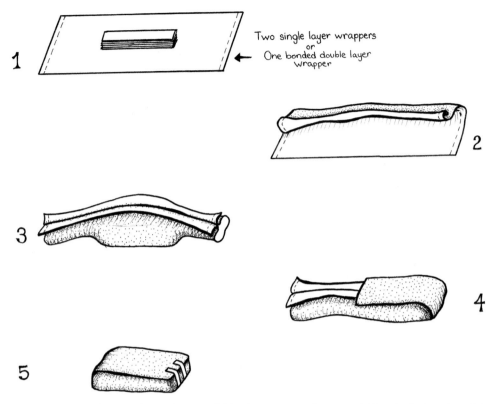

Figure 9.6   This illustrates the simultaneous fold technique using the square-fold method. The edge of the wrapper is placed parallel to the edge of the table. The instrument tray (or linen pack) is placed in the center of the wrapper, parallel with the edge of the wrap. The edge of the wrapper is folded over the top of the contents covering the entire item. This edge is folded back on itself to form a cuff. The upper edge of the wrapper is folded over the contents, covering it completely, and folded back on itself to form another cuff. The upper and lower wrapper folds on the left side of the contents are folded in toward midline to facilitate making a snug fold over the contents of the pack and then folded back over itself to form a cuff. The upper and lower right wrapper folds on the right side of the contents are folded in toward midline to make a snug fold over the previous fold. The open edges are tucked under and secured with indicator tape. Illustration provided by Kayla Kohlenberg, Ithaca, NY.

sequence; it's a pack within a pack. Simultaneous wrap means the pack is wrapped once, but it requires a double layer of synthetic nonwoven bound on two or four sides or double-layer reusable material.

There are two techniques for wrapping packs; both are used with sequential or simultaneous wrap methods. They are square fold (also called the parallel fold) and the envelope fold. See Figures 9.6–9.9 for step-by-step descriptions of each of these methods and techniques.

The correct size wrap should be chosen; the wrap should be large enough to cover the contents without an excess of material that could hinder sterilant penetration. Wraps should be snug to prevent low spots where moisture can accumulate. They should not be too tightly wrapped because this can result in puncture or strike-through. Regardless of the wrap chosen, the pack needs to be examined carefully for damage prior to sterile presentation. If any damage is observed, the pack must be considered contaminated and must be reprocessed.

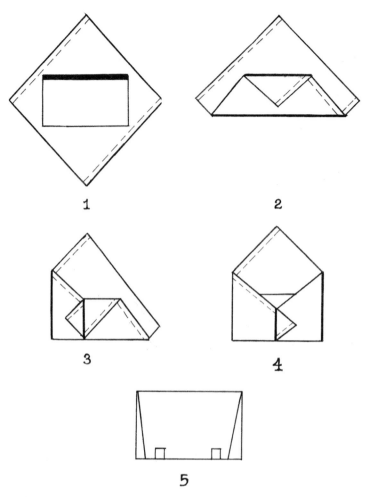

Figure 9.7 This illustrates the simultaneous fold technique using the envelope-fold method. The wrapper is placed on the table with one corner of the square pointing to the front of the table. The tray (or linen pack) is placed in the center of the wrapper, parallel to the edge of the table. The corner pointing toward you is brought up to cover the contents, and the tip is folded back on itself to form a tab. The left corner is folded over the pack, folding the tip back on itself to form a tab. The right corner is folded over the left fold and the tip folded back on itself to form a tab. Bring the top corner down over the previous folds and tuck the corner under the folds formed by the left and right folds. A small "tab" may be formed by exposing the tip of the corner of the wrapper. The pack is secured with indicator tape. Illustration provided by Kayla Kohlenberg, Ithaca, NY.

Textile product packs (e.g., drapes, gowns, surgical towels) should be prepared with preconditioned textiles that have been inspected to ensure their effectiveness. The textile manufacturer should be consulted for their validation information on sterilization cycle parameters, according to the pack size and density. Textiles must be placed in a manner that allows proper air removal, steam penetration, and steam evacuation. To ensure there is steam sterilant penetration in your typical textile pack, a sample test pack is created by placing a biologic indicator in the center, processing the sample test pack in a typical cycle with other packs, and achieving a negative biologic reading. More information on the use of biologic indicators is found in Chapter 10.

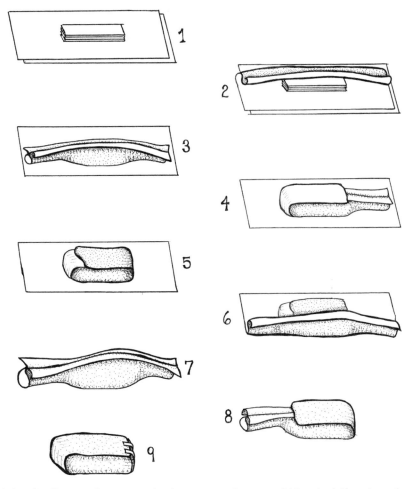

Figure 9.8 This illustrates the sequential technique using the square-fold method. The edges of two single-sheet wrappers are placed parallel to the edge of the table. The instrument tray (or linen pack) is placed in the center of the wrapper, parallel with the edge of the wrap. The edge of the innermost wrapper is folded over the top of the contents, covering the entire item. This edge is folded back on itself to form a cuff. The upper edge of the innermost wrapper is folded over the contents, covering it completely, and folded back on itself to form another cuff. The upper and lower wrapper folds on the left side of the contents are folded in toward midline to facilitate making a snug fold over the contents of the pack and then folded back over itself to form a cuff. The upper and lower right wrapper folds on the right side of the contents are folded in toward midline to make a snug fold over the previous fold. The open edges are tucked under. The above steps are repeated with the remaining wrapper. This outermost wrapper is secured with indicator tape. Illustration provided by Kayla Kohlenberg, Ithaca, NY.

Wrappers should not compress the contents of the textile pack. Historically, a textile pack would not exceed 12 pounds and would measure 12 inches wide by 12 inches high by 20 inches long; this standard was developed for muslin drapes and wrappers. Today, we are using products composed of different materials. The manufacturers of the various textiles should be consulted as to the instructions on pack preparation and density parameters.

Peel pouches are used for small, lightweight items. The pouches allow for visualization of the instruments. The paper side allows air, steam, or other sterilant penetration. Peel pouches are

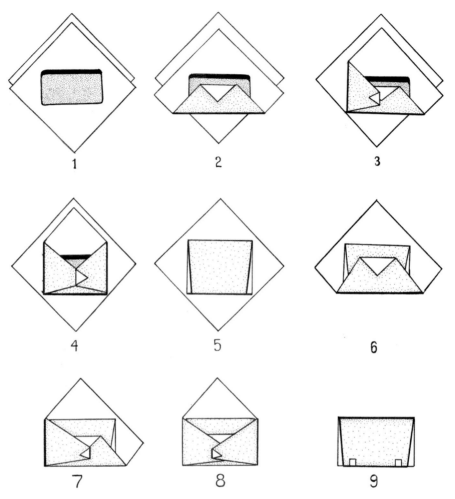

Figure 9.9 This illustrates the sequential-fold technique using the envelope-fold method. The edges of two single-sheet wrappers are placed on the table with one corner of the square pointing to the front of the table. The tray (or linen pack) is placed in the center of the wrapper, parallel to the edge of the table. The corner pointing toward you is brought up to cover the contents and the tip is folded back on itself to form a tab. The left corner is folded over the pack, folding the tip back on itself to form a tab. The right corner is folded over the left fold and the tip folded back on itself to form a tab. Bring the top corner down over the previous folds, and tuck the corner under the folds formed by the left and right folds. The above steps are repeated with the remaining wrapper. This outermost wrapper is secured with indicator tape. Illustration provided by Kayla Kohlenberg, Ithaca, NY.

available in various width rolls or in assorted sizes of premade pouches with a "chevron"-sealed end. Premade peel pouches allow for easy aseptic presentation. If sharp or pointed instruments are placed in a pouch, a tip protector should be used to prevent the ends from poking through the paper or plastic of the pouch.

Items should be placed in the pouch so the handle or finger-rings end will be presented when it is taken by the sterile person. The correct size pouch for the instrument size is an important consideration when choosing a pouch. The pouch must allow for sterilant penetration, air removal, and proper drying.

Pouches should not be overfilled because this can stress the integrity of the preformed seams. (If the finger rings are pressing against the sides of the pouch, the pouch size is too small.) Conversely, too much pouch can also compromise the pouch integrity. (Items can slide around freely, causing a puncture or break in the preformed seals of the pouch.) As with a tray, examine the pouch for moisture following sterilization. This moisture can compromise the seal's integrity or the barrier capability of the pouch material and therefore the sterility of the contents. The density may be too great for the pouch; the contents should be divided into two pouches to reduce the problem.

There are three methods of sealing paper–plastic pouches: heat seals, self-adhesive, and sealing tapes. With the heat-seal method, the manufacturer of the pouch should be consulted to see which heat sealers are compatible with their product. The seal may not bond or it may burn through if the correct heat sealer or sealer parameters are not compatible. It is critical to follow the sealer manufacturer's recommendations for the temperatures settings, applied pressure, and contact time for the seal. For paper-to-plastic seals, the edges of the pouch are placed within the preheated jaws of the sealer, pressure is applied for the recommended contact time, and the jaws are released. The seal is observed for bubbles, gaps, folds, or creases; the presence of these defects can allow for bacterial contamination following sterilization.

Self-adhesive pouches contain an adhesive portion and a removable strip at one end of the pouch to allow for sealing. To seal, remove the protective strip and carefully fold over the opening of the pouch. As with the heat-sealing method, check the sealed area for gaps, wrinkles, folds, or creases.

Sealing tape (e.g., autoclave tape) can be used to seal pouches or roll-style packaging material. Proper taping techniques includes first folding the corners inward so that the side edges of the top corners are parallel to the bottom edge of the pouch. Make sure the plastic is folded onto plastic, not paper-to-paper. Seal with tape, overlapping the edge of the pouch by about $\frac{1}{4}$ inch, and secure. Check to see the tape has completely covered the open edge of the pouch and is securely adhered to the plastic. Observe that there are no gaps, creases, or wrinkles. See Figure 9.10 for an illustration of this technique.

Double pouches can help in aseptic presentation of multiple items or those that have multiple parts. Double pouches are prepared by placing the items in one pouch, sealing it appropriately, then placing it inside a second, slightly larger pouch and sealing it. Arrange the pouches paper side–to–paper side, plastic-to-plastic to allow visibility of the contents, air removal, sterilant penetration, and proper drying. Choosing the proper sequential sizes of pouches is essential when double pouching is done. The inner pouch should not be folded over because this can

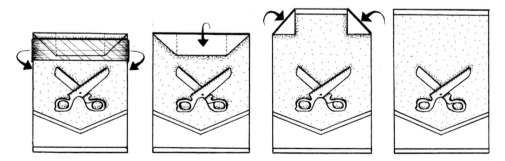

Figure 9.10   This illustrates the placement of a ring-handled instrument in a pouch being sealed by the proper tape-seal technique. Illustration provided by Kayla Kohlenberg, Ithaca, NY.

interfere with air removal and sterilant penetration. Double packaging in paper–plastic peel pouches should also not be performed unless the manufacturer of the pouch has provided you with documentation that the pouch has been validated for this type of use. The reason for this is the plastic laminate is impervious to the sterilant and may prevent the sterilant from reaching the surface of the item that is physically touching the plastic side (AAMI, 2009).

LABELING

Labeling of all pouches and trays is always done prior to sterilization. Label information should include at least a brief description of the contents (e.g., spay pack, orthopedic tray), date of sterilization, and sterilizer and load information. Labeling helps with rotation of stock and identifies items that are minimally used. Labeling can be done with marking pens on the indicator (autoclave) tape or with commercially available preprinted adhesive labels.

Marking pens used should be nontoxic, indelible, nonbleeding, and non-fading. Writing on the paper side of pouches or wraps (whether woven or nonwoven) should be avoided as it could cause damage to the contents (AAMI, 2009). Labeling of self-adhesive pouches can be done on the folded-over paper portion that is on the plastic side of the pouch. If preprinted labels are used, they should also be placed on the folded over portion of the pouch. They should not be put on the paper side; this may interfere with steam penetration and venting of the pouch. If preprinted labels are used in labeling of packs wrapped with SMS nonwoven flap wrap, the label is placed on the autoclave tape. (The label will not stick to the nonwoven wrap after sterilization.)

PACKAGE CLOSURE

The purpose of package closure is to seal the pack contents securely, maintain sterile integrity, and to prevent resealing of an opened pack. Tapes other than those specified for the specific sterilization process (e.g., "autoclave" or "Steam") should not be used. The adhesive may not hold when exposed to the high temperature and moisture. Sharp items like safety pins, staples, or even paper clips should not be used; they cause puncture holes that allow for bacterial contamination. Rubber bands or tape should not be used to hold instruments together in a grouping; this can interfere with the sterilant contact beneath the bands.

LOADING THE STERILIZER

When loading a sterilizer, the manufacturer's written instructions should be followed. Creating written procedures describing the load content placement following the manufacturer's recommendations helps facilitate consistent outcomes. Proper loading of a steam sterilizer will allow for satisfactory air removal, penetration of steam into each pack or pouch, and steam evacuation. Some general guidelines include the following:

- Avoid overloading, because steam cannot penetrate tight spaces.
- Items capable of holding water (e.g., basins or solid bottom trays) should be placed so air can get out and steam can get in. These are placed on their edges, all in the same direction.

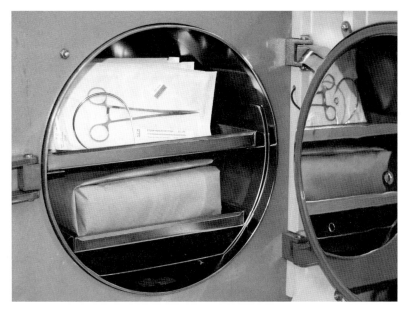

Figure 9.11   This shows the correct placement of peel pouches and a wrapped instrument tray in a tabletop sterilizer. Photograph is provided courtesy of SPSmedical, Rush, NY.

- Items that can produce condensate (e.g., basins) need to be placed on the bottom shelf so that any drips will not fall on other packs in the load.
- Packs or pouches should not touch the chamber walls. Figure 9.11 shows proper placement of pouches and trays in a tabletop steam sterilizer. Figure 9.12 shows proper placement of pouches and trays in a larger chamber-size steam sterilizer.

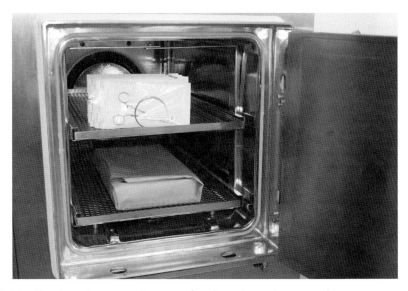

Figure 9.12   This shows the correct placement of peel pouches and a wrapped instrument tray in a larger steam sterilizer with shelves. Photograph is provided courtesy of SPSmedical, Rush, NY.

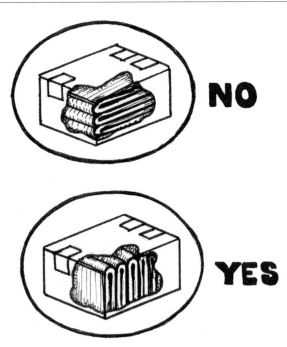

Figure 9.13 Illustration of the placement of towels within a pack. The folds are placed perpendicular to the shelf of a sterilizer for appropriate steam penetration. Illustration provided by Kayla Kohlenberg, Ithaca, NY.

- Textile packs should be positioned with the layers perpendicular to the shelf. Figure 9.13 shows the arrangement of towels within a wrapped pack for proper placement in the sterilizer.

Your hand should be able to fit easily between the textile packs when they are placed on the sterilizer shelf.

- Wrapped instrument sets with perforated bottom trays or rigid containers should be placed so the bottom of the tray is parallel to the shelf. Figure 9.14 illustrates the placement of peel pouches and perforated bottom trays on shelves of a steam sterilizer.
- Stand paper/plastic peel pouches on edge using a basket or rack, enabling the sterilant to reach the paper side of the pouch (the plastic side cannot be penetrated by air or steam). Arrange the peel pouches paper-to-plastic, paper-to-plastic so the paper side of one pouch is next to the plastic side of the adjacent pouch. Placing them flat with either the paper side down or the plastic side down can cause moisture to remain inside the pouch or on top of the plastic. Figure 9.15 shows the proper placement of peel pouches on edge in a rack ready to be placed on a steam sterilizer shelf.
- All pack and peel pouch contents should be dry. If items are moist going in, they will be wet coming out.

Sterilization parameters for high-temperature items are discussed in greater detail in Chapter 10. Low-temperature sterilization parameters are discussed fully in Chapter 11.

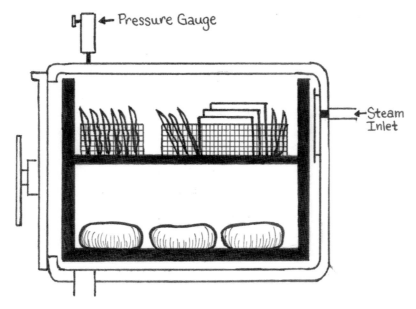

Figure 9.14 This illustrates the correct placement of peel pouches and a wrapped instrument trays in a larger steam sterilizer with shelves. Illustration provided by Kayla Kohlenberg, Ithaca, NY.

UNLOADING THE STERILIZER

When the cycle is complete, the sterilizer door should be cracked to allow residual moisture to escape and to start equalizing the temperature inside the chamber and the room. For a gravity unit, this may be 25–30 minutes; for a prevacuum unit, it is about 10 minutes. For heavier items, it may be longer. Load contents should appear to be free of any liquid or water droplets. If droplets are observed, each item in the load needs to be checked after it is taken out of the chamber.

Do not touch the pack or pouches at this point. They are very warm and still may contain steam vapor. If they are touched, this moisture can carry microorganisms from your hand through

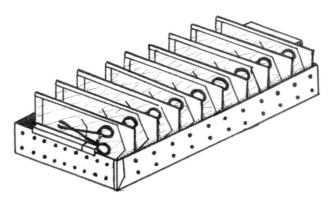

Figure 9.15 This illustrates the proper placement of peel pouches in a tray ready for sterilization. Illustration provided by Kayla Kohlenberg, Ithaca, NY.

the wrap material to the tray or peel pouch contents. Package materials are only an effective barrier when they are dry. After the initial period of time with the door cracked, remove the cart or carry-tray of instruments; do not touch the individual items. Place this cart or carry-tray in an area where the packs and pouches can be allowed to cool to room temperature. The carry-trays should be placed on open wire shelves. Do not place the warm packs on a solid or cold surface; condensation will occur beneath the packs, rendering the packs unsterile.

The packs or pouches should remain on the cart or carry-tray in an area that is free of traffic and away from air conditioning or heating vents. Items can be touched when they have cooled to room temperature; this takes anywhere from 30–60 minutes, depending on the density of the trays or items within a tray. Handle the packs as little as possible. This corresponds with the conditions for using event-related sterilization parameters.

STERILE STORAGE

Historically, the sterile maintenance of a pack or peel pouch was thought of as "time related." The package was considered sterile until it reached that expiration date. It was then taken out of circulation and went through the entire cleaning, assembly, wrapping, and sterilization process. This is a time-, labor-, and material-intensive process. Human health care organizations (e.g., Joint Commission on Accreditation of Healthcare Organizations [JCAHO], Association for periOperative Registered Nurses [AORN]) now recognize that the shelf life of a packaged sterile item is "event related" not "time related." Event-related sterility maintenance is based on the potential for microbial contamination of its contents, as caused by an event rather than by the passage of time. Event-related sterility depends on the quality of the wrap material, monitoring of the sterilization processes, handling procedures of the items, the number of times an item is handled, and storage and transportation conditions. However, if a commercially prepared sterile product has an expiration date, it must be followed. This is a reflection of potential deterioration or instability of the package contents, rather than the sterility (e.g., latex or medications).

Basic Components in Event-Related Sterility Maintenance

The principal conditions that affect the maintenance of a sterile package are moisture and liquid contamination; dirt, dust, or debris; and physical damage (e.g., cuts, tears, punctures). Once a sterilized package has been allowed to cool in a controlled environment, a "sterility maintenance" or dust cover can be put on the pack. This provides an extra protection level for the item, particularly those that are used infrequently or may be exposed to uncontrolled environmental factors (e.g., leaving the facility). Dust covers are applied just as soon as the pack is completely cool and dry. Dust covers are plastic material made specifically for this purpose; they are at least 2–3 mm thick. Dust covers are not a sterile wrap, nor do they provide a microbiological barrier. The cover cannot be removed and the pack placed on a sterile table; the tray wrapper needs to be removed first; then the tray can be presented aseptically. The label on the tray (on the closure tape) identifying the tray should remain visible through the dust cover. The dust cover should be securely sealed with tape or by a heat seal.

The area where sterile items are stored should be clean, dry, and have no open pipes or ducts that can shed dust or debris. The temperature should be maintained between 64°F and 75°F (18°C and 24°C) with a relative humidity below 70–75%. The room ideally should be under positive air pressure as compared to adjacent rooms, with at least four air exchanges per hour.

Packages should be stored at least 2 inches from exterior walls, windows, and windowsills where condensation might form. Moisture causes tape and labels to lose their adhesiveness;

condensate on the wrap material can wick through with microorganisms to compromise sterility; and moisture provides an opportunity for fungal growth. Sterile packages should not be stored near sinks, exposed water pipes, or air conditioning drains. Ideally, storage should be located away from heavy traffic areas.

Sterile packages can be stored on open- or closed-shelf storage systems. With open-shelving system, the shelves have open wire racks to prevent dust accumulation. The items stored on open shelves are more exposed to physical and environmental hazards. The shelves for the sterile items should be 8–10 inches above the floor and at least 18 inches below the ceiling. This allows for adequate air circulation and easy cleaning. The bottom shelf of an open-shelf system should have a physical barrier to prevent floor cleaning agents, mops, and spills from contaminating the sterile items.

Heavy items should be stored where they can be easily handled—not dragged across the shelf—generally on middle to lower shelves. Sterile-stored items should be arranged so packages are not crushed, bent, or compressed. If air inside a package is forced out, it can potentially rupture the closure system and seams; it also creates a slight void in the pack. When the compression is released, a slight suction can draw in contaminated air (AORN, 2009).

When compared with the open-shelving system, the closed-cabinet system limits dust accumulation, reduces the amount of handling, and minimizes accidental contact with the sterile items. Cabinets are appropriate for storage of seldom used items, delicate items, or expensive items.

If your sterile storage area is also used for presterilized products from an outside source, these products need to be removed from the outside shipping containers (corrugated cardboard boxes) before being stored in the sterile storage area. Shipping containers are exposed to unknown and potentially high microbial contamination, including bacterial spores and fungus (AAMI, 2009). After these products are removed from the shipping container, they can be transported in a clean container (e.g., plastic) to the sterile storage area.

The arrangement of sterile stock should be for efficiency, ease of locating items, and appropriate stock rotation. Shelf items can be organized alphabetically by name or grouped together by specialty areas. All sterile items need to be rotated by a "first-in, first-out" system. This ensures the oldest pack or peel pouch is used first and prevents some packs from being left longer than others. The rationale is that if a pack has been exposed to environmental and physical abuse longer, the potential for contamination is greater. One system follows a right-to-left flow: when new items are placed on the shelf to the right, the older item is moved to the left; the packs on the left are to be taken first for use. Another system uses a back-to-front system: when new items are placed in the back, the older items are moved to the front; the items in the front are taken for use. Once an arrangement system is established, everyone who handles sterile packs and pouches must follow the system.

Transporting a sterile pack from the storage area to the end user should be done in a manner that will protect the pack from puncture, moisture, dust, or excessive humidity. Packs should not be dragged or pushed against any surface as this causes friction or abrasion, which can cut or snag a tray. Shelf liners on open wire shelving units provide a cushion between the tray and the shelf. For heavier packs, specialized transportation trays can assist in handling sterile trays. When packs are on the transport tray, the tray is handled, not the heavy pack. Figure 9.16 shows a larger pack positioned on a transport tray.

Packs that are carried by hand should be held parallel to the floor, not "cradled."

When packs are removed from the shelf, they should be examined for cuts, tears, moisture, and compromised seals. The indicator tape should be checked to see if the item has been subjected to a sterilization process. Any sterile item that has been dropped to the floor should be considered contaminated. The jarring and compression of landing can force dust and airborne

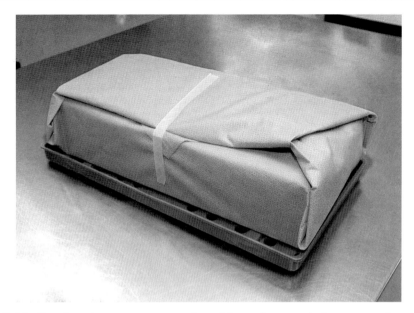

Figure 9.16 This photo shows a transport tray that will be used to carry the large wrapped tray from the prep table to the sterilizer shelf. Photographed by Dewey Neild of Dewey Neild Photography, Ithaca, NY.

microorganisms into the pack. If a cart is being used to transport sterile items from storage to another area, it should be covered or closed and equipped with a solid bottom. The cart should be cleaned routinely and have proper maintenance.

The importance of careful handling of sterile packages cannot be stressed enough. Bumping into, leaning on, or even excessive rearranging all can compromise the sterility of a pack. Table 9.2 is a summary of criteria for event-related sterile storage.

Table 9.2 Criteria for Event-related Sterility

Event-related sterility depends on the quality of the wrap material, monitoring of the sterilization processes, handling procedures of the items, the number of times an item is handled, and storage and transportation conditions.

The temperature should be maintained between 64°F and 75°F (18°C and 24°C) with a relative humidity below 70–75%. The room ideally should be under positive air pressure as compared to adjacent rooms with at least four air exchanges per hour.

Packages should be stored at least 2 inches from exterior walls, windows, and windowsills where condensation might form.

Sterile packages can be stored on open- or closed-shelf storage systems.

The arrangement of sterile stock should be for efficiency, ease of locating items, and appropriate stock rotation.

Transporting a sterile pack from the storage area to the end user should be done in a manner that will protect the pack from puncture, moisture, dust, or excessive humidity. Packs should not be dragged or pushed against any surface, as this causes friction or abrasion that can cut or snag a tray.

If a cart is being used to transport sterile items from storage to another area, it should be covered or closed and equipped with a solid bottom. The cart should be cleaned routinely and have proper maintenance.

CONCLUSION

The choices of wrap, configuration, preparation, wrapping, and storage of packs all pose concerns and challenges that need to be addressed by each facility. There is no one-size-fits-all when it comes to preparing and storing sterilized items. Creating detailed policies and procedures for each step can help eliminate inconsistencies and minimize risk of contamination. Training and education of staff members that handle sterile equipment is vital to any facility. Following established best-practice guidelines assures our patients are not going to be hurt.

REFERENCES

[AAMI] Association for the Advancement of Medical Instrumentation, American National Standards Institute. 2009. ANSI/AAMI ST79:2006: Amendments A1 and A2. Packaging, preparation, and sterilization. In: *Comprehensive Guide to Steam Sterilization and Sterility Assurance in Health Care Facilities*, ANSI/AAMI, Arlington, VA, pp 57–79.

[AORN] Association of periOperative Registered Nurses. 2009. Selection and use of packaging systems for sterilization. Recommendation I-XII. In: *Perioperative Standards and Recommended Practices*, AORN, Denver, CO, pp 637–646.

[IAHCSMM] International Association of Healthcare Central Service Material Management. 2007. Sterile packaging and storage. In: *Central Service Technical Manual, 7th ed.*, IAHCSMM, Chicago, IL, pp 237–264.

10 High-Temperature Sterilization

Linda Caveney

High-temperature or thermal sterilization is the most common method for sterilization of heat-stable medical devices. Sterilization is defined by standards (AAMI, 2009) as the complete destruction of all forms of microbial life. With the thermal energy from moist heat, steam sterilization is a relatively quick, low-cost, safe, nontoxic, and effective way to render a product free of microorganisms. This chapter will review the structure and makeup of a steam sterilizer, the basic types of steam sterilizers, the basics of steam sterilization processing, quality assurance procedures for monitoring the sterilization cycle, and sterilizer maintenance.

STRUCTURE AND MAKEUP OF A STEAM STERILIZER

The first pressure steam sterilizer was developed in 1880 by Charles Chamberlain (IAHCSMM, 2007). It resembled a pressure cooker and allowed the use of pressurized steam to reach temperatures higher than the boiling point of water, killing larger numbers of heat-resistant bacteria. Steam sterilizers now come in a variety of sizes, from tabletop units to large units capable of holding floor rolling carts.

On larger hospital steam sterilizers, a jacket surrounds the sides, top, and bottom of the chamber. The jacket's function is to circulate steam around the outside wall of the chamber to assist in the drying of sterilized items. For these larger units in hospital facilities, steam is piped in from an external source to the jacket; tabletop units generate their own steam and generally do not include a jacket. See Figure 10.1 for a cross-section of a larger steam sterilizer and Figure 10.2 for a cross-section of a tabletop steam sterilizer.

In either system, the door of the sterilizer has a safety mechanism that activates when the chamber is pressurized and can only be unlocked when there is no internal pressure. The door gasket maintains a tight seal to prevent steam from escaping the chamber or air from entering the chamber.

A chamber drain allows the air to be forced out during the conditioning phase. The drain contains a screen to keeps items from unintentionally being forced through. A thermostatic trap is located in the drain line; it contains a heat sensor that measures the steam temperature and automatically controls the flow of air and condensate from the sterilizing chamber. The drain is considered the coolest spot in the sterilizer. (See Figure 10.1 for location of drain line.)

Veterinary Infection Prevention and Control, First Edition. Edited by Linda Caveney and Barbara Jones with Kimberly Ellis. © 2012 John Wiley & Sons, Inc. Published by John Wiley & Sons, Inc.

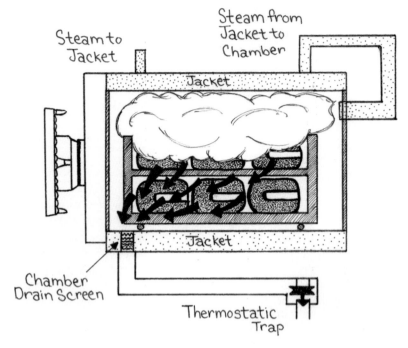

Figure 10.1 Cross-section of a typical steam sterilizer with a steam generation source. Illustration by Kayla Kolenberg, Ithaca, NY.

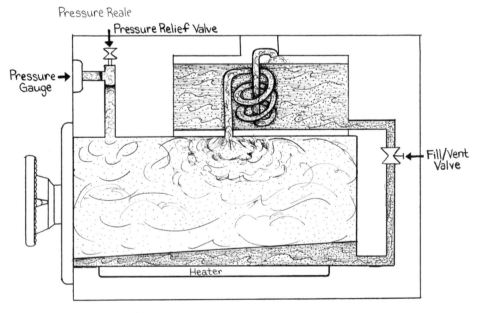

Figure 10.2 Cross-section of a tabletop steam sterilizer Illustration by Kayla Kolenberg, Ithaca, NY.

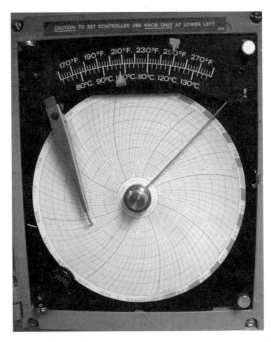

Figure 10.3   Tracing on a round recording chart from a steam sterilizer with mechanical controls.

Instrumentation and controls on the front of the sterilizer provide mechanical monitoring of the sterilization conditions, to ensure necessary sterilization parameters have been met for a preset cycle. The documentation from these controls can be in the form of a chart recorder or a printout from a microprocessor. Chart recorders are the older systems; they operated on the principle of liquid expanding when it is heated (in a liquid-filled bulb and capillary system) to move a pen that made tracings on a recording chart. See Figure 10.3 for an example of a round recording chart.

Newer systems use electronic controls (such as thermocouples or resistive thermal devices) to produce a visual readout (electronic display) and a paper printout. See Figure 10.4 for an example of a digital printout.

Although tabletop units may simply contain a pressure gauge with a special "hand" that moves to indicate the highest temperature/pressure that was reached during a cycle, others incorporate state-of-the-art electronics with data log printouts. See Figure 10.5 for gauges on a tabletop sterilizer and Figure 10.6 for a printout on a tabletop sterilizer.

Whichever recording system is used, it should be checked to see that all sterilization parameters were met. If they were not, the load is not sterile.

BASIC TYPES OF STEAM STERILIZERS

Steam sterilizers are chosen to meet the needs of each facility. Knowledge of the types available can assist in making the correct choice, based on the types of items that need to be steam sterilized. There are two basic sterilization cycles: terminal and flash. Terminal refers to the

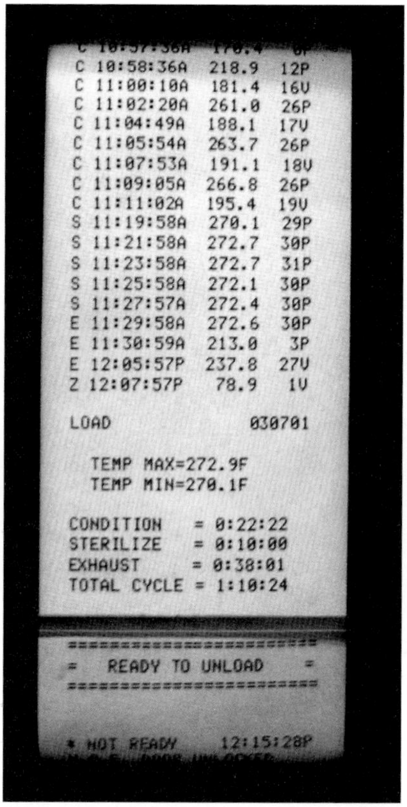

Figure 10.4 Example of a digital printout from a steam sterilizer with a microprocessor. Photographed by Dewey Neild, Dewey Neild Photography, Ithaca, NY.

process of sterilizing an item that is packaged or wrapped, then stored for later use. Flash is the process of sterilizing an unwrapped item for immediate use.

Sterilizer cycle "phases" differentiate the various types of sterilizers. These phases of the sterilization cycle involve conditioning, exposure, exhaust, and drying. Steam sterilizers are identified by the method of air removal; they are called gravity air displacement sterilizers or dynamic air removal sterilizers.

Gravity Air Displacement Sterilizer

Gravity air displacement sterilizers are generally small to medium size units that rely on gravity to remove air from the chamber. The initial conditioning phase introduces steam into the chamber. Because air is heavier than steam, a steam layer is created above the air. As more steam is introduced, the space available for the air in the chamber decreases and the air is pushed down the drain at the bottom of the sterilizer. It is critical to load the packs and items so that air is allowed to flow out of them, in a downward direction, under the influence of gravity. When steam contacts the cool surface of metal instruments within a pack, it warms them. This heat transfer changes the steam back into a liquid state because it no longer has the energy (in the

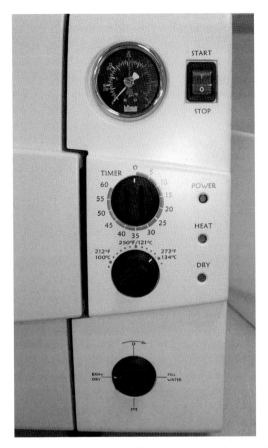

Figure 10.5 Mechanical gauge on a steam tabletop sterilizer. Photograph provided courtesy of SPSmedical, Rush, NY.

form of heat) it had in the vapor state. This produces condensate (liquid water). If condensate is not drained from the load or chamber, it will interfere with the drying process at the end of a cycle. During the conditioning phase, air and condensate both escape from the chamber by going down the drain or out the steam trap. The chamber drain line closes during the last portion of the conditioning phase. Steam continues to enter the chamber (which is now a closed space) so the pressure begins to rise along with the temperature of the steam.

Once the temperature reaches the selected sterilization set point, the exposure timing phase (actual sterilization) of the cycle begins. At the conclusion of the exposure phase, the chamber drain is opened, releasing steam pressure in the chamber to atmosphere. When the chamber pressure reaches 0 psi, the dry cycle begins.

The drying cycle uses the heat of the items and the chamber walls to revaporize any liquid. To remove the vapor from the load and chamber, filtered air is admitted into the chamber, mixing with the vapor and exhausting through the drain line. If the condensate from the conditioning and sterilizing phases were not drained sufficiently, the moist conditions in the chamber during the drying phase may overburden the drying cycle and cause the load to be wet at the end of the standard drying time.

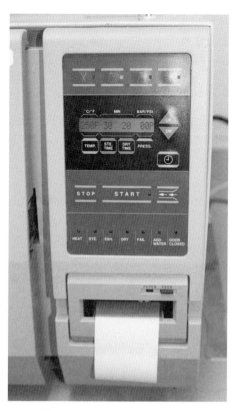

Figure 10.6 Printout on a steam tabletop sterilizer. Photograph provided courtesy of SPSmedical, Rush, NY.

Tabletop Sterilizers

Tabletop sterilizers are commonly gravity displacement sterilizers and are found in small facilities. Distilled water is poured into the bottom of the chamber or into a special port. Water is electrically heated until it turns into steam. Steam rises to the chamber's top as more steam is produced. When the steam enters the tabletop sterilizer's drain, a thermally operated valve closes. This causes the steam to build up pressure until the operating temperature is reached. Exposure time begins. At the end of the sterilization cycle, an exhaust valve is opened to allow the steam to escape. In most tabletop models, the steam passes through a coil in the water reservoir, where it condenses back into water. Once the pressure has dropped, the door can be opened. Drying of items in most tabletop sterilizer is accomplished by cracking open the door to allow excess steam and moisture to escape. When the drying cycle begins, heating units energize to assist in the drying of the packs or trays. After drying, packs should be allowed to cool first before placing them on a shelf or table. The specific operating instructions from the manufacturer of the steam sterilizer should be followed for your specific make and model sterilizer.

Dynamic Air Removal Sterilizers

Dynamic air removal or "prevac" sterilizers use a vacuum pump or water ejector to actively remove air during the conditioning phase of the cycle. Steam is injected into the chamber (just as it is in a gravity air displaced sterilizer), and after a set period of time, the chamber drain valve closes. More steam enters the chamber and pressure builds to a preset point. Then the chamber drain opens and the pressurized steam/air is exhausted through the drain, aided by the use of a water ejector or vacuum pump. The pressure continues to drop to 0 psi; at this point, the vacuum pump continues to run, drawing a vacuum inside the sterilizer chamber. This vacuum assists in the air removal from the chamber and the packs. The vacuum pump continues evacuating air from the chamber until a minimum preset vacuum is reached and held for a certain period of time. At the end of the time period, steam is injected into the chamber to again build pressure. This cycle of pressure and vacuum is referred to as a pulse. Because not all air is removed in a single pulse, the process is repeated. Most prevac sterilizers in the United States have four pulses during the normal conditioning phase of a sterilization cycle. This makes a prevac sterilizer more efficient at removing air and less dependent on the load position and makeup compared with gravity sterilizers. The pulses during the conditioning phase of the cycle increase the speed of operation and reduce the chance of air pockets in the chamber or packs. Dynamic air removal sterilizers usually operate at higher temperatures than gravity sterilizers.

To ensure that complete air removal is occurring, a specialized air-removal test should be preformed daily. This is called the Bowie-Dick test. The creators of this test (J. Bowie and J. Dick) determined that, if residual air remained in a sterilizer after the vacuum phase and there was only one package in the chamber, the air would concentrate in that package (Reichert and Young, 1997). A passed Bowie-Dick test indicates that steam penetration and complete air removal has occurred. Commercially made test packs can be purchased to run this test. Some newer dynamic air removal sterilizers also have a preset leak test cycle. Note that the leak test cycle and the Bowie-Dick test evaluate only the efficiency of the air removal and not the sterilization efficacy. See Figure 10.7 for an example of a Bowie-Dick test sheet.

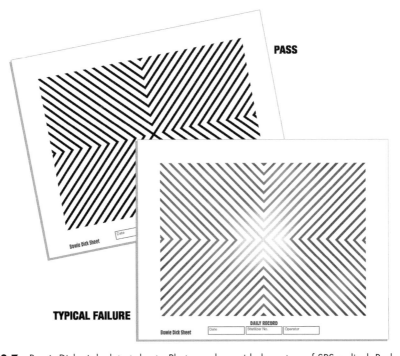

Figure 10.7   Bowie-Dick air leak test sheets. Photograph provided courtesy of SPSmedical, Rush, NY.

The Bowie-Dick test should be performed each day the sterilizer is used, before the first processed load. It provides a rapid means of detecting air leaks and inadequate air removal, which could result in insufficient steam penetration and sterilization failure. The cycle to run a Bowie-Dick test is specified by the sterilizer manufacturer. The general recommended exposure time is 3.5 minutes; a 4-minute exposure time can also used. Exposure time should not exceed 4 minutes at 273°F (134°C). Drying time can be omitted as it will not affect the outcome of the test. Any color change on the test sheet, such as the center being paler or any nonuniform color change, indicates that there was an air pocket present during the cycle due to a sterilizer malfunction. Actions following a failed Bowie-Dick test should be to retest with another Bowie-Dick test or have service performed by a service technician. If the sterilizer fails the Bowie-Dick test, it cannot be made functional by increasing the exposure time. Once serviced, a Bowie-Dick test is repeated.

Flash Sterilization Process

"Flash" refers to a cycle or a process rather than the actual sterilizer. This can be done in either a gravity displacement sterilizer or a prevacuum sterilizer, which can be used to quickly process a dropped instrument at the point of use. For example, a single, unwrapped, nonporous instrument (made of metal and without a lumen) is placed in a mesh-bottom pan or specialized container. The gravity displacement flash sterilizer cycle is typically 3 minutes at 270°F (132°C). There is normally only a 1-minute dry time, and the item being sterilized may not be completely dry. Specialized prevacuum sterilizers use a preset flash cycle. It goes through a standard sterilization cycle (3 minutes at 270–274°F for items made of metal and without a lumen) with limited drying time (usually 1 minute). As with the gravity flash sterilizer, the dry time is limited and the instruments may not completely dry. Refer to Chapter 12, section on flash sterilization, for more details.

STEAM STERILIZATION PARAMETERS

Whichever sterilizer is chosen for use, there are four conditions required for the sterilization process: contact, temperature, time, and moisture.

Items to be steam sterilized must first go through the cleaning and decontamination process as described in Chapter 8. Failure to remove all organic material or detergent residue may block the steam from coming into direct contact with all surfaces of the instrument. If the item or device is not clean, it will not be sterile. See Table 10.1 for some common causes for steam sterilization failure.

Temperature is another critical parameter; the temperature needs to be high enough to kill heat-resistant organisms and bacterial spores. The temperature of saturated steam is determined by pressure. The two most common temperatures for steam sterilization are 250°F (121°C) with a gauge pressure of 15 psi and 270–275°F (132.2–134°C) with a gauge pressure of at least 30 psi.

Steam sterilization cycles are based on a time–temperature relationship. Exposure time refers to the length of time at the preset temperature (250 or 270°F) that has been scientifically validated to kill all microorganisms (IAHCSMM, 2007), thus achieving sterilization.

Table 10.1 Common Causes for Steam Sterilization Failures

Inadequately cleaned object: any organic matter can protect microorganisms from direct steam contact.

Pack is wrapped too tightly: air can become trapped inside a pack and cannot escape, forming an air pocket that prevents the temperature from rising to sterilization levels.

Loads are too crowded in the sterilizer: air can become trapped and steam is unable to penetrate into all areas.

Trays or solid-bottom containers incorrectly positioned: these items should be placed so that air and condensed steam (moisture or water droplets) can be removed.

Clogged strainer in the drain line: small drain strainers in the sterilizer's drain line can be plugged with lint, autoclave tape, or other items such as small peel pouches.

Adapted from IAHCSMM, 2007 and AAMI, 2009.

Moisture is the other component for sterilization. Dry saturated steam is essential for steam sterilization. Saturated steam is steam that contains the maximum amount of water vapor (97–99% relative humidity). If steam is not saturated (<97% relative humidity), the items in the sterilizer load will be exposed to conditions similar to hot air, which will not kill all microorganisms in the preset cycle time.

Tables 10.2 and 10.3 are the minimum exposure cycle times for gravity displacement and dynamic air removal steam sterilizers. Sterilizer manufacturers' recommendations for sterilization exposure times may vary. More complex medical devices may need longer exposure times; manufacturers of these devices should provide recommended exposure times for their items. Note that specific cycles for some devices may differ from those preset on the sterilizer.

The following are the standard cycles recommended by the Association for Advancement of Medical Instrumentation (AAMI), the guidelines for steam sterilization and quality assurance in the human health care field.

Table 10.2 Minimum Cycle Time for Gravity-Displacement Steam Sterilization Cycles

Item	Exposure Time at 250°F (121°C)	Exposure Time at 270°F (132°C)	Exposure Time at 275°F (135°C)	Drying Times
Wrapped instruments	30 minutes	15 minutes		15–30 minutes
			10 minutes	30 minutes
Textile packs	30 minutes	25 minutes		15 minutes
			10 minutes	30 minutes
Wrapped utensils*	30 minutes	15 minutes		15–30 minutes
			10 minutes	30 minutes
Unwrapped nonporous instruments		3 minutes	3 minutes	0–1 minute
Unwrapped porous and nonporous mixed load		10 minutes	10 minutes	0–1 minute

Source: AAMI, 2009.
*Utensils include solid-bottom trays and basins.
Note: This table represents the variation in sterilizer manufacturers' recommendations for exposure at different temperatures. For a specific sterilizer, consult only that manufacturer's recommendations.

Table 10.3   Minimum Cycle Times for Dynamic-Air-Removal Steam Sterilizer Cycles

Item	Exposure Time at 270°F (132°C)	Exposure Time at 275°F (135°C)	Drying Times
Wrapped instruments	4 minutes		20–30 minutes
		3 minutes	16 minutes
Textile packs	4 minutes		5–20 minutes
		3 minutes	3 minutes
Wrapped utensils*	4 minutes		20 minutes
		3 minutes	16 minutes
Unwrapped nonporous items	3 minutes	3 minutes	N/A
Unwrapped porous and nonporous mix	4 minutes	3 minutes	N/A

Source: AAMI, 2009.
*Utensils include solid-bottom trays and basins.
Note: This table represents the variations in sterilizer manufacturers' recommendations for exposure at different temperatures. For a specific sterilizer, consult only that manufacturer's recommendations.

LOAD CONFIGURATION PRIOR TO STEAM STERILIZATION

Chapter 9 covered the proper preparation, assembly of a tray or individual items, and load configuration prior to the sterilization process. The following is a quick review.

- Instrument placement within a tray is essential to allow proper air removal, steam penetration to all surfaces, and condensate drainage.
- The load within the sterilizer must allow air circulation and drainage of condensate.
- Refer to the sterilizer manufacturer's recommendations for loading of the steam sterilizer.

Proper technique for unloading the sterilizer also was covered in Chapter 9. The following is a quick review:

- Crack open the door of the steam sterilizer to allow evaporation and drying.
- Do not touch the pack or individual items when they are warm. Allow items to cool to room temperature before handling.
- Handle the sterile pack or package as little as possible.

WHEN WET PACKS OCCUR

"Wet packs" refer to trays or packages that have been processed in a steam sterilization cycle, but retain moisture in the form of dampness, droplets, or puddles on the outside of a pack or contained within a pack. Wet packs are considered contaminated and must be reprocessed.

There are many possible contributing factors for wet pack problems. Begin by determining the types of wet packs that are occurring (e.g., internal moisture vs. external droplets), as well as the type of load that was run, time of day, and who operated the sterilizer. Other considerations include sterilizer operation, the pack preparation process, poststerilization handling, and, if applicable, utility steam supply. See Table 10.4 for wet pack causes and recommendations.

Table 10.4   Wet Pack: Probable Causes and Suggestions for Correction

Wetness Location

Internal wetness – Too many instruments or excessive density of devices within a set can cause excessive condensation. Another source of internal wetness can be metal items within a tray that allow water to pool, or items that trap steam, which later turns into water. Items not completely dry before being wrapped will retain their moisture after a standard drying cycle. Some foam products used with a tray may hold condensate.

> Suggestion: Use absorbent tray liners to wick excess moisture or divide the tray contents into smaller sets. Check with the manufacturer of certain medical devices to see whether they recommend extended sterilization or drying time for their products. These recommendations must be followed even if the device is placed in a tray with other instruments. Position items within a tray to allow adequate air removal as well as steam penetration and evacuation.

Outer wetness – Excessive condensation can "drip" out of a tray onto packs located on lower shelves. Condensate also can form on the sterilizer shelf itself and drip down on a pack or peel pouch. This can be observed once the sterilizer door is opened.

> Suggestion: Check to see that the packs, textiles, or peel pouches have been placed correctly within the sterilizer, in accordance with manufacturers' recommendations, to ensure air removal and steam penetration.

Moisture between folds – Using wrappers that are too large for an item or pack causes excessive folding of the wrap around the tray or item. This creates more layers the steam has to penetrate and can prevent evacuation of steam.

> Suggestion: Use the correct wrapping technique with the appropriate size for the item being wrapped.

Moist linen packs – Linens packed too tightly can cause excess moisture to be retained. As linens are folded and then wrapped, cooler air can be held within the layers of linens.

> Suggestion: Cloth textiles should be folded properly without excessive compacting as they are wrapped. They should be loaded into the sterilizer so they are perpendicular to the shelf. Packs can be loaded into the sterilizer and allowed to warm (preheat) for 5–10 minutes prior to starting the cycle to lessen the potential for condensation formation.

Location in the Sterilizer

Top shelf – If the steam inlet seal is malfunctioning, it can allow steam to enter the chamber and condense at the point of entry. The inlet is typically on the top of the sterilizer; this source of condensate would be noticed on the packs on the top shelf of the load.

> Suggestion: Have a sterilizer service technician check the seal on the steam inlet to correct the problem.

Bottom shelf – As steam exits the sterilizer via the chamber drain, it condenses. If there is a blockage in the drain, the condensate would "back up" and be found on the items on the bottom shelf.

> Suggestion: Check to see whether the drain strainer is blocked or have a sterilizer service technician inspect and test the check valve in the drain line.

Near the door – A defect in the door gasket can cause pressure loss, which in turn causes steam to condense. Moisture would be found on the exterior of the packs.

> Suggestion: Contact your sterilizer service technician to replace the door gasket and verify the integrity of the seal.

(Continued)

Table 10.4 *(Continued)*

Load Configuration

* *Load size* – Overloading the sterilizer increases the potential for condensate to form. An increase in density of packs placed within a load can alter drying of contents.

> Suggestion: Follow manufacturer's recommendations for load configuration. With sterilizers that have two shelves, place linen packs on the upper shelf, spaced so that your hand can fit between packs. Peel pouches should be placed on edge with the paper side of one pouch facing the plastic side of the adjacent pouch. Perforated bottom trays should be placed with the bottom of the tray parallel to the shelf. Items that can hold water (solid-bottom pans, bowls) should be placed tilted on edge and oriented in the same direction, preferably on the bottom shelf in the sterilizer with multiple shelves. Never stack items or trays.

* *Rushing a load* – After the drying cycle of the sterilizer, the remaining steam can condense from the "shock" of 70°F room air temperature rushing into the sterilizer and contacting the instruments in the packs where temperatures still exceed 160°F.

> Suggestion: Cracking the door about 6 inches following the dry cycle will allow the load to cool slowly, letting the heat escape and the cooler air to gradually enter the sterilizer. The drying process continues until the items within the sterilizer equalize to the room air temperature.

* *Cooling of the load after sterilization* – Steam vapor remains after the completion of the dry cycle; if items are removed before thoroughly cool, moisture will remain.

> Suggestion: After the items are removed from the sterilizer, heat continues to radiate from them until they are completely cool. Sterilizer contents should sit in a low-traffic area, away from any air vents, allowing ample time for the pack contents to dry and cool to room temperature. Do not rush this process.

Sterilizer Systems

* In facilities with a centralized steam boiler, several factors (alone or in combination) can affect sterilizer performance: variations in steam pressure, boiler location relative to the sterilizer, supply line size, trap location, and performance.

> Suggestion: Sterilizers should have dedicated lines to deliver the high-quality steam that is required for sterilizers. When pressure is down, the potential for condensate rises. As recommended by the manufacturer of the sterilizer, regular preventative maintenance of the sterilizer—and steam supply system—should be performed and documented by a qualified service technician.

General Recommendations

* Document the occurrence of each wet pack; this includes the date, load, description of the wet item, degree of wetness, location of the item in the sterilizer load, and other potentially significant comments (e.g., rushed load, low sterilizer pressure, improper assembly of trays). This log can help in the investigation and lead to solutions that will reduce or eliminate the occurrence of wet packs.

* Follow the general daily and weekly cleaning and maintenance schedule outlined by the manufacturer in the operations manual. After repairs have been performed on the sterilizer, a biologic indicator within a process challenge device should be run three consecutive times in an empty chamber. For tabletop models, after repair has been performed, a biologic indicator within a process challenge device should be run three consecutive times in a full load (AAMI, 2009).

Adapted from the following sources: AAMI, 2009; Brown and Bliley, 2008; IAHCSMM, 2007; Reichert and Young, 1997.

STERILITY ASSURANCE

Proper sterilization of instruments and packs is a critical aspect of infection control. The goal of sterility assurance is to determine whether something is sterile without contaminating it. Sterilization by steam requires these conditions: sufficient temperature, sufficient moisture, proper time, and sterilant contact. Verifying that these conditions have been met is the basis for the quality assurance program. Quality assurance involves conscientious attention to all of the following:

- Mechanical/electrical controls
- Chemical indicators/integrators
- Biological indicators
- Sterilizer maintenance
- Record keeping

Mechanical/Electrical Controls

Mechanical or electric controls are the physical monitors on a sterilizer that display the temperature and pressure. These readings are generally taken from a monitoring device in the chamber drain and do not necessarily reflect conditions inside the pack (Dix, 2006). Several sterilizer manufacturers use analog or mechanical controls (usually the older-style sterilizers), whereas newer sterilizers have digital or electronic controls. Controls provide a recording chart or printout of the temperature and time of each cycle; the digital printout may also indicate the pressure readings. Typically, tabletop sterilizers do not have a recording device built in; the operator should routinely monitor the time and temperature gauges during a cycle to verify that sterilization parameters have been met.

After each cycle is run, the recording chart or printout should be checked (and initialed) to see whether all the sterilization parameters were met. If not, anything processed in that load cannot be considered sterile and must be reprocessed and resterilized.

Chemical Indicators/Integrators

Chemical indicator (CI) is a system that shows a change in one or more predefined process parameters on the basis of a chemical or physical change that results from exposure to the sterilization process (IAHCSMM, 2007). CIs are classified by the FDA as Class II medical devices. For pack monitoring, there are two types—internal or external—depending on whether they are placed inside a tray or used externally on the outside of a tray or package. CIs are an important part of the sterilization quality assurance program; used in conjunction with the mechanical monitors and with biological indicators, they assist in determining the effectiveness of the sterilization process. There are six classes of CIs as described in the ANSI/AAMI's Comprehensive Guide to Steam Sterilization and Sterility Assurance in Health Care Facilities (AAMI, 2009).

Class I or process indicators are external indicators used to show a processed versus unprocessed item. They are generally in the form of tape, labels, or preprinted indicators on the paper portion of a peel pouch. Class I indicators react only to the temperature component of steam sterilization.

Class 2 or indicators for use in specific tests (i.e., Bowie-Dick test) are intended to test specific procedures. Bowie-Dick tests are used to show air leaks, inadequate air removal, and inadequate steam penetration in dynamic air removal (prevacuum) sterilizers by a pass/fail method. A commercially available Class 2 test pack is placed in a preconditioned, empty chamber of a dynamic air removal sterilizer. The pack is placed horizontally in the front, bottom section of the sterilizer rack, near the door and over the drain. A specific cycle is run; it is generally 3.5–4 minutes at 273°F (134°C). After the cycle, the test pack is removed. A drying cycle is not done. The test sheet is removed from the test pack and examined. Compare the test sheet to the "color standards sheet" provided by the test pack manufacturer to see if the patterns are identical. If they are not, there is a malfunction in the sterilizer and it should be serviced before using. After service, another Bowie-Dick test should be performed.

Class 3 or single variable indicators are designed to react to one of the critical variables and intended to indicate exposure to a sterilization process at a stated value of one variable (i.e., change color when a specific minimum temperature at that location in the sterilizer load has been reached). They are not sensitive to the other parameters of sterilization (i.e., time and sterilant).

Class 4 or multivariable indicators will respond to two or more critical variables and are intended to indicate exposure to a sterilization process at a stated value of the chosen variables. See Figure 10.8 for a variety of Class 4 multivariable chemical indicators.

Class 5 or integrating indicators respond to all critical variables with the stated values having been generated to be equivalent to, or exceed, the performance requirements of a biologic indicator. These indicators monitor the sterilization process over a specified range of sterilization temperatures (e.g., 245–280°F). As previously stated, their performance has been correlated to the performance of a biologic indicator under the label conditions of use. Figure 10.9 shows examples of Class 5 integrating indicators: unprocessed, failed, and passed.

Class 6 emulating indicators are cycle verification indicators that react to all critical variables of specified sterilization cycles, with the stated values having been generated from the critical variables of one specific sterilization process. Thus, a 4-minute dynamic air removal cycle at

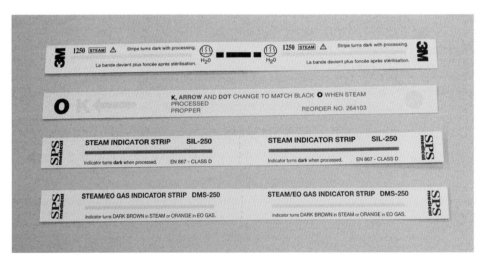

Figure 10.8 Various styles of Class 4 indicators available. Photograph provided courtesy of SPSmedical, Rush, NY.

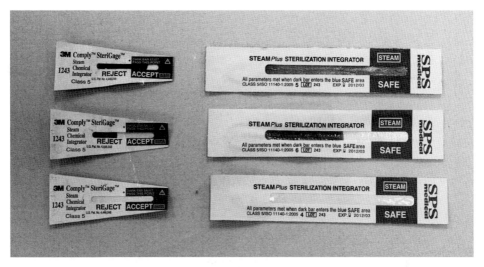

Figure 10.9 Various styles of Class 5 integrating indicators showing unprocessed, failed test, and passed test strips. Photograph provided courtesy of SPSmedical, Rush, NY.

270°F requires one type of indicating strip, whereas a 15-minute gravity cycle at 270°F has another indicator.

Following "best practice" standard guidelines, a Class 3, 4, or 5 indicator should be used for internal monitoring of sterilization variables. These indicators should be placed in the center of every tray or linen item that is being processed.

Biological Indicators

Biological indicators (BIs) involve the use of live bacterial spores. They are considered the highest level of sterility assurance because they test the sterilizer's ability to kill nonpathogenic but highly resistant organisms. These spores are specific for each type of sterilization process. Biologic indicators are incubated at a specific temperature, depending on the process to be monitored, and for a specific amount of time, depending on the manufacturer's recommendation for that product. After the preset time, the media is observed for color change or turbidity, depending on the BI used. A "control" is incubated with each BI that is processed through a sterilization cycle. This is simply an unsterilized BI. The control would show a "positive" result as the spores would grow in the media at the proper incubation temperature and amount of time. The sterilizer-processed BI should show no visible change, a "negative" indication that all the spores were killed by the sterilization process. A negative BI result shows that all conditions required for sterilization were met. For steam sterilization (either gravity or dynamic air removal), *Geobacillus stearothermophilus* spores are used. A biologic indicator consists of these spores in or on a carrier (self-contained BIs are accompanied by incubation media). Available forms of BIs include the following:

- Spore strip with a known spore population. After processing, the strip is placed in a tube of sterile culture media and then incubated for a predetermined amount of time at a specific temperature.

- Sealed glass ampules contain spores mixed with media. After processing, the ampule is incubated for the predetermined amount of time. No media color change or turbidity within the ampule indicates a "negative" result.
- Self-contained vials are glass ampules of sterile media surrounded by a plastic vial with a spore strip inside. After processing, the BI is activated by crushing the vial to allow the spores into the media; then the vial is incubated for the predetermined amount of time. No media color within the vial indicates a "negative" result. These are the most commonly used.

Some types of BIs contain spores with an enzyme early readout capability. "An active enzyme is impregnated on a carrier strip located between the walls of the outer and inner containers, and a substrate that reacts with the active enzyme is contained within the sealed inner tube. The enzyme system gives a rapid indication of the effectiveness of a sterilization cycle, which is then confirmed by measurement of spore outgrowth over a longer period of time" (U.S. Patent 6,897,059). Figure 10.10 shows examples of various configurations of BIs available.

BIs are commonly found inside a commercially available "test pack" called a process challenge device (PCD). This PCD is used to assess the effective performance of the sterilization process by providing a challenge to the process that is equal to or greater than the most difficult item routinely processed (AAMI, 2009).

The BIs in the commercially available PCDs can come in different combinations, with a Class 5 integrating CI. PCD should be run in a full load at least once a week as well as in any load that contains implantable devices. If extended sterilizer cycles are used, the manufacturer of the PCD should be consulted to see whether the BI was validated for increased cycle times.

For tabletop sterilizers, a representative of the same type of package or tray routinely processed in the sterilizer is chosen to serve as the PCD for sterilizer efficacy monitoring (AAMI, 2009). The PCD selected should contain the normal items in the tray and a minimum of one BI and one CI. The BIs are handled the same as commercially available PCDs. PCD representative package should be run in a full load once a week or when the load contains implantable items.

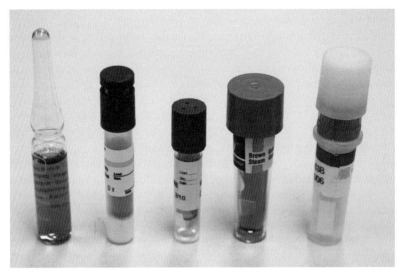

Figure 10.10   Various configurations of biological indicators. Photograph provided courtesy of SPSmedical, Rush, NY.

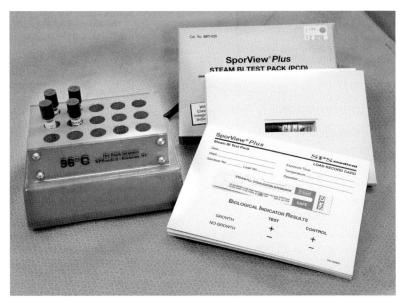

Figure 10.11 This photograph shows a block-style incubator for the biological indicators and one style of premanufactured process challenge device. Photography by Dewey Neild of Dewey Neild Photography, Ithaca, NY.

There are no universally accepted standardized PCDs for tabletop gravity-displacement type sterilizers (AAMI, 2009).

The PCD should be placed in an area of the sterilizer that is considered the most difficult area to reach sterilization parameters. The sterilizer manufacturer's instruction manual can be consulted for this information. Typically, this is the front bottom section of the sterilizer near the drain. The PCD is placed in this spot, along with your regular sterilizer load of trays, packs, and textiles. After completion of the sterilization cycle, the PCD should be cooled with the other items in the load. Once cool, the BI should be removed. Crush the vial (if applicable), or place the exposed spore strip placed in media vial (if applicable) and place in the incubator according to the manufacturer's instructions at the specified temperature. Figure 10.11 shows a block-style incubator for the incubation of the BI. Also included in the figure is a commercially available PCD.

The incubation temperature for steam BIs is 131–140°F (55–60°C). A control BI, from the same lot, should be incubated along with the sterilized, processed BI. After the manufacturer's recommended incubation time, results of both the processed BI and the control should be read and recorded. The control BI should always be positive, showing the spores are viable and have grown in the media. If the control fails to grow, that lot number may contain nonviable (dead) spores, and another test should be done using a different lot number. The processed BI should not have any viable spores (killed in the sterilization process) growing in the media. If the processed BI is "positive," the other items (trays and packages) processed in the same load as the positive BI are held, as they may not be sterile; all of the following should be reviewed: placement of the PCD, reading on the sterilizer mechanical controls, and the status of the internal CI in the same test. If there is any doubt on any of the above questions, the items in the load should be considered not sterile and will need to be reprocessed and resterilized. Whenever you are not sure, the load contents should be reprocessed and resterilized. If the sterilizer malfunctioned, it should be serviced before further loads are run. A PCD should be run to verify the sterilizer is again functioning properly.

Table 10.5 provides a summary of steam sterilization monitoring, including the frequency with which the tests should be performed.

Sterilizer Maintenance

Every sterilizer manufacturer provides the owner of a sterilizer with a manual that includes the care and maintenance instructions for that sterilizer. This includes the following:

- Routine maintenance is done by the users, such as cleaning of gaskets, chamber drains/ screens, internal chambers, and external surfaces. Routine maintenance should be done on a daily or weekly schedule as indicated by the manufacturer's written instructions.
- Cool the chamber before performing any cleaning or maintenance.
- Clean the inside of the chamber only with products specified by the sterilizer manufacturer. This should be done with nonabrasive, nonlinting products. The cleaning schedule recommended by the manufacturer should be followed.
- Inspect door gaskets and wipe with a damp, nonlinting cloth. Look for signs of wear, defects, or deterioration.
- If applicable, clean the chamber drain strainer. A clogged strainer will not properly remove air and condensate from the inside of the sterilizer.
- Preventative maintenance is periodic maintenance as recommended by the manufacturer and performed by a qualified service technician. This can include inspection, maintenance, and replacement of components subject to wear, such as filters, steam traps, drain pipes, valves, and door gaskets. A record should be kept for each piece of equipment, documenting parts that were replaced, dates, name of service personnel, and the results of necessary postmaintenance testing (PCD or Bowie-Dick tests). Maintenance records should be updated each time before the sterilizer is returned to use.
- Scheduled maintenance is lubrication of appropriate parts and replacement of expendable parts, performed by qualified sterilizer service technicians. Frequency of scheduled maintenance is determined by the use of the specific sterilizer and the age of the unit. Maintaining a log of the maintenance can help determine replacement schedules for specific parts.
- Calibration is a periodic check of pressure- and temperature-sensing gauges, cycle timers, controls, and recording devices as performed by a qualified person and specified by the manufacturer's recommendations. Equipment used for calibration should conform to the primary standards of the National Institute for Standards and Technology (IAHCSMM, 2007). Proper calibration is essential for effective and reliable sterilization.

Record Keeping

This involves keeping records of sterilizer performance, as well as the mechanical controls of the sterilizer, the BI results, and the Bowie-Dick test results (if applicable). Documentation of the maintenance on the sterilizer should also be kept with the date of servicing, reason for the request, task performed, parts replaced, and who performed the maintenance. Keeping a record of the date, load, mechanical controls, BI, and CI from any load that contains implantable devices provides evidence that the sterilization parameters have been met. Documentation establishes accountability. It states unequivocally that something has been done, so there is no question.

Table 10.5 Steam Sterilization Monitoring Frequency Guideline

Type of monitoring	Type of sterilizer	Test	Frequency	Test for
Equipment control	Dynamic air removal	Bowie-Dick test	Daily or following any service, relocation, or any problems/issues with trays	Complete air removal, run by itself in sterilizer
Equipment control: mechanical	Gravity displacement and dynamic air removal	Verify digital printout, recording chart, or gauges on sterilizers	Every load	Verify temperature, time, and pressure
Exposure control	Gravity displacement and dynamic air removal	Class I chemical indicator	External on each item sterilized	Indicates processed vs. nonprocessed items
Pack control	Gravity displacement and dynamic air removal	Chemical indicator: Class III, IV, V, or chemical integrator	Inside every item or device being sterilized	Indicated conditions for sterilization have been met
Load control	Gravity displacement and dynamic air removal	PCD containing a biologic indicator and a Class V integrating indicator or for tabletop sterilizers, a BI and Class V integrator within a representative of the same type of tray routinely processed	Once a week, in any load containing implantable devices, or after any major repairs (monitoring of 3 consecutive cycles in an empty chamber with PCD; for tabletop sterilizer, monitoring of 3 consecutive cycles fully loaded chamber with a BI and Class V integrator within a representative of the same type of tray routinely processed)	Effective performance of the sterilization process

Adapted from AAMI, 2009.

CONCLUSION

Steam sterilization is a relatively quick, low-cost, safe, nontoxic, and effective means to render a heat-stable item free of microbial contamination. To verify that an item has been effectively exposed to the steam sterilization process, certain criteria need to be met, monitored, and documented. This is all essential to sterility assurance. Written protocols for all phases of sterilization need to be established, consistently followed, and updated frequently as new equipment and technologies become available.

REFERENCES

[AAMI] Association for the Advancement of Medical Instrumentation. 2009. ANSI/AAMI ST79:2006. Amendments A1 and A2. *Comprehensive Guide to Steam Sterilization and Sterility Assurance in Health Care Facilities*. American National Standards Institute, Arlington, VA, pp 68–118.

Association of periOperative Registered Nurses (AORN). 2009. *Perioperative Standards and Recommended Practices*. RP: Sterilization. Recommendation I–XVI. AORN, Denver, CO, pp 647–670.

Brown JM, Bliley J. 2008. How to solve wet packs, and evaluate water issues. *Mater Manag Health Care* 17:50–52.

Dix K. 2006. The SPD'S ground zero quality assurance for sterilization. *Infection Control Today* [Reprinted by SPS Medical with permission from Virgo Publishing].

[IAHCSMM] International Association of Healthcare Central Service Material Management. 2007. *Central Service Technical Manual, 7th ed.* IAHCSMM, Chicago, IL, pp 285–319.

Reichert M, Young JH. 1997. *Sterilization Technology for the Health Care Facility, 2nd ed.* Aspen Publication, Gaithersburg, MD, pp 146–150.

Rutala WA, Weber DJ. 2004. Disinfection and sterilization, in *Disinfection and Sterilization in Healthcare Facilities*, pp 10–11. Available at: http://disinfectionandsterilization.org.

Rutala WA, Weber DJ, Healthcare Infection Control Practices Advisory Committee (HICPAC). 2008. *Guideline for Disinfection and Sterilization in Healthcare Facilities*. CDC, Atlanta, GA, pp 58–61.

11 Low-Temperature Sterilization

Linda Caveney

Many of today's medical devices cannot withstand the high temperatures of the steam sterilization process. Chemical alternatives to steam sterilization are available to sterilize heat-and moisture-sensitive items. But all of these chemicals have toxic properties and need to be handled with extreme caution.

The low-temperature sterilization systems commonly used in practices today are ethylene oxide (EtO), hydrogen peroxide (H_2O_2), and ozone (O_3). One liquid sterilant that is available is peracetic acid, used in the Steris System I unit. Cidex (a glutaraldehyde-based product) can also be used as a liquid sterilant, although exposure time is extremely lengthy (10 hours). This chapter reviews the requirements and uses of these low-temperature systems.

BASIC REQUIREMENTS FOR ALL LOW-TEMPERATURE SYSTEMS

There are seven basic requirements for any of the low-temperature systems to be effective in the hospital environment. Failure to meet any of these seven requirements (effectiveness, safety, monitoring, quality assurance, penetration, material compatibility, and approval) can cause significant risk to the patient or staff member.

Many veterinary practices have a container for placement of commonly used surgical instruments that is referred to as "cold sterilization." This is not a correct use of the word "sterilization," as the solution used to soak these instruments in is generally a low-level disinfectant with an anti-rust component. This solution is not monitored by a test strip to ensure it contains the minimum effective concentration to deliver the desired outcome. Also, each instrument placed in the container needs to be thoroughly scrubbed and cleaned with a detergent, rinsed, dried, and then placed to soak in the disinfectant solution. There is no assurance that this is done by everyone placing items in the solution. Addition of water and debris from just passing it under running tap water and placing in the container will dilute the solution, and the debris that was not removed will cause the active ingredient in the solution to be ineffective. Some solutions state they can be used for up to 14 days once made. Someone needs to monitor the date when the solution was created and should be changed. This does not mean that it will remain effective as organic debris, water, or evaporation can alter the solution.

Veterinary Infection Prevention and Control, First Edition. Edited by Linda Caveney and Barbara Jones with Kimberly Ellis.
© 2012 John Wiley & Sons, Inc. Published by John Wiley & Sons, Inc.

Effectiveness

In the United States, the Food and Drug Administration (FDA) requires each of these sterilants to undergo rigorous tests on a broad range of microorganisms. Each method of sterilization (EtO, H_2O_2, and O_3) uses different sterilizing agents and processing protocols. When used according to the products label, any of these sterilants is capable of providing the same sterility assurance level (SAL) as that of terminal steam sterilization (10 to −6).

Safety

There should be no toxic residue left on the package or device after the sterilization process. Also, the equipment must be safe for the person operating it. All of the low-temperature sterilants possess toxic properties and must be handled only by individuals who have been properly trained. Personnel should be required to wear appropriate personal protective equipment (PPE) designed to protect their skin, eyes, mucous membranes, and clothing from splashes. Health care facilities using liquid chemical solutions must follow OSHA's Medical and First Aid Standard (29 Cr 191.151), which requires suitable facilities for eye washing (AAMI, 2005a–c).

Monitoring

OSHA originally established specific guidelines for the use of EtO, based on data developed in the 1980s. Subsequently, OSHA now has developed permissible exposure limits (PELs) for all low-temperature sterilants. PELs for particular agents indicate both the maximum airborne concentration of the chemical agent to which the employee can be exposed and the duration (time) of exposure (IAHCSMM, 2007). PELs are expressed as an 8-hour time weighted average (TWA)—the total allowable average airborne exposure a worker is exposed to during an 8-hour shift of a standard 40-hour workweek (IAHCSMM, 2007).

To supplement the PELs, the National Institute for Occupational Safety and Health (NIOSH) has also developed parameters for "Immediately Dangerous to Life or Health" (IDLH) concentrations of potentially toxic, low-temperature standard sterilants. Clinics or practices that use any of the low-temperature sterilants are required to follow OSHA regulations.

Quality Assurance

As with the steam sterilization process, the low-temperature sterilization process should be monitored with physical, chemical, and biological indicators. Each of these indicators should be used to assess whether the item or load has successfully been exposed to the sterilant.

Penetration

The sterilant must be able to penetrate the packaging material and must reach the most difficult areas of the device being exposed to the process (e.g., small lumens, tightly matted surfaces). If the sterilant cannot reach these areas, the sterilization process will not be effective. For example, the properties of EtO inactivate microbes by a process of alkylation; it is able to reach the most remote surfaces where microbes are located and inactives them. Other chemical agents used (H_2O_2, O_3) inactivate microbes by the process of oxidation. Oxidation is less specific, reacts easily, and can be depleted before all surfaces (e.g., small lumens) can be reached (IAHCSMM, 2007).

Material Compatibility

The chemical agent being used must be compatible with the device being sterilized. The manufacturer of the medical device should be consulted for recommendations on which low-temperature sterilization processes can be used on their device. The packaging material used must also be compatible with the sterilization process. The packaging material must be permeable to the sterilant; allow release of gasses; provide a barrier to dust, liquid, and microorganisms; allow easy aseptic presentation; and have proven seal integrity.

Approval

Whichever sterilization process is used, it must be a registered or a cleared system under the appropriate regulatory agency.

ETHYLENE OXIDE

EtO has been used in the medical field since the 1960s as the sterilant of choice for low-temperature sterilization. It has exceptional penetration abilities and is compatible with many materials used in medical devices.

There are two forms available for use: mixed EtO blends and 100% EtO. For larger EtO sterilizers, the mixed EtO blends are supplied in large tanks. These combine an inert gas with the EtO to make it nonflammable and nonexplosive. Prior to 1996, chlorofluorocarbons (CFCs) were combined with EtO in a 12/88 gas mixture (12% EtO, 88% CFC). Since then, modifications were made to the blend, bringing it into compliance with the Clean Air Act of 1996. Hydrochlorofluorocarbons (HCFCs) were substituted for CFCs, and the mixtures most commonly found are under the brand names of PENNGAS 2 or Oxifume 2000 and 2002.

These blends come in large tanks that require connections to the gas sterilizers. (Minimal modifications were made to gas sterilizers, enabling them to switch to the newer gas blend formulas.) 100% EtO is available in small cartridges or ampules with enough EtO to sterilize one load. Chamber sizes of 100% EtO systems vary depending on the sterilizer manufacturer.

EtO evaporates easily and is able to be maintained in the vapor state, which makes it capable of spreading out and filling a sterilization chamber. In the presence of moisture, EtO combines chemically with specific protein structures or genetic materials, making these molecules lose their size and shape.

EtO molecules are small, allowing them to reach the most remote areas of a device. This is also the reason for the long aeration period following the sterilization cycle. The aeration process removes the residual EtO from materials in the load. With larger sterilizers, at the end of the exposure cycle, one or more vacuum pulses remove the EtO from the chamber. Warm air is then circulated through the sterilizer chamber; EtO molecules migrate to the surface of the material and are carried away by the warm, moving air. When packages are loosely arranged in the chamber, air can easily circulate around them and remove the residual EtO.

Safety of Ethylene Oxide

EtO is a toxic gas and is classified as a known carcinogen. EtO is highly flammable in its pure state (100% ampule or cartridge). The EtO sterilizer should be located in a well-ventilated room with a minimum of 10 air exchanges per hour. Recommendations of the sterilizer manufacturer and the EtO supplier should be followed.

Furthermore, OSHA standards need to be heeded. As activities are performed involving the handling of EtO, monitoring devices are attached to the staff members' clothing in the breathing zone (within 1 foot of the person's nose) for sampling of air. These devices are sent off to assess the results of exposure. Area monitoring devices can provide real-time monitoring of airborne EtO in the general vicinity, but they may not reveal breathing zone measurements. Employers must inform the staff members of the results of the monitoring devices, and employers must keep these records for 30 years after the employee has completed the last EtO-related task (IAHCSMM, 2007).

EtO residues can remain on a device after typical mechanical aeration cycles; the device manufacturer should provide recommendations for temperature, exposure, and aeration times. In accordance with the Clean Air Act of 1990, the EPA regulates EtO emissions from commercial establishments, and from hospital sterilizers in some states. Catalytic converters placed on EtO sterilizers' exhaust systems convert the gas into a nonhazardous emission. Smaller sterilizer units are not required to have special exhaust systems (other than exhausting it to an external area).

General Operation Procedures

There are about four manufacturers of 100% EtO sterilizers and about four manufacturers of EtO/HCFC sterilizers. Choosing the appropriate sterilizing unit to use is based on many factors. For the most part, the EtO/HCFC units are for larger hospital application, although many human health care facilities have the smaller 100% EtO sterilizers as well as other low-temperature alternative sterilizers. Smaller facilities use the cartridge or ampule systems. In one 100% system, a cartridge is placed inside the chamber along with the packaged contents; then a vacuum is pulled and the cartridge is punctured, allowing the gas to escape into the chamber. In a 100% ampule system, items are placed in a sterilization liner bag; a gas-release bag with an ampule inside is placed in the liner bag. A purge probe is inserted and secured with a connector attached to the sterilizing unit, which pulls a vacuum. The ampule top is snapped off inside the gas-release bag and the cycle is started.

Whichever system is chosen, there are four process parameters needed to achieve EtO sterilization: temperature, time, concentration, and relative humidity. There are two temperature regimes used for exposure: warm-temperature cycles are 130–140°F (55–60°C), whereas cool-temperature cycles are 100–122°F (37–50°C). Higher temperatures create faster reaction rates (e.g., inactivation of bacterial spores). Time is related to the temperature of the cycle. The concentration of EtO is generally greater than what is needed.

A relative humidity of 35% is considered optimal for destroying microbes. Some units use a higher relative humidity (between 60% and 80%). Regardless of the system chosen, follow the sterilizer manufacturer's and the gas supplier's recommendations. Also, consult the medical device manufacturers for their recommendations.

Total exposure and aeration times vary, depending on the sterilizer type, temperature of the cycle, mechanism for removal of residual EtO, and the construction of the medical device. Aeration is critical to removing residual EtO, because the chemical could be harmful to the patient.

Quality Assurance Monitoring

As with steam sterilization, quality assurance monitoring must be done through physical, chemical, and biological indicators. None of these performance monitors itself proves sterility; the combination of results from each monitor provides a higher degree of assurance that the parameters of sterilization have been met (IAHCSMM, 2007). Physical monitoring includes reviewing the operating pressure controls (if applicable), temperature controls, humidity sensors, and timing charts. External chemical indicators should be used on the outside of each pack or peel pouch to show that these items have been exposed to the process.

Internal chemical indicators should be placed inside each pack to determine whether the sterilization process parameters have been met inside the pack contents.

Biologic indicators (BIs) are used for sterility assurance monitoring, just as they are with the steam sterilization process. The organism used within the EtO biologic is *Bacillus atrophaeus*. The BI of choice is placed in each sterilizer load, incubated at 100°F (37°C) for 48 hours, and then read. A control should also be incubated and read. A record for each sterilizer load should be kept, noting the date, load contents, cycle parameters, BI results, and control results.

HYDROGEN PEROXIDE GAS PLASMA

The first hydrogen peroxide gas plasma system was marketed in the United States in 1993 under the name STERRAD System by Advanced Sterilization Products. Figure 11.1 shows a Sterrad NX, and Figure 11.2 shows a Sterrad 100S.

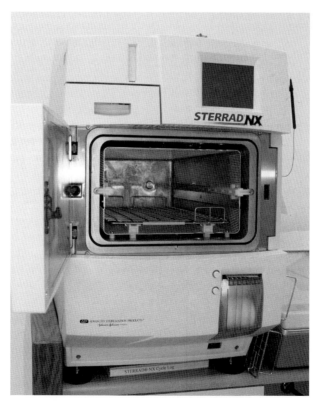

Figure 11.1   This shows the Sterrad NX low-temperature hydrogen peroxide gas plasma sterilizer. Photograph provided courtesy of SPSmedical, Rush, NY.

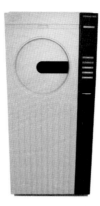

Figure 11.2 This shows the Sterrad 100S low-temperature hydrogen peroxide gas plasma sterilizer. Photograph provided courtesy of SPSmedical, Rush, NY.

The AMSCO V-PRO 1 by Steris and the Steris VHP MD Series are low-temperature sterilizing systems that use vaporized hydrogen peroxide under vacuum conditions. Note that neither of the Steris systems is FDA approved at the time of this writing.

General Background Information

The Sterrad system works by first evacuating the sterilization chamber, and then injecting hydrogen peroxide solution from a cassette into a chamber, where it vaporizes. The vapor diffuses through the chamber, exposing all surfaces of the load to the sterilant, and initiating the inactivation of microorganisms. When a radiofrequency electrical field is applied to the chamber, a gas plasma of hydrogen peroxide is created, and microorganism-killing free radicals are generated. (Free radicals from the plasma field interact with microorganisms' essential cell components, fatally disrupting their metabolism; Rutala et al., 2008).

Excess gas is removed in the final stage of the process, and the sterilization chamber is returned to atmospheric pressure by introduction of high-efficiency filtered air. The by-product of the cycle is water vapor and oxygen, which are nontoxic and need no aeration. The type of seed gas and the depth of the vacuum are critical for the effectiveness of the process.

The Steris VHP MD and Amsco V-PRO 1 series use vaporized hydrogen peroxide. One method uses a deep vacuum to pull liquid hydrogen peroxide (30–35%) from a disposable cartridge through a heated vaporizer and into the sterilization chamber. A second method is the flow-through approach in which the vaporized hydrogen peroxide is carried into the sterilization chamber by a carrier gas (such as air) using either a slight vacuum or slight positive pressure. The by-products of the cycle are water vapor and oxygen. There is no gas plasma involved in this process. The Steris VHP has not been cleared by the FDA for sterilization of medical devices in health care facilities in the United States (Rutala et al., 2008).

Hydrogen peroxide acts as a strong oxidizing agent. This is how it inactivates microorganisms relatively quickly; cycle times are about 52–75 minutes, depending on the unit. The temperature for hydrogen peroxide gas plasma cycle is 100–112°F (37–44°C). The process does not require aeration.

Compatibility

A wide range of medical devices are compatible with the hydrogen peroxide sterilization process. Manufacturers of the medical devices provide recommendations for correct reprocessing of their product. Because of their absorption properties, items made of cellulose (e.g., paper or linen) are not compatible with the hydrogen peroxide sterilization process. Special Mylar or Tyvek pouches are available for hydrogen peroxide sterilization. Nonwoven polypropylene wrap (SPUNGUARD) also is compatible with this sterilization process.

Furthermore, there are lumen size, length, and number of lumens restrictions per sterilization cycle. Equipment with dead-end lumens may not be compatible with this process. Check with the sterilizer manufacturer for these specific guidelines.

Effectiveness and Penetration

Hydrogen peroxide does not have the same penetrating abilities as EtO, in part because it is difficult to keep the molecule in the gas phase. To increase the penetrating ability of this vapor, deep-vacuum conditions as well as multiple pulse additions of the sterilant and increased concentrations are required. Still, the hydrogen peroxide may not reach all surfaces at remote locations (due to being absorbed or reacting), and sterilization failure may occur. It is important not to overload a chamber.

Safety

The sterilizer manufacturer has designed the unit to minimize the risk of exposure to the concentrated hydrogen peroxide by containing it in a cassette system. The cassette is placed directly into the unit; hands do not come into contact with the hydrogen peroxide. There have been reported chemical burns from hydrogen peroxide residuals within a load, following mechanical problems. The established OSHA permissible exposure limit for hydrogen peroxide is 1 part per million over an 8-hour TWA (AAMI, 2005a–c).

Quality Assurance Monitoring

As with steam and EtO sterilization, quality assurance monitoring must be done through physical, chemical, and biological indicators. None of these performance monitors alone proves sterility; the combination of results from all indicators provides a higher degree of assurance that the parameters of sterilization have been met.

Physical monitoring of hydrogen peroxide sterilizers operates on a fixed automatic cycle that is controlled by a microprocessor. All critical parameters are monitored throughout the cycle, and a printout is created. If any of the process parameters fail to meet the established limit, the cycle is canceled and the printout records the malfunction. In that case, all the contents of the load must be repackaged and resterilized.

The chemical indicators should be used on the outside of each pack or peel pouch to indicate exposure to hydrogen peroxide process. An internal chemical indicator should be used, documenting the penetration of hydrogen peroxide at challenging areas within a pack or peel pouch.

The BI (Cyclesure 24BI) for Sterrad process validation contains *Geobacillus stearothermophilus* spores. The BI is placed in a 3 × 8-inch or larger Tyvek pouch. Place the pouch in the most challenging spot in the chamber (typically close to the rear of the chamber) and on top of a wrapped instrument tray. After the cycle, remove the pouch. Wearing gloves, press the cap down on the vial. Crush the vial while holding the vial in the upright position. Place the processed vial in an incubator with the temperature of 55–60°C. Also, place a control vial that has had the cap pressed down and vial crushed in the incubator. After a 24-hour period, check the results of the BIs and record them in a log. The process vials should read negative; the unprocessed vial should be positive. Dispose of the positive vial after autoclaving at 250°F (121°C) for 30 minutes.

OZONE

Ozone (O_3) is a relatively new low-temperature sterilant. The 125L by TSO3 is an FDA-approved ozone sterilizer. Ozone is a powerful oxidizing agent; it is generated within the sterilizer. An initial vacuum is pulled, then moisture is added as the load is warmed. This cycle is repeated a second time to provide better load penetration. Ozone is generated and allowed to diffuse through the load to kill microorganisms by oxidation. Figure 11.3 shows the TSO3 Sterizone sterilization process.

In general, the cycle time is about 4 hours; no aeration time is needed. The items are ready for use or storage when removed from the sterilizing unit. The temperature for sterilization is approximately 95°F (32°C).

As with hydrogen peroxide vapor sterilization, there is a restriction on lumen size and length in ozone sterilization. The process is not intended for use with flexible endoscopes or any

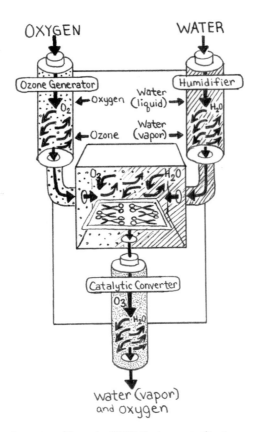

Figure 11.3 This is an illustration of how the TSO3 Sterizone sterilization process works. Illustration by Kayla Kolenberg, Ithaca, NY.

implants. Latex and textiles cannot be processed with ozone. Check with the device manufacturer for recommendations on cycle compatibility with ozone sterilization. Tyvek packaging is recommended for use with ozone sterilization.

Safety

Because the ozone is generated within the sterilizer, no handling of the sterilant occurs. It is very reactive, so it converts back to oxygen easily. The by-products of the cycle are oxygen and low-humidity water vapor. OSHA has established the permissible exposure limit of 0.1 ppm over an 8-hour TWA. There are no personnel monitoring devices available to measure ozone concentration.

Quality Assurance Monitoring

As with the other low- or high-temperature sterilants, physical, chemical, and biologic monitoring must be preformed to prove the effectiveness of the sterilizing process. The sterilizer monitors the cycle parameter (time, temperature, ozone concentration, and relative humidity), records them, and provides a printout of this information. Chemical indicators specific for ozone should be used on the outside of packs to show that an item has been exposed to the sterilization process; and an internal chemical indicator to determine whether the sterilant penetrated to the most challenging area of the pack.

Use BI specific for ozone sterilization, containing the microorganism *Geobacillus stearothermophilus*. Incubate between 131°F and 140°F (55°C and 60°C) along with a control BI. A final reading of the result at 48 hours should be documented in a log.

LIQUID PERACETIC ACID

The Steris System I sterile processing system was approved by the FDA in 1988 for sterilization of immersible medical, surgical, and diagnostic devices including flexible and rigid endoscopes (Reichert and Young, 1997). The system uses Steris 20 sterilant, which contains 35% liquid peracetic acid, together with buffering, anticorrosion, wetting, and surface-active powder agents. Peracetic acid is an oxidizing agent at low temperatures. The total processing time is about 30 minutes. Figure 11.4 shows a Steris System I with a flexible scope in place.

General Operation

The Steris System I consists of a processor and multiple interchangeable trays with adaptors for various scopes. A special container system is used for rigid scopes. A clean, leak-tested scope is placed in the tray with the appropriate Steris quick-connect attached for lumened devices. A Steris process chemical indicator is placed in the tray/container, and a container of the Steris 20 sterilant is set in place in the processor. The unit is closed, and the cycle is started. The unit fills with sterile filtered water, diluting the sterile concentrate to a use dilution of 0.2% peracetic acid. After a 12-minute exposure time at 122–132°F (50–56°C), there are four sterile rinses to remove the residual sterilant. The process does not require aeration, and the items are ready for immediate use.

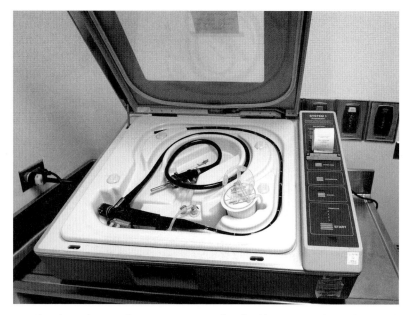

Figure 11.4   This shows the use of a Steris System I with a flexible scope in place. Photograph by Dewey Neild, Dewey Neild Photography, Ithaca, NY.

Material Compatibility

Peracetic acid has proved to be compatible with plastics, rubber, and the composition of most medical devices. The device manufacturer should be consulted as to their recommendations for sterilization with peracetic acid.

Penetration

When using a liquid sterilant, it is critical that the device is thoroughly cleaned. The device manufacturer's recommendations on cleaning (and for scopes, leak testing), must be followed prior to sterilization. The sterilant must come in contact with all surfaces in order to render the item sterile. The presence of biofilm or organic material on a device will inhibit the sterilant from coming in contact for the appropriate amount of time.

Packaging

There is no packing involved in the Steris System I processing; items are ready for immediate use. Processed items cannot be stored in a sterile manner with this system.

Safety

In the use dilution of 0.2%, peracetic acid has an approximately neutral pH, is nontoxic, and can be disposed of in a regular sanitary sewer. The process is self-contained within the Steris System I unit.

Quality Assurance Monitoring

The physical, chemical, and biologic monitoring of the peracetic acid process will measure the effectiveness of the cycle. The critical parameters for the sterilization process are monitored internally and documented by a printout for each cycle. If a process parameter cannot be met, the cycle will be immediately cancelled. The failure message and diagnostic information will be printed out. Chemical indicators are placed within the tray or container to assess where the conditions of sterilization have been met. The Verify Biological Monitoring Kit is used for routine monitoring of the Steris System 1 sterilant concentration. It provides confirmation that the Steris 20 sterilant (in its use dilution) is sufficient to sterilize the BI, which contains *Geobacillus stearothermophilus* spores on a strip. The strip is placed in the processing tray along with a chemical indicator. Testing can be done with or without a device. Complete a regular processing cycle. Wearing gloves, retrieve the chemical indicator and interpret the results. Aseptically transfer the biologic indicator to the media vial provided in the kit. Label the vial "test," and place the vial in an incubator for 24 hours at a temperature of 131–140°F (55–60°C). A control strip should be placed in a vial labeled "control" and incubated. After a 24-hour period, the control should show a growth and color change; record the result as a pass. The BI test vial should show no growth, indicating the BI was sterilized. If the test vial showed growth, have a microbiology lab identify the organism by gram stain. The test organism is a gram-positive to gram-variable spore-forming rod. Identification of organisms indicates accidental environmental contamination or actual sterilization failure. If growth was identified as a gram-positive rod, the sterilizer operation is suspect. The unit should be evaluated by a service technician before further use.

CONCLUSION

EtO blend of 12/88 was the most widely accepted method for sterilizing of heat-sensitive medical devices since the 1960s and was considered the "gold standard." The main disadvantage of EtO has been the long aeration time (12–16 hours) and environmental concerns regarding the depletion of the ozone layer. Since the mid-1990s, the old 12/88 EtO blend is no longer available, and newer blends (along with newer technologies) have evolved. There are many choices available now, each having advantages and disadvantages. Numerous factors—such as worker and environmental safety, cycle time, type of medical device, package compatibility, and cost—all need to be evaluated when choosing the correct process for a particular application.

REFERENCES

125L Ozone Sterilization. TSO$_3$ Products-Sevices. Available at: http://www.tso3.com.

Andersen Products, Haw River, NC. Anprolene Gas Sterilization. Available at: http://www.anpro.com.

[AAMI] Association for the Advancement of Medical Instrumentation. 2005a. Annex E: Peracetic acid-hydrogen peroxide solutions, in *ANSI/AAMI ST58:2005: Chemical Sterilization and High Level Disinfection in Health Care Facilities*. American National Standards Institute, Arlington, VA, pp 77–81.

AAMI. 2005b. Annex H Hydrogen peroxide gas plasma sterilization, in *ANSI/AAMI ST58:2005: Chemical Sterilization and High Level Disinfection in Health Care Facilities*. American National Standards Institute, Arlington, VA, pp 89–91.

AAMI. 2005c. Annex I: Ozone sterilization, in *ANSI/AAMI ST58:2005: Chemical Sterilization and High Level Disinfection in Health Care Facilities*. American National Standards Institute, Arlington, VA, pp 92–94.

Association of periOperative Registered Nurses (AORN). 2009. *Perioperative Standards and Recommended Practices*. RP: Sterilization. Recommendation V–VIII. AORN, Denver, CO, pp 653–657.

[IAHCSMM] International Association of Healthcare Central Service Material Management. 2007. *Central Service Technical Manual, 7th ed*. IAHCSMM, Chicago, IL.

Reichert M, Young JH. 1997. *Sterilization Technology for the Health Care Facility, 2nd ed*. Aspen Publication, Gaithersburg, MD.

Rutala WA, Weber DJ. 2004. Disinfection and sterilization, in *Disinfection and Sterilization in Healthcare Facilities*. Available at: http://disinfectionandsterilization.org

Rutala WA, Weber DJ, Healthcare Infection Control Practices Advisory Committee (HICPAC). 2008. *Guideline for Disinfection and Sterilization in Healthcare Facilities*. CDC, Atlanta, GA, pp 61–66.

Steris System 1, publication ID #M1866EN.2—0-07.Rev E GPSI Printed 05/2005, 5000. Steris Corporation, Mentor, OH. Available at: http://www.steris.com.

Sterrad Systems, Advanced Sterilization Products, Division of Ethicon, Inc., a Johnson and Johnson Company. Available at: http://www.sterad.com.

Warburton PR. 2008. The myths of sterilant gas safety exposed. *Infect Control Today* [reprinted with permission from ICT, Virgo Publishing].

12 Processing of Complex Medical Equipment and Specialty Processing

Linda Caveney

ENDOSCOPES

Flexible, semi-rigid, and rigid endoscopes (scopes) have become a popular diagnostic tool in the veterinary field in recent years. Bronchoscopy, gastroscopy, and colonoscopy are performed routinely. Rigid scopes are being used for laparoscopy and arthroscopy.

It has been documented in the human field that transmission of infections can occur from failures during cleaning/disinfecting/sterilization (AORN, 2009). It is critical that staff who handle the scopes be properly trained to follow strict guidelines in the cleaning and disinfection process. Knowledge of all components of the scope, including the working parts, helps eliminate costly repairs. The following is a review of current guidelines to assist in the development of procedures for the endoscopes in your practice. The Society of Gastroenterology Nurses and the Associates and Association for Professionals in Infection Control and Epidemiology are good references for further information on the use and processing of scopes.

Components of a Flexible Endoscope

A standard flexible endoscope is composed of a handpiece with an air/water valve, suction valve, deflecting knobs and locks, and an accessory channel attached to a flexible insertion tube containing optical fibers ending with a maneuverable tip. Optical fibers in the light-transmitting cable are generally permanently attached to the handpiece at one end and to the light source at the other end. Components are covered with an impervious material that can be bent gently, but not sharply, to maneuver inside the body. There are two basic types of endoscopes: the fiberoptic scope (as described above) and a videoscope. With a fiberoptic scope, the image is transmitted from the distal tip of the insertion tube to the eyepiece through the lenses and both image-guide and light-guide optical fibers. A videoscope's image is transmitted electronically to a video monitor from a charge-coupled device (CCD) chip in the distal tip of the insertion tube. For most veterinary use, the fiberoptic scope has considerable cost advantages.

Flexible endoscopes can range in length from 36–60 inches or longer. Diameters of the scopes range from 14 mm to <1 mm. Most scopes >2 mm in diameter have channels for irrigation, suction, and inserting instruments. The biopsy channel has the largest opening so that delicate, flexible forceps can be inserted (from the handpiece to the distal tip) for taking samples. Accessory connectors on the light-transmitting cable include the light-guide (source)

Veterinary Infection Prevention and Control, First Edition. Edited by Linda Caveney and Barbara Jones with Kimberly Ellis.
© 2012 John Wiley & Sons, Inc. Published by John Wiley & Sons, Inc.

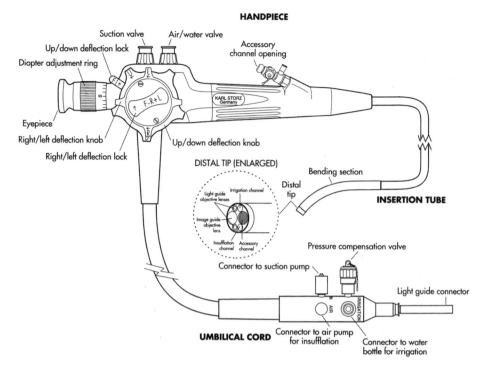

Figure 12.1   Diagram of a typical gastrointestinal fiberscope showing the handpiece, insertion tube, and umbilical cord. This illustration was published in *Small Animal Endoscopy*, 2nd ed., Todd R. Tams, DVM. Endoscopic Instrumentation. Copyright Elsevier, 1999.

connector, a suction pump, water container for irrigation, an air pump, and a venting connector to allow penetration of ethylene oxide gas sterilant and for testing for internal leaks. See Figure 12.1 for a diagram of a typical gastrointestinal fiberscope.

The complexity of the scope and the instruments used in conjunction with the scope produce a great potential for contamination by hidden organic debris and microorganisms. Manufacturers of the scope as well as scope instrumentation manufacturers should be consulted for the proper processing of their equipment.

Reprocessing Steps

In general, there are four main steps in the reprocessing of flexible endoscopes: cleaning, disinfection, drying, and storage. Each step can be divided into a sequence of specific processes as recommended by the scope manufacturer. The manufacturer's instructions should always be your first resource for reprocessing your specific endoscope. The manufacturer's sales representation can also be a reference to specific information on a particular scope. The sequence and equipment may differ slightly, depending on the scope type and manufacturer. The following are general procedural guidelines for reprocessing of flexible endoscopes.

Cleaning of Flexible Endoscopes

First and foremost is the cleaning of the scopes. The longer the proteins and other organic materials are allowed to dry, the harder they will be to clean from the scope, both inside and out.

It is best practice to clean the scope within 30 minutes after use. Check to see which enzymatic cleaning solution is compatible with the scope manufacturer's recommendations. Follow the scope manufacturer's recommendations on what type of water should be used to dilute the enzymatic detergent (i.e., RO, distilled, or tap). Preclean the scopes exterior with an enzymatic detergent. Repeatedly turn the valves while flushing and aspirating enzymatic solution through the channels to remove the organic materials (blood, tissue). Always following the dilution recommended by the enzymatic detergent manufacturer. This precleaning is conducted in the area where the procedure takes place. The scope is then taken to an area where further cleaning occurs. The enzymatic solution used in the precleaning should then be discarded; they are not microbiocidal or microbiostatic.

Leak Testing

The next step in cleaning is the leak test. The leak test is a procedure to ensure that the scope's flexible covering and internal channels area are watertight. Performance of the pressure/leak test is specific for each scope; follow the manufacturer's recommended guidelines. Before you start, inspect the joints and seams to see whether any tears or holes are present. If there are any detected, do not continue and send the scope out for repairs.

If no defects are present, the next step is to remove any valves or attachments. Examine the water-resistant cap for damage before using. If any defects are observed, the pressure will not hold; the cap should be replaced. Attach the leak tester to the ETO venting connector or to the leak tester connector of the water-resistant cap as recommended by the manufacturer. See Figure 12.2 for a leak tester connected to a fiberscope.

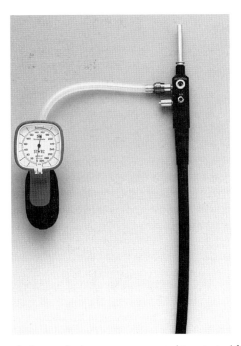

Figure 12.2   This photograph shows a leakage tester connected to a typical fiberscope. This illustration is copyright of Elsevier (Tams, 1999).

Pressurize the scope with air to the recommended pressure, then place the distal tip in plain water and angulate the distal tip carefully. The control knob of the endoscope should not be immersed in water at this time because the "O" rings are not designed to operate under water with excessive pressure. A continuous stream of bubbles from the scope indicates a leak. If air bubbles are visible, do not submerge the scope further. If no bubbles are seen, submerge the rest of the scope in water. Start by observing the control knob (a continuous stream of bubbles will appear if the "O" ring is damaged). Check to see if there are holes in the scope's internal channels. Some bubbles will exit a channel opening at the valve ports, air/water inlets, suction port, light-guide connector, biopsy port, or channel openings at the distal tip. Air in these channels can be expected to form bubbles when first submerged in the water; this is not necessarily a leak (with a leak, there will be a steady, continuous stream of bubbles). Flushing the channels with water can clear the air out of them. Observe the entire length of scope for any bulging areas as this may be a weak point in the tube where a hole may later occur. If a continuous stream of bubbles appears, do not deflate the leak tester until the entire scope has been removed from the water.

Remove the scope from water and drain the channels. Release the pressure and verify by listening for the sound of air being forced out. Follow Table 12.1, the Leak Testing Flow Chart, for proper handling of scopes.

Proceed with manual cleaning of the endoscope. Manual cleaning is the most critical step in the processing of the scope. As with any piece of medical equipment requiring a high level of disinfection or sterilization, meticulous cleaning to remove any and all organic material and microorganisms enables the disinfectant or sterilant to come directly in contact with all surfaces.

Detach all removable parts, soak, then scrub or brush them to remove organic debris. Immerse the scope in fresh enzymatic detergent solution and thoroughly clean the external surface with a soft cloth or sponge that is specially made for scope cleaning. Clean the internal channels by alternately brushing and flushing with enzymatic solution to remove organic materials from the channels. A back-and-forth motion with a brush can damage the internal channel. The correct size brush for the lumen of the internal channel should be used. The brush should be long enough to exit the channel, be cleared of debris, and then removed from the lumen. The brush should be cleaned of debris and rinsed each time it is placed into the scope lumen. Refer to Figure 12.3 for examples of the types of brushes available for this procedure.

If these procedures are not completed meticulously, the difficult-to-clean areas can develop a build-up of denatured proteins—the beginning of biofilm that is nearly impossible to remove. Use the manufacturer's recommended adapters to clean the air and water channels. The brushes used to clean the lumens also need to be cleaned, disinfected, and dried before being used on another scope. If organic materials cannot be removed completely from the brush, it should be discarded. One-time-use disposable brushes are available in various sizes for cleaning scope channels.

Disinfecting the Flexible Endoscope

The next step in the process is disinfecting or sterilizing the scope. The reprocessing recommendation by the CDC is based on the Spaulding classification system, according the intended use of the item and the risk of disease transmission of that item.

"Critical" items in the Spaulding classification are those that penetrate skin or mucous membranes or enter a sterile body system. Those devices must be sterilized. Flexible endoscopy biopsy forceps and arthroscopes fall into this category.

Table 12.1   Leak Test Flow Chart

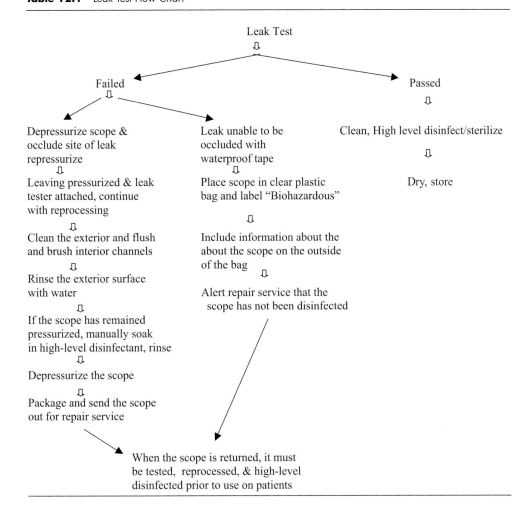

"Semicritical" items contact intact mucous membranes. These items require a minimum of high-level disinfection. FDA-listed high-level disinfectants kill mycobacterium, vegetative bacteria, nonlipid and lipid viruses, fungi, and a few kinds of bacterial spores. Gastrointestinal and colonoscopies fall into the semicritical category.

The endoscope manufacturer will recommend which disinfectants are compatible with the materials contained in each type of scope. There are three main chemical compounds used for high-level disinfection: glutaraldehyde, orthophthaladehyde (OPA), and peracetic acid.

Glutaraldehyde has been around the longest. It is a 2% alkaline solution that is compatible with most endoscope materials. Sterilization can be achieved with extended exposure time (generally a minimum of 10 hours with glutaraldehyde). Always check with the manufacturer for recommended exposure times for high-level disinfection or sterilization. Glutaraldehyde has some disadvantages, however: noxious odor, a relatively short (14–28 days) product use life after activation, and the fact that dilution of the glutaraldehyde reduces the kill claims. Furthermore, it contains fixatives that can build up on scopes, it has no cleaning ability, and glutaraldehyde

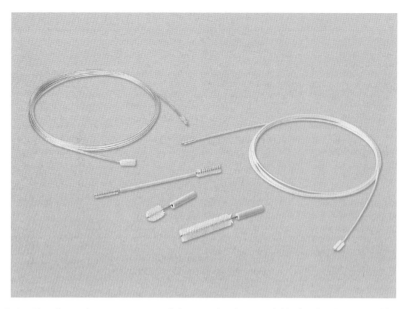

Figure 12.3 This shows the various types of cleaning brushes available for the cleaning of flexible endo-scopes. Photograph provided courtesy of Spectrum Surgical, Stow, OH.

requires profuse amounts of sterile water for rinsing. Glutaraldehyde, like other liquid chemical disinfectants, requires the minimum effective concentration (MEC) to be monitored with test strips during its reuse period. If it falls below the manufacturer's guideline for MEC, it needs to be discarded, even if the 14- or 28-day use period is not up.

Glutaraldehyde is an irritant to eyes, skin, and the respiratory system. OSHA guidelines recommend its use in a covered container system, in a well-vented area, and at a maximum ceiling exposure limit of 0.05 ppm. An eye wash station must be available within 10 seconds' travel time. Nitrile gloves should be worn while handling glutaraldehyde (latex gloves do not provide adequate protection).

OPA is a newer high-level disinfectant. It is a 0.55% solution effective at room temperature. Its odor is not as noxious as that of glutaraldehyde, but it should still be used in a well-ventilated area. It requires no activation and has a 14-day reuse life. OPA solution needs to have the MEC checked before each use. If it falls below 0.3%, it should be discarded.

OPA also needs to be rinsed with large volumes of water for a minimum of 1 minute. The rinse water should not be reused. OPA cannot be used as a sterilant. Always check with the manufacturer of the scope to ensure compatibility with the OPA solution.

Peracetic acid is used in an automatic endoscope reprocessing systems. These systems contain 35% liquid peracetic acid diluted with a buffer, surfactant, and an anticorrosive dry powder to its 0.2% use dilution. The processing cycle is 12 minutes at 122–133°F. The automatic system's cycle includes rinsing with water that has passed through a 0.2-micron filtration membrane. Automatic systems process one scope at a time with the solution being used only once. Biological and chemical indicator monitoring procedures are specifically designated for use with this system. Chapter 11 describes the use of peracetic acid processing system further.

Always check with the scope manufacturer before using a system that uses peracetic acid as its main ingredient.

An automated system's printout of the cycle parameters (along with the biologic and chemical indicators) provides the quality-assurance documentation for sterilization. However, specialized trays and different scope adapters limit the type and configuration of the items that can be processed in automated systems. Neither the water bottle nor their delivery systems are approved for sterilization in such systems. Consult the manufacturer as to the best method of sterilization of those components.

There are some automatic endoscope reprocessors (AERs) that are capable of cleaning, high-level disinfecting, and rinsing flexible endoscopes. Scopes are placed in the AERs after they have been manually cleaned and the lumens have been brushed and flushed. An advantage of an AER is that it can reprocess two or more endoscopes at one time. Also, it can limit the exposure to the high-level disinfectant because they are in a closed processing system.

Once the choice of high-level disinfectant is made, the scope is immersed in the disinfectant solution for the time recommended by the solution's manufacturer. Do not coil the scope too tightly. The basin needs to be large enough to accommodate the scope, with sufficient solution to cover it. Use cleaning adapters to fill the lumens with disinfectant solution until no bubbles remain. Also place all removable parts in the disinfectant solution. Cover the basin to minimize chemical evaporation. Follow the manufacturer's recommendations for exposure (contact) time: set a timer to remind you when to remove the scope, because excessive exposure can damage the scope components. When the immersion time is up, flush all lumens with air to remove the disinfectant solution. The scope must be thoroughly rinsed to remove all traces of the disinfectant from the external surface and internal channels. Thoroughly rinse the scope and all removable parts with filtered water that is free of waterborne organisms that can contaminate the scope. Check with the manufacturer of the scope as to the type of water that should be used for rinsing (i.e., RO, distilled, sterile). This rinse water should be discarded after flushing each scope; it should not be reused for any purpose. If any of the scope's reusable parts are heat stable, they should undergo the same cleaning, rinsing, and drying before being packaged for sterilization and proper storage. After the last rinse is complete, a final drying step is needed.

Drying the Flexible Endoscope

The scopes should be dried with medical-grade forced air. Drying the exterior and using forced air in the channels minimizes moisture that promotes bacterial growth. Proper storage of the endoscope is also an important step to prevent bacterial growth, minimize retention of moisture, and protect it from damage.

Storage of Flexible Endoscopes

Scope should be stored with the insertion tube hanging vertically, with the weight of the control body supported, and with the angulation locks in the "off" position. Scopes should be stored in a dust free, well-ventilated cabinet. Control valves, as well as distal hoods or caps, should be removed during storage. Scopes should be properly carried to avoid damage from contact with walls or other objects. Always hold the scope loosely coiled, protecting the distal tip. Figure 12.4 illustrates a proper storage cabinet system for flexible endoscopes.

Documentation

A record or log should be kept for all endoscopic procedures. It should contain the date, patient information, disinfectant verification (MEC), type of procedure, and any noted problems. If any

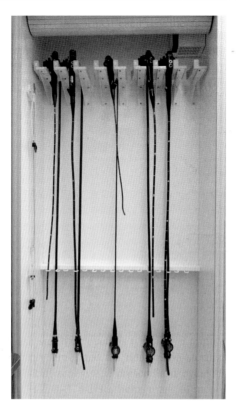

Figure 12.4 This photograph shows one system for proper storage of multiple flexible endoscopes. Photographed by Dewey Neild, Dewey Neild Photography, Ithaca, NY.

problems are noted, the scope should be sent out for repairs. Some common problems identified by scope manufacturer repair facilities are found in Table 12.2.

Additionally, each scope should have its own log. This log should also include information about repairs and preventative service specific for that scope. Table 12.3 is an example of a log kept for an endoscope repair log sheet.

Rigid Scopes

The size and variety of rigid scopes available today facilitate their use by many medical specialties. The differences are in the widths, working lengths, and angles for viewing. The number of procedures that are done using rigid scope has grown as the size of the shaft has been reduced. These instruments are very complex and fragile, especially the smaller arthroscopes. Mishandling can result in time-consuming and costly repairs. The cameras and cables used with the scopes also are fragile and need careful handling.

Components of a Rigid Scope

The optical portion of the rigid scope is called a telescope. It provides both the image and the transmission of light. An optical lens train (a series of precisely aligned lenses, spacers,

Table 12.2   Common Endoscope Reprocessing Errors

Precleaning	Failure to preclean special channels (elevator wire or auxiliary water channel)
	Not using proper adapter in cleaning air/water channels
Leak Testing	Forgetting to leak test or leak test correctly
	Using damaged water-resistant cap during testing
	Forgetting to pressurize the scope prior to immersion
	Not fully angulating the distal tip during leak test
	Not following manufacturer's guidelines for reprocessing a damaged scope
Manual Cleaning	Not diluting the enzymatic detergent according to manufacturer's recommendations
	Reuse of disposable brushes and other accessories
	Failure to use manufacturer's recommended cleaning adapters or using damaged adapters
High-Level Disinfectant	Not testing the minimum effective concentration of disinfectant according to manufacturer's instructions
	Failing to fully immerse instrument in disinfectant solution
	Not following manufacturer's recommended length of time to achieve adequate high-level disinfection
Storage	Forgetting to remove all valves and caps during storage
	Not ensuring that scopes are hung with all locks in free position
	Crowded and unsecured scope storage area

Adapted from Dix, Kathy, 2008. Scope Cleaning and Repair; Top 10 Ways to Keep Scopes Happy. *Infection Control Today*. 12(3):46–52.

and mirrors) occupies the center portion of the telescope and provides the image. Glass-fiber bundles that are distributed around the lens train provide illumination from the light source. These components are contained inside a metal shaft. The rigid scope has an eyepiece with ocular lens at one end and an objective lens at the other. See Figure 12.5 for a longitudinal cross-section of the lens system.

Table 12.3   Example of an Endoscope Repair Log Sheet

Scope Model: V-Bronchoscope   Serial Number N11579   MFG: Storz   Purchase Date: 6-10-99

Date sent for repair	Sent to (repair co.)	Description of problem	Initials of staff identified problem	Repair findings	Return date	Cost
7-10-00	Storz	Blurry picture, positive leak test	ABS	Fluid invasion	7-15-00	$7000.00
10-2-00	Storz	No picture, positive leak test	NC	Fluid invasion	10-8-00	$7000.00
10-31-00	Storz	Hazy picture, positive leak test	NC	Fluid invasion	11-5-00	$7000.00

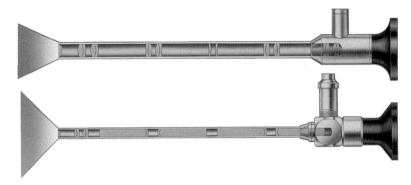

Figure 12.5 This shows a comparative cross-section of a conventional optical lens system compared with the Hopkins rod lens system (on bottom). Illustration provided courtesy of Karl Storz, Tuttlingen, Germany.

A light source is connected to the scope just distal to the eyepiece by a light-transmitting cable. The illumination sources most commonly used are xenon or halogen (when light intensity and color reproduction are not critical).

All rigid scopes should be placed in a perforated, protective case for transport, sterilization, and storage. See Figure 12.6 for an example of a specially designed tray for rigid scopes.

The steps in reprocessing rigid scopes are basically the same as for flexible endoscopes. Refer to the manufacturer's guidelines for selection of cleaning, disinfectant, and sterilization products. Failure to follow the manufacturer's recommendations can result in damage to the instrument or lenses. Disconnect light cables and cable adapters; remove the camera head (if applicable) before reprocessing.

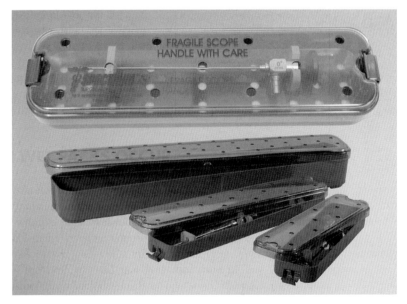

Figure 12.6 This photograph shows various trays available for rigid scope processing. Photograph provided courtesy of Spectrum Surgical, Stow, OH.

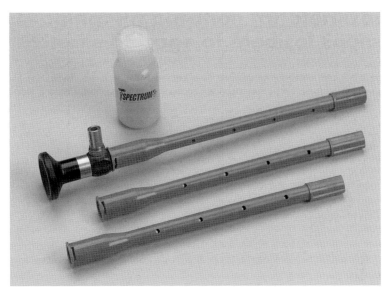

Figure 12.7   This photograph shows a protective rigid scope sleeve that can be used during transport from point of use to the processing area. Photograph provided courtesy of Spectrum Surgical, Stow, OH.

Reprocessing Steps

The first step for reprocessing rigid scopes is the precleaning at the point of use. Remove all organic material and irrigation fluids with a soft cloth and water. Carefully transport the scope to the designated area for further cleaning. Figure 12.7 shows a protective sleeve that can be used for transport of a scope to the cleaning area.

Use a soft cotton cloth and approved enzymatic solution to remove any residual organic debris. Detergents are not generally recommended as they contain surfactants that leave a residual film on the telescope portion of the scope. Rinse with warm water and dry with a clean soft towel. Clean the lenses and fiber optic inlet post with a cotton-tipped applicator dipped in 70% isopropyl alcohol. The scope should be inspected for scratches or dents. Avoid touching the ocular or objective lenses; fingerprints hinder the view and debris can scratch the lenses.

To inspect the optical clarity of the lens, view a nonglare piece of white paper with print on it. Look through the lens with the paper held 3 inches from the distal tip. Move the scope tip closer until the paper is only $^1/_4$ inch away. The image should be crisp and clean. Discoloration or haze may be from improper cleaning, disinfectant residue, or a cracked or broken lens. Additionally, moisture in the shaft or external damage to the shaft that has broken the glass fibers can affect clarity. Reclean the lens and repeat the procedures. If the view is not clear, the scope will need to be sent for repairs.

To inspect the optical fibers, hold the scope in your hand, point the distal tip toward a bright light (overhead or a window), and look through the eyepiece. The light carriers are the glass fibers in the perimeter of the scope. Black dots, irregular areas, or shadowed areas may indicate broken fibers that inhibit the transfer of light. Inspect the eyepiece for damage. Place the scope in a trocar by aligning the locking pin with the notch. Check for proper visual alignment by confirming a clear view.

Disinfection/Sterilization

Under most circumstances, rigid scopes will need to be sterilized. Refer to the scope manufacturer's recommendations to determine how the scope should be processed. Most scopes can be processed with low-temperature sterilization by ethylene oxide gas, peracetic acid (Steris System 1), or hydrogen peroxide gas plasma (Sterrad). This low-temperature sterilization can prolong the life of the lenses. There are newer scopes that can be steam sterilized.

Documentation

A record should be kept for all procedures in which a particular rigid scope is used. It should contain the date, patient information, sterilization method and verification, type of procedure, and any noted problems. Additionally, each size and type of scope should have its own log. This log should also include information about repairs and preventative service specific for that scope.

Summary

Flexible endoscopes and rigid scopes are valuable diagnostic and therapeutic tools for patient care. Strict adherence to accepted "best practice" guidelines is critical for the safety of the patients. General guidelines are available from the Association for Professionals in Infection Control and Epidemiology and The Society of Gastroenterology Nurses and the Associates. Manufacturer representatives from the scope you have can and should be relied on as a source of information regarding each scope.

All staff members who handle any of the scopes or have any role in scope reprocessing should be extensively trained; their competency should be reviewed annually. Transmission of pathogenic disease has been linked to staff taking shortcuts in the reprocessing procedures.

POWERED SURGICAL INSTRUMENTS

Powered surgical instruments are those devices powered by electric motor, compressed gas (pneumatic), or battery. They come in a variety of sizes, compactness, and design complexity. The materials these devices are made of vary. The products used for cleaning need to be compatible with the specific material. This section will review the general recommendations for processing of powered surgical equipment. Powered surgical instruments and all attachments should be decontaminated, lubricated, assembled, sterilized, and tested before use according to the manufacturer's written instructions. Always refer to your specific manufacturer's guidelines and recommendations for the cleaning and sterilization of their equipment. Many manufacturers will provide training on the proper techniques for handling and processing of their devices.

Electric-Powered Equipment

Electric-powered equipment generally consists of a motorized handpiece (used in the surgical field), a cord on the other end of the handpiece that attaches to a power unit, and a cord from the power unit that plugs into an electrical outlet. The handpiece as well as the cord it is connected to need to be sterilized. An arthroscopy shaver is an example of an electric-powered device. It is essential that fluid does not enter the handpiece or the cable end that attaches the handpiece to the power unit. Manufacturers generally recommend having these attached during the cleaning process. Do not immerse any pieces during cleaning, and use only the products and lubricants recommended by the manufacturer. Use a nylon bristle brush designed for medical equipment to clean the distal tip. Dry the handpiece and the cord (going to the power unit) with a lint-free towel.

Common problems associated with this type equipment are damage during sterilization, condensation entering the handpiece when seals wear out, and electric contacts wearing out (IAHCSMM, 2007).

Pneumatic (Air)-Powered Equipment

Pneumatic-powered equipment use compressed gas (CO_2) or medical-grade nitrogen to power them. An air hose connects the handpiece at one end to a pressure regulator on either a stand-alone cylinder (tank) or to a regulator mounted in a wall or column for piped-in gas on the other end. There are two gauges on the regulators: one telling the supply (tank or piped-in) pressure and the other measuring the pressure in the handpiece. Different types of powered equipment require different operating pressures. Extreme care should be taken to follow the manufacturer's recommendations for proper pressure during operation. Damage of the equipment or injury to the user or patient could result if the recommended pressure is not used. The air hose should be inspected regularly for cuts and other damage.

During the cleaning process, it is important that fluid not enter the hose, handpiece, or any attachments. Manufacturers generally recommend connecting the hose to the handpiece during cleaning. The hose, handpiece, and attachments should never be immersed in any solution, nor should they be placed in an ultrasonic cleaner. Some handpieces need to be lubricated; follow the manufacturer's recommendations on the specific lubricant and amount.

Among common reasons why power equipment needs to be repaired are corrosion of the internal components from steam condensation, immersion in water solutions, biofilm build-up caused by improper cleaning, mishandling that causes physical damage, and lack of preventative maintenance. See Figure 12.8 for an example of internal damage done to a pneumatic drill.

Battery-Powered Equipment

This style of power equipment is the least cumbersome of all available power systems; battery-powered devices allow freedom of movement over the sterile field. The downside of the battery style is the cost. Furthermore, batteries and chargers for different systems typically are not interchangeable. The manufacturer's instructions for sterilization must be closely followed. Steam damage can cause batteries not to hold their charge. In some styles, the batteries cannot be sterilized; doing so can cause the battery to malfunction.

As with the other power equipment, the handpiece, attachments, and batteries should never be immersed in any solution or even water. An already-dead battery can be connected while cleaning the handpiece; this protects the electrical components from moisture.

General Recommendations for Powered Handpieces

- If possible during the procedures, remove as much tissue debris with a sponge moistened with sterile water; do not use saline.
- Remove the burs, bits, and blades at the end of the procedure.
- Remove any attachments from the handpiece and disconnect the hose from the power source.
- Leave the hose attached to the handpiece to prevent water from entering the motor.

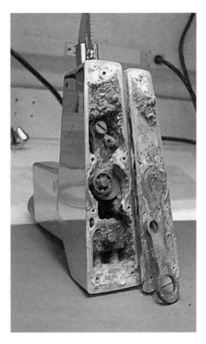

Figure 12.8 This illustrates the corrosion found in a powered saw following incorrect processing. Photograph provided courtesy of Spectrum Surgical, Stow, OH.

- Use a soft bristle brush to clean any depressions.
- Operate the moving parts to ensure all areas are cleaned and no resistance is noticed.
- Use a stiff brush of the appropriate diameter and length to clean the cannulations (if applicable).
- Inspect the hose or cable for any defects.
- Lubricate the handpiece with the right amount and type of lubricant, as recommended by the manufacturer, in the sites specified by the manufacturer.
- Dry all components with a lint-free cloth.
- Package and sterilize the equipment as recommended by the manufacturer. Special racks or positioning devices may be needed.
- Check the manufacturer's instructions carefully for sterilization guidelines. Many of the new powered handpieces need to be sterilized in extended cycles. Extended sterilization cycles are traditionally longer than those recommended for general use trays and packs. Many of the chemical indicators and the biologic indicators are not valid in these special cycles. Always check with the manufacturer for the appropriate cycle times, temperature, and length of drying. Table 12.4 gives a general idea of the variation in cycle times of common veterinary drills and powered equipment.

Summary

Motorized equipment is very expensive. Proper use and handling along with standard preventative maintenance will ensure the equipment is available when it is needed. Always consult the manufacturer's recommendations for cleaning and sterilization guidelines.

Table 12.4 Recommended Sterilization Cycles for Power Equipment

Power Equipment	Autoclave Type	Sterilization Exposure Time	Comments
3M Mini Driver K-200	Gravity 270–272°F	25 min 8 min dry time	Do not run when not dry or hot
	Prevac 270–272°F	4 min 8 min dry time	Do not run when not dry or hot
Hall Surgairtome Two Air Drill	Gravity 270–272°F	20 min, 8+ min dry time	Do not flash
	Gravity 250–254°F	40 min, 8+ min dry time	Do not flash
	Prevac 270–272°F	4 min, 8+ min dry time	Do not flash
Slocum Pneumatic Oscillating Saw	Gravity 270–272°F	35 min	Do not run when warm
	Gravity 250–254°F	60 min	Do not run when warm
	Prevac 274°F	3–3.5 min	Do not run when warm
Synthes Small Battery Drive (532.010)	Prevac 270–272°F	4 min	Do not flash; no gravity recommendations

Adapted from operator manuals of the various manufacturers (Linvatec, Slocum, Synthes) listed above.

When either a scope or power equipment needs repair, it is important to have it provided by a reputable company. Cost is also a concern when getting these items repaired. Follow closely the manufacturer's guidelines when the item is covered under warranty. If you have not followed their recommendations, you may be voiding your warranty. Once the warranty period is over, you are not obligated to return the item to the manufacturer; you may find another service provider. Table 12.5 provides some guideline on how to select a repair provider.

PROCESSING OF OPHTHALMIC SURGICAL INSTRUMENTS

This section will review the general principles for cleaning and sterilizing intraocular instruments as well as specific recommendations for all intraocular surgical instruments. Recently, ophthalmic surgical instrument hygiene has become critically important because of occurrences of a condition called "TASS."

Toxic Anterior Segment Syndrome (TASS) is an acute inflammation of the anterior chamber of the eye that has been reported by the American Society of Cataract and Refractive Surgery. Veterinary ophthalmologists suspect that TASS occurs in postphacoemulsification (method of

Table 12.5 Selecting a Repair Provider

Compile a list of repair providers
Obtain references from other facilities that have used recommended provider
Ask the following questions of both repair providers and other facilities:
   How well does the repair provider respond to quick turn-around needs?
   What warranties does the repair provider offer for their work?
   Does the repaired equipment still experience unscheduled downtime after service?
   Are repair parts readily available?
   Are new or used parts installed?
   Are service and/or support personnel available to answer questions during surgical procedures?
   Does the service supplier offer user training program as needed?
   Does the service supplier maintain adequate liability and shipping insurance?

removing the cataract lens through the uses of an ultrasonic waves emitted from a handpiece that breaks up the lens so it can be removed by suction) in veterinary patients (Myrna et al., 2009). Signs are acute (presenting within 24 hours of surgery), and patients exhibit diffuse corneal edema, dilated pupil, and relatively mild discomfort. TASS is not bacterial, cultures will be negative, and the symptoms of TASS do not respond to antibiotics. Although usually associated with cataract surgery, TASS can occur after any type of anterior chamber surgery. The challenge of preventing TASS is complicated by the wide variety of substances that have been implicated as possible causes. Specialists hypothesize that TASS might be caused by extraocular substances that inadvertently enter the anterior chamber during or after the procedure (e.g., topical antiseptic agents, talc from surgical gloves); products that are introduced into the anterior chamber as part of the procedure (e.g., preservatives, inappropriately reconstituted intraocular preparations, intraocular lenses, contaminated irrigating solutions); or irritants on the surface of the surgical instruments as a result of inadequate or inappropriate cleaning (e.g., denatured viscoelastic solution [viscoelastic is a hydroxymethylcellulose material injected into the anterior chamber during the surgery to maintain depth of the chamber, protect the corneal endothelium, and stabilize the vitreous], enzymatic detergent residues, impurities of steam in the sterilization process, endotoxins from gram-negative bacteria in ultrasonic cleaners). Until the cause or causes of TASS can be determined, special attention should be paid to manufacturers' recommendations for cleaning and sterilizing ophthalmic surgical instruments.

General Principles for Processing Intraocular Surgical Instruments

As with all surgical instruments, the intraocular instruments should be kept moist. Viscoelastic solution can dry and harden within minutes. The detergents manufacturer's directions for use should be strictly adhered to. The detergent used should be compatible with the recommendations of the instrument manufacturer. Adequate rinsing of the instruments removes the detergent and the debris that was loosened in the cleaning process. Most instrument manufacturers recommend that the final rinse be with sterile distilled or sterile deionized water. The method of sterilization should be one that is approved by the instrument manufacturer as well as the sterilizer manufacturer. Written procedures for the cleaning and sterilization process should be developed and followed. Staff members should be trained on all steps in the cleaning and sterilization process.

Specific Recommendations for Cleaning and Sterilizing Intraocular Surgical Instruments

Allow adequate time for thorough cleaning and sterilization; shortcuts should never be taken to save time or money. Sufficient inventory of intraocular instruments should meet the needs of the surgical caseload. Flash sterilization should be avoided. Instruments should be immersed in sterile water immediately after the procedure; this will help prevent biofilm from adhering to the surfaces of the instruments. Cannulas should also be flushed with sterile water; this is particularly important if the instrument had any viscoelastic solution on or in them. Viscoelastic material can quickly harden and plug a lumen; ideally, viscoelastic cannulas should be single-use only.

Intraocular instruments should be cleaned separately from nonophthalmologic surgical instruments. This prevents them from being contaminated with cleaning chemicals that might be on other surgical equipment. Follow the ophthalmologic instrument manufacturer's recommendations on the use of enzymatic detergents. If enzymatic detergent use is not contraindicated, follow the detergent manufacturer's instructions for proper dilution and soak times.

Brushes used in the cleaning process should be designed for ophthalmic instruments only. Ideally, single-use syringes and brushes are recommended and should be discarded after each use. Reusable brushes should be cleaned and high-level disinfected or sterilized after each use. Cleaning brushes can contain contaminants that can be transferred during cleaning of the next instrument. Syringes used as cleaning tools should be discarded after each use.

Cleaning solution used should be discarded after each use. After cleaning with detergents, thoroughly rinse with ample amounts of tap water to remove any residue of the detergent. The final rinse should be with sterile distilled water or sterile deionized water. Follow instrument manufacturer recommendations for specific volume, temperature, and number of rinses or flushes. Do not reuse sterile rinse water; it should be discarded.

Filtered, medical-grade, oil-free compressed air forced through the lumen of intraocular instruments helps to eliminate moisture that can promote microbial growth. Check the instrument manufacturer's recommendations before subjecting the instrument to the ultrasonic cleaning process. If the instrument manufacturer recommends ultrasonic cleaning, the instruments should be processed in a freshly filled, degassed chamber with only ophthalmic instruments. The ultrasonic cleaner itself should be emptied, cleaned, disinfected, rinsed, and dried at least daily. If not contraindicated by the manufacturer of the ultrasonic cleaner, a final rinse with 70% ethyl or isopropyl is recommended.

The phacoemulsification handpiece and the irrigator/aspirator tips and handpiece should be cleaned and flushed according to the manufacturer's recommendations. Inspect and verify that all visocelastic solution material has been removed before sterilization. Additional cleaning and rinsing may be necessary to ensure complete removal of viscoelastic solution. Use the method of sterilization as indicated by the ophthalmologic instrument manufacturer as well as the directions provided by the sterilizer manufacturer.

Choose the appropriate steam sterilization cycle according to published guidelines from the instrument manufacturer and the sterilizer manufacturer. Glutaraldehyde is not recommended for sterilizing any intraocular instruments because of the toxic residues resulting from inadequate rinsing or contamination during poststerilization handling. The use of other low-temperature sterilization methods should be avoided unless, that is, the instrument manufacturer and the low-temperature sterilizer manufacturer have validated the method for the specific instrument with respect to efficacy of sterilization, potential ocular toxicity (e.g., from oxidation of metals), and instrument function (Hellinger et al., 2007).

Verification of sterilizer function should be conducted in accordance with published industry standards and directions from the sterilizer manufacturer. Maintenance of water filtration systems and the quality of water supplying the steam sterilizer should be verified yearly. At each facility, policies for cleaning and sterilizing intraocular surgical instruments should be written, reviewed periodically, and made available to all individuals involved in the handling, cleaning, and sterilization of intraocular equipment.

Regarding TASS: Other Recommended Practices

Identifying a causative factor in TASS is challenging because many factors have been found to be a potential source. Precise documentation of equipment use, sources, and expiration dates, and lot numbers for all materials that go into the eye can help identify the cause(s). Furthermore, limiting reuse of items designed for single use (e.g., cannulas, tubing) can help to minimize the possibility of the patient developing TASS.

Summary

Although TASS is not formally documented in veterinary patients, review of the surgical procedure and the processing of ophthalmic surgical instruments can help identify a causative agent in the event of an occurrence. Strict compliance with written policies and procedures and adequate staff training ensure successful patient outcomes.

FLASH STERILIZATION

Flash sterilization is a modification of conventional steam sterilization (either gravity or pre-vacuum) in which the flashed item is placed in an open tray or specially designed covered, rigid container to allow rapid penetration of steam (Rutala, 2008). The time required for flash sterilization depends on the type of sterilizer (gravity vs. dynamic air removal) and the type of item (porous vs. nonporous, lumen vs. nonlumen).

Historically, flash sterilization was used only in an "emergency" (e.g., when a one-of-a-kind item was dropped from the sterile field). The cycles were designed for one instrument at a time, for an unwrapped object at a temperature of 270°F (132°C) for 3 minutes with 27–28 pounds of pressure.

Today the reasons for flash sterilization range from not having adequate time to process the instruments through the standard wrapped cycles, to budgetary constraints (not having money to purchase multiple specialty instrument sets), to scheduling back-to-back procedures that need the same instruments, and using loaner trays from device manufacturers or other facilities (IAHCSMM, 2007).

Recommended Guidelines for Flash Sterilization

Several human health care agencies have established standards, guidelines, and recommendations for use of flash sterilization or point-of-use processing of steam-sterilizable items. The Association for the Advancement of Medical Instrumentation (AAMI, 2009) outlined certain criteria in the "Comprehensive Guide to Steam Sterilization and Sterility Assurance in Health Care Facilities," approved by American National Standards Institute:

- Work practices should ensure proper cleaning, decontamination, inspection, and placement of instruments in trays for flash sterilization.
- The area's physical layout should provide for direct delivery of the sterilized item to the point of use.
- Procedures should be developed, followed, and audited to ensure aseptic handling and personnel safety during transport to point of use.
- Items should be used immediately after flash sterilization.

The recommendations are not laws, but they are nationally recognized as best practice for professional standards.

The Association of periOperative Registered Nurses (AORN, 2009) publishes its recommended practices and guidelines based on the AAMI standards and the best perioperative practice. AORN states that flash sterilization can be performed only in select clinical circumstances:

- Flash sterilization should only be used in select clinical situations and in a controlled manner.
- The use of flashed items should be kept to a minimum.
- Flash sterilization should be done when there is not enough time to process the item by the preferred wrapped method.
- Flash sterilization should not be used as a substitute for inadequate instrument inventory.
- Only flash sterilize an item if the device manufacturer's instructions for flash sterilization are followed.
- Placement of the instruments in the container or tray should allow for steam penetration.
- There is a procedure for aseptic transfer to the sterile field.
- Documentation and monitoring results should be maintained to allow tracking of the processed item to the individual.

AORN recommends that flash sterilization be performed only if all the following criteria are met:

- The device manufacturer's written instructions on cycle type, exposure times, temperature setting, and drying times are available and followed.
- The items are disassembled and thoroughly cleaned with detergent and water to remove soil, blood, body fats, and other substances.
- Lumens are brushed and flushed under water with a cleaning solution and thoroughly rinsed.
- Items are placed in a closed sterilization container validated for flash sterilization, or tray, in a manner that will allow steam to contact all surfaces of the instruments.
- Measures are taken to prevent contamination during transfer to the sterile field.

When an item needs to be flashed for immediate use, time pressures may cause staff to skip vital steps needed for the delivery of a flashed item. Any contaminated instrument needs to be properly cleaned and dried before it can be flashed. Cleaning is the most critical step prior to any sterilization process and must be done according to the device manufacturer's recommendations. The recommended cleaning agents, tools, and water quality should be the same as for instruments that are processed for terminal (wrapped) sterilization. The instruments must be in the open position or disassembled and placed in a perforated or mesh-bottom tray that allows for proper air removal and good steam circulation. It is unacceptable to attempt to clean instruments for flashing in a scrub sink or hand sink.

Rushing to use an item that in not cooled completely may cause burns to patients, or using sterile water or saline to cool an item may affect the metal of the item.

Full trays of instruments should not be flash sterilized. The total metal mass increases the heat-up time, which will increase the total cycle time. If using a preprogrammed cycle, this will only heat the instruments, not render them sterile.

Sterilization monitoring should be the same as that of wrapped cycles. Physical parameters (time, temperature, and pressure) are verified by reviewing the recorded (by gauges, graphs, or printouts) information to check the proper function of the sterilizer.

Table 12.6 Typical Flash Steam Sterilization Parameters

Type of Sterilizer	Load Configuration	Time	Exposure Temperature	Drying Time
Gravity Displacement	Metal or nonporous items only (no instruments with lumens)	3 minutes	270–275°F (132–135°C)	0 – 1 minute
	Metal items with lumens and porous items (rubber) sterilized together	10 minutes	270–275°F (132–135°C)	0 – 1 minute
	Complex devices (power equipment) [Manufacturer's instruction should be consulted and followed.]	10 minutes	270–275°F (132–135°C)	0 – 1 minute
Dynamic Air-Removal (Pre-Vac)	Metal or nonporous items only (no instruments with lumens)	3 minutes	270–275°F (132–135°C)	N/A
	Metal items with lumens and porous items sterilized together	4 minutes	270°F (132°C)	N/A
	Metal items with lumens and porous items sterilized together	3 minutes	275°F (135°C)	N/A

Adapted from AAMI, 2009.

An internal chemical indicator (CI; preferably a Class 5 integrating indicator) should be placed along with the instruments on the inside of an open, perforated-bottom flash tray. An external CI should be used on a rigid reusable sealed containment tray to determine whether it has gone through the sterilization process. If a rigid container is used, two CIs should be used, one in two opposite corners. The indicator will show whether the physical parameters of steam sterilization were achieved within the container or tray; a Class 5 integrating indicator will monitor all parameters of the cycle (time, temperature, and the presence of steam).

Biological testing of the flash sterilizer cycles using a process challenge device (PCD) should be performed at least weekly, preferably every day the sterilizer us used. If multiple flash sterilization cycles are used (i.e., 4 minutes and 10 minutes), only the shortest cycle needs to be tested. If a gravity and a dynamic air removal cycle are used, each cycle type needs to have a PCD run to test the cycle. If different trays or rigid containers are used, you need to test each with a BI at least weekly, but preferably every day the sterilizer is used.

Table 12.6 provides the recommended cycle times for flash sterilization.

The device manufacturer's sterilization recommendations should be followed for each sterilization method.

Some medical devices cannot be flashed in gravity displacement sterilizers. If they are to be flash sterilized, it must be in a dynamic air removal sterilizer.

After the cycle, the item must be transported directly to the point of use—in a way minimizing the potential exposure to contaminants. If an open, perforated-bottom tray was used, there will be condensate present within the tray. Staff should don a pair of sterile gloves. Sterile towels can be used as a potholder when removing the tray from the sterilizer. A sterile towel or a sterile flat metal tray can be placed over the instruments, using aseptic technique to take the tray to the point of use.

Neither the open flash tray nor the rigid reusable sealed containment tray should be placed directly onto the sterile field; a scrubbed person can carefully remove the item from the tray with sterile forceps or gloved hands. The item will be hot. The item must be cooled prior to use on a patient because it could cause a burn to the tissues.

AORN standards do not recognize flash sterilization for implants because of the increased risk of surgical site infection. AAMI specifies that implantable medical devices should not be flash sterilized. In a clinical setting, sometimes flashing of an implant is unavoidable. Each facility should develop written guidance regarding what the emergency situations are. One definition is "life or limb" threatening. When this occurs, a BI with a Class 5 chemical indicator should be run with the load. The implant should be held until the BI results are known. If the item is implanted before the BI results are known, documentation must be completed for premature release of implantable device. The FDA defines implantable devices as those that are placed into a surgically or naturally formed body cavity with the intention of remaining there for 30 days or more.

Flash sterilization monitoring is an essential part of quality assurance. Record keeping of each flash cycle should contain all or most of the following information:

- Date of the flash sterilization.
- Identification of the sterilizer.
- Name of the person who cleaned the item.
- Load or cycle number.
- Specific instrument.
- Exposure time and temperature (read from the chart or printout).
- Patient name and medical record number.
- Name of the person running the load.
- Name of the person removing it from the sterilizer and transporting it to the point of use.
- Process indicator used (Class 4 or 5).
- Date and result of the latest BI.
- Reason for flash sterilization.

Summary

Flash sterilization can be performed safely if staff members are trained properly and if everyone follows established guidelines. Flash sterilization should be closely monitored and used only when absolutely necessary.

PROCESSING OF MEDICAL EQUIPMENT CONTAMINATED WITH PRIONS

Prions are defined as small proteinaceous infectious particles. They are transmissible pathogenic agents that cause disease with a long incubation period, from 2 months to 20 years. Prions are most frequently found in the brain, dura mater, and spinal cord; they can cause death within several months after initial onset of symptoms. Prions cause the animal diseases of scrapie in goats and sheep, bovine spongiform encephalopathy (BSE, or "mad-cow disease") in cattle, feline spongiform encephalopathy in domestic cats, chronic wasting disease in elk and mule deer, as well as Creutzfeldt-Jakob disease (CJD) in humans. These diseases go under the general heading of transmissible spongiform encephalopathy, or TSE.

It is extremely important to note that the usual procedures for disinfection and sterilization of reusable medical devices and instruments will not inactivate prions. Scientific literature and various health care authorities have made recommendations for processing of equipment, but these are all subject to ongoing review and modification. The CDC should be relied on for the most updated and current recommendations on processing devices contaminated with high-risk tissue (brain and dura mater) (AAMI, 2009).

In human health care, disinfection and sterilization recommendations are based on risk categories that are dependent on the probability that the individual has TSE, the level of infectivity of tissue of the individual, and the route of exposure to the tissue (IAHCSMM, 2007). The distribution of infectivity ranges from high concentration to low or no infectivity detected. High-infectivity tissue includes central nervous system tissue—brain and dura mater, spinal cord—as well as the eye (cornea). Medium-infectivity tissue includes cerebrospinal fluid, lymph nodes, spleen, pituitary gland, and tonsil. Low-infectivity or no-infectivity tissue includes blood, bone marrow, heart, lung, liver, kidney, nasal mucous, and sputum.

Decontamination Guidelines for Equipment Contaminated with High-Infectivity Tissue

Guidelines vary for procedures to decontaminate equipment that has come into contact with high-infectivity tissue. The World Health Organization (WHO) made recommendations in 2003 for cleaning and sterilizing high-risk critical or semicritical medical devices using a combination of sodium hydroxide and sterilization of the immersed instruments. However, the WHO procedure can create dangerous vapors and will damage the internal chamber of the sterilizer and the instruments. AAMI recommendations state that under no circumstances should devices or instruments be processed by the WHO guidelines as it is dangerous to staff members.

When a patient is suspected of having prion disease, single-use instruments and devices should be used. Disposable gowns and surgical drapes, instruments with lumens (e.g., needles, suction tubing), and other single-use devices (e.g., biopsy sets) should be placed in biohazard sharps boxes after the procedure and incinerated. Any liquid from the procedure or cleaning should be solidified and incinerated.

Universal recommendations for handling of high-risk instruments include keeping them damp until they can be decontaminated; they should be decontaminated as soon as possible after they are used. Drying renders prions more resistant to steam sterilization. If the item can be adequately cleaned, it can then be decontaminated by:

1. Processing in a dynamic air removal sterilizer at 272°F (134°C) for 18 minutes.
2. Processing in a gravity displacement sterilizer at 250°F (121°C) for 60 minutes.
3. Immersed in 1 N sodium hydroxide (40 g sodium hydroxide in 1 liter water) for 60 minutes at room temperature followed by steam sterilization at 250°F (121°C) in a gravity displacement sterilizer for 30 minutes.

Following these decontamination procedures, the item can be cleaned, wrapped, and sterilized by the standard cycle.

If the high-risk item is unable to be cleaned, it should be discarded (incinerated).

If devices or instrumentation used are generally processed in low-temperature sterilization (e.g., ethylene oxide or hydrogen peroxide gas plasma), they should be discarded (incinerated) because ethylene oxide, hydrogen peroxide gas plasma, and peracetic acid are ineffective against prions.

If noncritical medical devices contaminated with high-infectivity tissue are cleanable, first clean according to your routine procedures. Then disinfect with a 1:5* dilution of sodium hypochlorite (5000 ppm of available chlorine) or 1 N sodium hydroxide (40 g sodium hydroxide in 1 liter water), using the solution least damaging to the instrument. Then process according to your routine procedure.

For environmental surfaces exposed to high-infectivity tissue, a disposable, impermeable material should be used to cover the surface before exposure. This material is then incinerated after use. The person cleaning the area should wear a disposable gown, gloves, mask, and eye protection. The area is first cleaned with a detergent, then the surface is disinfected with a 1 part sodium hypochlorite* to 5 parts water. Next, the entire surface should be cleaned by the routine procedure for surface decontamination. The gown, gloves, and mask should be incinerated following the cleaning process.

Decontamination Guidelines for Equipment Contaminated with Medium-, Low-, or Non-Infectivity Tissue

Guidelines for medium-, low-, or non-infectivity tissue exposure for critical, semicritical, or noncritical items need to be cleaned, disinfected, and sterilized according to routine procedures. This includes high-level disinfection or thermal or chemical sterilization. If the item cannot be cleaned, it should be disposed of.

Further Recommendations for Equipment with Possible Prion Contamination

Other general recommendations for surgical instruments that were used on a known or suspected patient include the following:

- No flash sterilization methods for reprocessing any of the devices exposed to high-infectivity tissue.
- Keep instruments moist to minimize drying of blood, tissue, or body fluids on the instruments.
- Avoid mixing instruments used on low- or non-infectivity tissues with those used on high-infectivity tissues.
- Become familiar with the safety guidelines when working with sodium hydroxide and high concentrations of sodium chloride.
- Avoid the use of power drills or saws as their design makes them difficult to adequately clean and they are too expensive to discard.

Summary

To restate the aforementioned caveat, at the time this book was written, these are the best-practice procedures for dealing with prion contamination. The CDC is the most reliable source for updated and current procedures.

Prions are resistant to regular disinfection techniques. If prion disease is suspected, special handling techniques for equipment and instruments should be implemented. Disinfection or disposal of items exposed to high-infectivity tissue should be clearly spelled out in the facility policy. Specialized training in the handling of chemicals used in the decontamination should follow OSHA guidelines.

---

*Check the amount of sodium hypochlorite present as concentrations can range from 3% to 6%.)

REFERENCES

[AAMI] Association for the Advancement of Medical Instrumentation. 2009. *ANSI/AAMI ST79:2006, Amendments A1 & A2, 2009. Comprehensive Guide to Steam Sterilization and Sterility Assurance in Health Care Facilities.* American National Standards Institute, Arlington, VA, pp 72–76.

[AAMI] Association for the Advancement of Medical Instrumentation. 2009. *ANSI/AAMI ST79:2006, Amendments A1 & A2, 2009. Comprehensive Guide to Steam Sterilization and Sterility Assurance in Health Care Facilities.* Annex C: Processing CJD-contaminated patient care equipment and environmental surfaces. American National Standards Institute, Arlington, VA, pp 131–135.

[AORN] Association of periOperative Registered Nurses. 2009. Sterilization, recommendation IV, in *Perioperative Standards and Recommended Practices.* AORN, Denver, CO, pp 650–653.

[AORN] Association of periOperative Registered Nurses. 2009. Cleaning and processing endoscopes, in *Perioperative Standards and Recommended Practices.* AORN, Denver, CO, pp 595–609.

Conmed/Linvatec. 3.1 Cleaning and Sterilizing 3M K-200 series. *Mini-Driver Operating and Maintenance Manual.*

Dix K. 2008. Scope cleaning and repair, top 10 ways to keep scopes happy. *Infect Control Today* 12(3):46–52.

Hellinger WC, et al. 2007. Special Report: Recommended practices for cleaning and sterilizing intraocular surgical instruments. *J Cataract Refract Surg* 33:1095–1100.

[IAHCSMM] International Association of Healthcare Central Service Material Management. 2007. *Central Service Technical Manual, 7th ed.* IAHCSMM, Chicago, IL, pp 198–206.

Myrna K et al. 2009. Letter to the Editor: Toxic anterior segment syndrome and are we missing it? *Am Coll Vet Ophthalmol* 12(2):138.

Rutala WA, Weber DJ, Healthcare Infection Control Practices Advisory Committee (HICPAC). 2008. *Guideline for Disinfection and Sterilization in Healthcare Facilities.* CDC, Atlanta, GA, p 60.

Slocum Enterprises. Pneumatic Oscillating Saw-Catalog No. 7140S. *Operating Instructions.* Slocum Enterprises, Inc. Eugene, OR.

Tams TR. 1999. Endoscopic instrumentation, in *Small Animal Endoscopy, 2nd ed.* pp 1–16. Mosby, St. Louis, MO.

Whittemore Enterprises. *Whittemore T.P.L.O. Saw Manual & Care Instructions.* Whittemore Enterprises, Rancho Cucamonga, CA.

13 Surgical Textiles, Linens, and Laundry

Linda Caveney

The use of reusable fabrics (as opposed to one-time use disposables) in the veterinary field is very widespread. The history of the fabrics, common applications, and how to launder then appropriately are covered in this section.

HISTORY OF TEXTILES

The first reusable woven material used in surgery was muslin (100% unbleached cotton cloth) called T-14 (Reichert, 1997). The T number is the sum of the threads per inch in both woven directions. A barrier is formed by creating a tortuous path of two layers of muslin through which microorganisms cannot penetrate on their own (Reichert and Young, 1997). For surgical wrappers, the two layers are sewn together at the edges to make one drape or cloth wrapper. A disadvantage of 100% cotton material is that it generates high levels of lint and can withstand only about 30 reprocessing (laundering and sterilization) cycles. Also, in surgical and sterilization applications, muslin absorbs liquids and therefore does not provide a barrier to microorganisms; they are carried through the fabric by the liquid. In the late 1960s, a blend of 50% cotton and 50% polyester (known as T-180 percale) was introduced into the medical field. It was slightly more durable (allowing 40 reprocessing cycles) but still was not a barrier to liquids.

Today, there are a wide variety of synthetic fabrics available with different levels of barrier performance. Barrier performance is defined as a boundary between clean and unclean area or between an aseptic field and a contaminated area. Barrier protection characteristics are especially important when selecting surgical drapes, gowns, and wrappers because of the potential for liquid strike-through (penetration of a liquid or microorganisms through a fabric causing the otherwise sterile field to become contaminated). The type and characteristics of these items are dependent on the task and degree of anticipated exposure. Table 13.1 reviews the barrier level of fabrics.

GENERAL RECOMMENDATIONS FOR REUSABLE SURGICAL LINENS

There are pros and cons when choosing between using disposable and reusable textiles. The human health care field has accepted the Association for the Advancement of Medical

Veterinary Infection Prevention and Control, First Edition. Edited by Linda Caveney and Barbara Jones with Kimberly Ellis.
© 2012 John Wiley & Sons, Inc. Published by John Wiley & Sons, Inc.

Table 13.1   Barrier Level of Fabrics

Barrier Level	Fabrics
None	T-140 muslin T-180 percale
Low	T-280 cotton, tightly woven Quarpel-treated T-175 50%cotton/50%polyester, tightly woven, Quarpel-treated
Medium	100% polyester, tightly woven, chemically finished
High	Synthetic laminate coated fabric

Source: Reichert and Young, 1997.

Instrumentation (AAMI) guidelines for performance properties—minimum strength, barrier protection, and fluid resistance—in selecting the appropriate product. AAMI uses an industry-established system of classification based on four liquid barrier performance tests: Spray Impact test (simulates resistance to "arterial spurting"); Hydrostatic Pressure test (a fabric's resistance to liquid being forced through it under a defined amount of pressure); American Society for Testing and Materials' ASTM F1670 (measures resistance of materials to penetration by synthetic blood at 2 psi under ambient pressure); and ASTM F1671 (measures resistance of materials by viral penetration at 2 psi and ambient pressure). These standards are used to assess the protective capabilities of a product, generally those used in surgery. AAMI performance levels range from 1 (least protective level) to 4 (most protective level). For surgical procedures in which exposure to blood and other body fluids is anticipated, an AAMI Level 3 gown is appropriate. AAMI PB70—Standard and Reusable Apparel—sets the criteria for reusable textile apparel. The manufacturer of reusable products must provide processing information, and this must be followed by the user. Ask the manufacturer for data that define the test methods used for evaluating the barrier properties; are these conducted under actual hospital laundry and sterilization capabilities? The manufacturer should provide information on what detergents and other chemicals can be used, the recommended wash cycle, water temperature, and recommended drying temperature and cycle time. Also important is finding out whether the fabric should be washed within a designated time period (from end of the procedure to the wash cycle) to assure that blood or other body fluids are removed. It is also essential to ask how the loss of effective barrier and repellency properties are tested—how can failures be recognized? Manufacturers state the number of times an item can undergo laundering and sterilization cycles before showing reduced performance characteristics; generally this is up to 50 times but ask what are the recognizable factors for reuse or downgrading to a nonprotective category of use. Once the item has been tested in accordance to the manufacturer's recommendation and demonstrates reduced performance, it can no longer be relied on to provide adequate barrier protection and is pulled from use.

Whether choosing disposable or reusable textiles, there are direct and indirect costs involved. For reusable textiles, there is the cost of purchasing the items and determining the correct inventory; bins and/or carts for clean and soiled items; labor involved in all steps of the process; laundry equipment and agents or cost of off-site laundry contracts; and maintenance of equipment and the textiles themselves. For disposable gowns, draping, and wrappers, there is the cost of purchasing the items; storage; developing a system for inventory control; disposal containers; and the cost of disposing of soiled items. Table 13.2 provides a comparison summary of disposable versus reusable linens.

Table 13.2   Choice of Reusable vs. Disposable Surgical Linens

Disposables	Reusables
Constant cost for purchasing	Large start-up expense for items and collection receptacles
Readily available	Needs to be sorted, folded, wrapped, and sterilized by staff
Guarantee of consistent barrier quality	Variability in barrier quality dependent of use
Ease of disposal	Handling of potentially contaminated gowns and drapes could spread microorganisms
Adds to landfills	Adds pollutants to water and air
Consumes more energy and materials to produce	Cleaning of reusable items consumes water, chemicals, and energy
Made of spun-bonded–melt-blown polyethylene; polyethylene film laminated beneath the nonwoven fabric in critical areas	Made of densely woven fabric-pina cotton with 270–280 threads per square inch or tightly woven 100% polyester
Cannot be resterilized	Limited number of laundering and sterilization cycles before finish deteriorates
	Continual need for repair and replacement
Need storage space	Need designated area for processing of reusable items: clean and dirty area for sorting, clean area for folding and wrapping, storage for wrapped unsterile items, as well as clean storage area for sterilized items.
	If processed on site, equipment/preventative maintenance cost

The use of reusable linens is far more labor intensive as compared with the use of disposable counterparts. The process starts with the sorting of all the textile products (surgical drapes, gowns, wrappers). Visual inspection of the critical zones of gowns, drapes, sterilization wraps, and table covers includes checking to see whether stain or residue removal is necessary; checking for physical defects, such as cuts, holes, punctures, small tears in the fabric, or missing components (i.e., ties on surgical gowns) that need repair; or if there is chemical or thermal damage that needs to be repaired. Detecting holes or other physical defects can easily be accomplished with a "light table." When textiles are passed over the top surface of a table with a built-in light source, small holes can be seen when light shows through. Otherwise, a light-colored table and a bright overhead light can be used to help identify small holes or punctures. A hole 1 micron or larger will allow bacteria to penetrate. An average microorganism is 0.5–1 micron, although there are many smaller than this average size.

If holes are identified, the option of a fabric heat-sealed patch of the same quality material as the items can be used to cover the hole. If the item is double ply, the patch is applied to both sides of the item. If the item is single ply, a patch is applied only to one side of the item. Sewing a patch on is not recommended because stitches make holes for microorganisms to go through. The hole made by a stitch is approximately 20 microns; this is 20 times larger than the average size microorganism. A limit should be set as to the number of patches that are acceptable. There is no "magic number" or percentage of coverage area that can be set for each reusable textile. The position of the patch (whether it is in the critical zone or on the periphery of the item), the number of layers of patched fabric, the shape and size of the patch itself, and the sterilization method used all need to be assessed in determining whether the item is acceptable or should be pulled from use. Patching material can prevent steam penetration so only the outside surface of the fabric is sterilized. Patches may also interfere with the drapability of the item.

Physical defects that can compromise the function of the item are things such as loose threads or missing ties or snaps. These items are sent for mending (repair by sewing). Sewing is used in the noncritical zones of the surgical product. If it creates needle holes near the critical zone, a patch can be applied to cover the holes. After the repair, the item is again sent for laundering.

Chemical or thermal damage can affect the function of a surgical item. Damage can occur while being used in the surgical procedure (contact with surgical cement or glue) or during the laundry cycle, when there is direct contact with concentrated chlorine bleach or overheating in the drying process. Depending on the severity, extent, and size of the damaged area, the item may or may not be able to continue to be used. If it can be repaired by patching, it can still be used.

Stains or discolorations of the surgical products can be caused by multiple factors; many may not represent a significant problem or affect the performance of the item. Medical stains caused by iodine-based products used in surgical prep, scarlet red or methyl blue, do not affect the performance but they may not be acceptable because of the perception of the lack of cleanliness. Color fade because of repeated laundering, ink or marker stains, or color change from autoclave tape are all acceptable as they do not affect the function or performance of the item. Dark brown or rust-colored stains resembling blood, raised residue, colorless oil stain, or scorched or melted fabric are examples of discoloration that should be reevaluated for either relaundering using special stain removal methods or discarded (items with raised residue that cannot be removed without damage to the integrity of the item).

Inspection also entails monitoring the number of laundry cycles an item has been through. Follow the textile manufacturer's recommendations for laundering agents and number of cycles; recommendations are backed by scientific testing of the barrier claims of the fabrics and should be followed closely.

Reusable textiles need to undergo steam sterilization. The steam penetration may be hindered by newer, tightly woven materials with moisture-retardant features. Sterilization may not be achieved within the normal sterilization phase because of the slow penetration of the steam. Each facility should conduct a test using a biological indicator placed in the center of the pack with the greatest density. If the biologic indicator is positive, the pack configuration or the sterilization cycle will need to be altered and retested with the new configuration of cycle time.

All reusable fabric materials should be laundered after they have been through a sterilization cycle. A condition called "superheating" can occur if reusable fabric material is again put through another sterilization cycle without proper laundering (AORN, 2009a,b). Superheating occurs when the material is dried during the first sterilization cycle. Processing the cloth again makes it take longer for the steam to penetrate through (because the fabric is taking on the moisture of steam); therefore, the inside of the pack will not achieve the proper temperature in the recommended time of the sterilization cycle. Reusable fabrics need to be rehydrated during the laundry cycle so this does not occur.

All fabrics that undergo the laundry process and storage should be held at room temperature (64–72°F) with a relative humidity range of 35% to 70%.

Actual laundry cycle recommendations are provided by the material's manufacturer. These include the time for each laundering process, action of repeated changes of water, water temperature, and chemical agents for each cycle. Another important factor is the temperature of the drying cycle. Some newer fabrics can "melt" when exposed to excessive heat. Recommendations should be followed to obtain the anticipated performance and life of the product. The manufacturer will also recommend the maximum number of reuses for the product based on laboratory testing. Commonly, a grid-type box is imprinted on the material; after each laundry cycle, another box can be checked to keep count of uses.

ENVIRONMENTAL AREA FOR LAUNDRY HANDLING

Veterinary facilities should have a designated area for handling and processing soiled laundry. This can either be separated by physical barrier or by negative air pressure in the soiled area compared with adjacent areas. Clean linen should be stored in a "clean" area, free from lint accumulation, positive air pressure with regards to adjacent areas, and with controlled temperature and humidity. Dirty and clean laundry should not be comingled.

HANDLING OF SOILED LINENS

Soiled textiles and fabric should be placed in bags or containers that can be securely tied or closed to prevent leakage as they are transported to the sorting/laundering area. Any bulk solids (e.g., feces, clumps of hair) should be removed from the item before the reusable materials are placed in collection container for laundering.

Care should be taken to remove all nontextile items (such as instruments or sharps) before textiles are placed in the collection container.

Soiled laundry can be sorted by either type of similar fabrics or type of goods (i.e., surgical gowns and linen, towels, blankets, lab coats).

If items have come from a patient with a known zoonotic disease, the collection container should be labeled with the name of the disease organism. Facilities can also determine a "discard rather than launder" risk policy. Reusable patient care items from patients with parvovirus, panleukopenia, or ringworm may result in further spread of the organisms and contamination of the facility during transporting and handling of these highly resistant organisms. This is evaluated by a risk-versus-benefit of the items. Patient bedding (which is heavily contaminated) may fall under this policy, whereas a reusable barrier pad used during patient examination (minimally contaminated) could be carefully contained in a plastic laundry bag or container, labeled, and transported to the laundry area for processing.

The staff member who does the sorting should always wear a minimum of gloves while handling these or any soiled items. An additional protective cover (i.e., lab coat or smock) should be donned while sorting of facility laundry. This attire is removed in the dirty area. If the person doing the sorting has other duties, a change of attire is highly recommended. Hand washing should be performed after either removing the protective attire and gloves prior to leaving the area or changing of attire and leaving the area.

LAUNDRY PROCESS

All reusable textiles should be laundered according to the manufacturer's recommendations. For the most part, a regular or commercial washing machine with hot water, detergents and bleach, timed cycles—followed by drying in a dryer on "heat" cycle—should render an item free of vegetative pathogens in the majority of cases (HICPAC, 2003).

The laundering process is a combination of mechanical, thermal, and chemical factors. Dilution and agitation in water removes a substantial quantity of microorganisms. Do not overload your washing machine; the agitation and dispersal of the detergent will be hampered if you overload your machine's capabilities. Soap/detergents suspend the particles in water and exhibit some microbiocidal properties. Hot water (160°F) for a minimum of 25 minutes is a very effective means of killing microorganisms. Chlorine bleach assures another level of safety in the killing of microorganisms. Chlorine bleach becomes activated in water temperatures of 135–145°F. Chlorine bleach is an economical, broad-spectrum germicide. Check the washing machine's manufacturer's recommendations as to the appropriate amount of bleach to add to a regular laundry cycle. Chlorine bleach alternatives can be used for those fabrics on which bleach cannot be used. Alternatives, such as activated oxygen-based laundry detergents, can provide color safety and antimicrobial activity. The oxygen-based products should be registered by the EPA to ensure adequate disinfection. Lower temperature wash cycles can save on the use of hot water and energy in the facility. Lower water temperatures (71–77°F) can reduce microbial contamination only if the wash cycles, detergent, and additives are carefully monitored and controlled. These low-temperature cycles depend heavily on the presence of chlorine or oxygen-activated bleach to reduce the microbial contamination. Consult the washing machine manufacturer and the laundry detergent manufacturer for specific application for your machine and detergent usage. Rinsing with the addition of a mild acid (known as "sour" in the commercial laundry world) will neutralize the alkalinity of the soap or detergent. The change in pH will also inactivate some microorganisms. A final extraction process is used to remove excess water; this is done by hydraulic pressure or centrifugal action. This facilitates a more rapid drying.

Damp textiles should not be left in machines overnight; this can be a breeding ground for microorganisms.

The drying process uses heat and air flow to dry damp textiles. The temperatures reached in drying will provide additional microbiocidal action. The individual temperature setting, heating times, and cool down times are adjusted depending on the performance and durability of the textiles being dried.

Once dry, each item is folded and sorted for distribution to use areas, storage, or holding area.

The storage area where the textiles are being stored prior to being assembled into finished packs should be controlled to prevent contamination. This is especially critical when open shelving or carts are used. This entails limiting traffic in the area, ensuring the area is properly ventilated, and the area is cleaned and kept free of dust and lint. A solid barrier for the bottom shelves protects against inadvertent contamination during cleaning (mopping).

AORN POSITION ON HOME LAUNDERING OF PERSONAL SURGICAL ATTIRE

The Association of Perioperative Nurses (AORN) does not recommend home laundering of surgical attire (Belkin, 2009). Commercial or hospital laundries follow strict guidelines throughout the entire laundry process and have documentation of all phases of the cycle. Although there is no concrete evidence to support or refute the practice, surgical attire becomes soiled or contaminated with microorganisms during wear. Taking worn or contaminated surgical attire home can result in spread of contamination to the home environment. AORN is aware that some facilities require employees to launder scrub attire; they do not support it. OSHA holds employers responsible for laundering those scrubs that have become contaminated with blood or other potentially infectious body fluids. This applies only to applicable members of the surgical staff.

Steps should be taken to minimize contaminants in the home environment by following some minimum criteria. Some of the suggested criteria for home laundering of surgical attire by AORN 2009 include the following:

- Use an automatic washer and hot air dryer.
- Use water temperature of 110–125°F (43.3–51.66°C).
- Use chlorine bleach.
- Use detergent according to manufacturer's recommendations.
- Launder surgical attire in a separate load from other items.
- Surgical attire should be the last load laundered.
- Keep laundry items completely submerged during the wash and rinse cycle to facilitate removal of soil or microorganisms. Avoid placing hands or arms in the laundry water.
- Thoroughly clean the door and lid of the washing machine before removing the surgical attire at the end of the cycle to prevent reintroduction of contaminants on cleaned attire when removing it from the washer to the dryer.
- Do not allow soiled items (or laundered wet items) to remain in the washing machine.
- Use the highest possible drying temperature that is safe for the material the scrubs are made of.
- Promptly remove the attire when dry to avoid heat desiccation of the materials.
- Protect the laundered items by placing them in a container or plastic bag to transport them to the practice.

LAUNDRY AREA ENVIRONMENTAL CLEANING

The floors and walls in the laundry should be constructed of material that can withstand routine wet cleaning as well as the heat and humidity of the environment. The ventilation system should be designed so that the air blows from the clean textile area to the soiled areas and is exhausted outside.

The dirty/sorting area as well as the clean area should be cleaned and disinfected daily or whenever either becomes visibly contaminated. All areas where laundry is processed should be kept free of lint and dust. Vents, walls, and ceilings should undergo a periodic vacuuming or blow-down process to reduce the build up of dust and lint. It is essential to have a sink for hand washing in the soiled area.

CONCLUSION

Textiles in a veterinary medical facility are considered hygienically clean when they are laundered with the proper amounts of detergent and bleach (or bleach alternatives) and subject to mechanical agitation in water of suitable temperature for the correct cycle time, then dried on high-heat cycles. Textile fabrics can be used with confidence on the next patient when a well thought out and executed protocol for reusable material infection control has been established and implemented. A combination of reusable textiles and disposable products is possible. Co-existence of both systems is directed toward making intelligent choices for quality patient care by proper use of materials that offer aseptic excellence and effectiveness rather than totally replacing one or the other.

REFERENCES

Association for the Advancement of Medical Instrumentation, American National Standard Institute Inc. *ANSI/AAMI ST 65:2008. Processing of reusable surgical textiles for use in health care facilities.* ANSI/AAMI, Arlington, VA, pp 7–47.

[AORN] Association of periOperative Registered Nurses. 2009a. Selection of gowns and drapes: recommendations I–VIII, in *Perioperative Standards and Recommended Practices.* AORN, Denver, CO, pp 361–365.

AORN. 2009b. Surgical attire: recommendation I, in *Perioperative Standards and Recommended Practices.* AORN, Denver, CO, pp 299–300.

Belkin NL. 2009. Chapter 101: Laundry, patient linens, textiles and uniforms, in *APIC Text of Infection Control and Epidemiology.* Association for Infection Control and Epidemiology, Washington, DC.

Disposable Products Enhance Infection Prevention Efforts. Available at: http://www.infectioncontroltoday.com. 2009. Article 244008. Virgo Publishing, Phoenix, AZ.

Hurley K. 2008. Potentials and Pitfalls of Infectious Disease Control for Practicing Veterinarians. Presented at Western Veterinary Conference, February 2008, Las Vegas, NV.

Reichert M, Young, JH. 1997. *Sterilization Technology for the Health Care Facility, 2nd ed.* Aspen Publication, Gaithersburg, MD.

The Healthcare Laundry Accreditation Council. 2006. *Accreditation Standards for Processing Reusable Textiles for Use in Healthcare Facilities.* HLAC, DuBois, PA.

[HICPAC] Healthcare Infection Control Practices Advisory Committee, U.S. Department of Health and Human Services, and CDC. 2003. *Guidelines for Environmental Infection Control in Health-Care Facilities.* CDC, Atlanta, GA.

14 Infection Control: The Surgical Environment and Ancillary Areas

Linda Caveney

The operating room is where aseptic surgical procedures take place. Surgical procedures put the patient at risk for surgical site infection (SSI) unless strict environmental and equipment care and maintenance are established. Patients are anesthetized for surgical procedures but often need radiographs before and after the procedure. It is common to simultaneously have patients being anesthetized for dental procedures, scoping, or other minimally invasive procedures that do not go into the operating room. Therefore, it is critical to have written protocols established for the protection of all patients. The policies should be reviewed periodically and updated as personnel and technology change. This chapter will review the recommended practices for the surgical environment, including general composition of an operating room, ventilation and air quality, traffic zones, surgical attire, recommended patient protection, and environmental cleaning of the operating room. This chapter also reviews the recommended practices for the areas of anesthesia and dentistry or dirty surgery, including environmental aspects, patient safety, and equipment cleaning and disinfection.

THE SURGICAL ENVIRONMENT

Controlling the operating room (OR) or surgical suite environment, education of key perioperative personnel in aseptic technique, and patient protection from SSIs are fundamental in achieving successful surgical outcomes. Development of effective strategies for preventing SSIs is the responsibility of all staff members, from those that do the cleaning to the surgeon. Continual assessment of new techniques and products to facilitate changes for quality improvement activities should be the mission of the facility for positive patient outcomes.

General Composition of the Operating Room

The surgical suite should be large enough to accommodate the required equipment—such as the anesthetic machine and monitoring equipment, IV pole, patient table, instrument table, mayo stand, gowning table, stools or chairs, and supply cabinet—while allowing movement of sterile personnel without getting contaminated. The floors, ceiling, and walls should be smooth, nonporous surfaces for ease of cleaning. These materials should be able to withstand frequent cleaning and disinfectant application. Cabinets containing supplies (e.g., scalpel blades, suture

Veterinary Infection Prevention and Control, First Edition. Edited by Linda Caveney and Barbara Jones with Kimberly Ellis.
© 2012 John Wiley & Sons, Inc. Published by John Wiley & Sons, Inc.

material, gauze sponges, etc.) that are located in the operating room should have tight-fitting doors that are kept closed unless items are being retrieved from them. The surgical lights should have maximum maneuverability and ideally should be located directly above the operating table suspended by a ceiling mount. Lights should be able to be easily cleaned. The patient table (operating table) should be made of stainless steel and have height and tilt adjustments. Specialized radiolucent tables are available with easy-to-clean surfaces to accommodate intraoperative imaging. A pad or mat on the table helps maintain body temperature and assists in positioning of the patient; pad/mat materials should be chosen for their ease of cleaning and disinfection after each surgical procedure. The use of water-circulating heating pads and hot air heating systems assist in sustaining the patient's temperature throughout the procedure. An instrument table or mayo stand should be made from stainless steel; it should be large enough to accommodate the instruments and equipment for the most complex surgical procedures.

Each room should have a sharps container for easy disposal of the surgical blades, needles, and other items deemed as "sharps" waste, whether used in the surgical procedure or by the anesthesiologist. Containers for other biological "red bag" waste should be available and used in compliance with all local, state, and federal regulations.

Ventilation and Air Quality

Air pressure balancing describes the pressure relationship of a room to the adjacent area or hall. It can be positive (excess air pressure in the room that causes air to flow out of the room), negative (air being drawn into a room from adjacent area or hall), or neutral. Operating rooms should be designed to provide positive air flow as compared with the adjoining rooms or hallways. Positive air flow decreases the likelihood of outside contaminated air entering the operating room. Each time the door is opened for passage of equipment or personnel, this pressure gradient is disrupted, allowing for contaminated air to flow into the OR. The ventilation in the operating room should operate at all times to maintain air movement relationship to adjacent areas. If the ventilation system is shut down for any reason, the cleanliness of the space may be compromised. Sudden activation of the system causes a rapid air turbulence that stirs settled particles, causing them to become airborne (Bartley and Olmsted, 2009). A simple way to check for positive air flow is to slightly open the door to the operating room from the adjacent area and hold a single-ply tissue in the opening. The tissue should move outward toward the adjacent area or hall.

The temperature and humidity of the operating room should be kept constant. The air temperature should be maintained at 66–70°F (18–21°C) with a minimum of 15–20 air exchanges per hour of filtered air, of which 20% should be fresh air (Kane, 2009). Air changes per hour (ACH) is the number of times the air volume of a given space is replaced in a 1-hour period and includes sufficient changes of fresh (outside) air to dilute the microbial contamination and gases (Kane, 2009). A minimum of two ACH of outside air is what is needed to remove odors. The humidity should be controlled to between 30% and 60%. The use of stand-alone humidifiers, dehumidifiers, and fans within the OR is not recommended. Table 14.1 provides a summary of APIC's recommendations for ventilation, temperature, and humidity in the OR as well as other patient care areas.

Filtration and Air-Cleaning Systems

Enhanced air filtration technology primarily focuses on the use of high-efficiency particulate air (HEPA) filters. HEPA filtration is defined as filtration efficiency of 99.97% in removing airborne

Table 14.1 Ventilation Requirements for Patient Care Areas

Area	Air movement relationship to adjacent area	Minimum air changes of outdoor air per hour	Minimum total air changes per hour	Relative humidity (%)	Design temperature [°F (°C)]
Operating rooms	Out	3	15	30–60	68–73 (20–23)
Intensive care	–	2	6	30–60	70–75 (21–24)
Scoping room	In	2	6–12	30–60	68–73 (20–23)
Procedure rooms	Out	3	15	30–60	70–75 (21–24)
Airborne isolation room	In	2	12	–	75 (24)
Radiology	–	–	6	–	75 (24)
Patient exam room	–	–	6	–	75 (24)
Dirty area for processing contaminated instruments	In	–	6	–	68–73 (20–23)
Clean area for sterile equipment	Out	–	4	30–60	75 (24)
Sterile pack storage	Out	–	4	Max. 70	–
Soiled linen area	In	–	10	–	–
Clean linen storage	Out	–	2	–	–

Adapted from Kane (2009).

particles 0.3 microns or larger in size (Kane, 2009). Most airborne infectious microorganisms are 0.3–0.5 microns in size. Installation of HEPA filters is typically within the heating, ventilation, and air conditioning systems. Routine preventative maintenance of the ventilation system should be scheduled according to the system manufacturer's recommendations. Maintenance includes inspection and cleaning of the ductwork, lumens, seams, coils, condensate pans, filters, to name a few, as recommended by the National Air Duct Cleaners Association (NADCA) (Kane, 2009).

Laminar airflow (LAF) refers to another type of air-handling system that produces little or no air turbulence while directing airflow. Typically, HEPA-filtered LAFs provide either vertical airflow from the ceiling to floor or horizontal airflow in a unidirectional manner across the OR from one wall to the other.

The use of ultraviolet germicidal irradiation (UVGI) may be of some benefit because it has bactericidal properties; however, a major drawback is all the air at the point of planned use needs to be exposed for sufficient time to kill microorganisms. UVGI can be used in conjunction with HEPA filters, but it is not recommended to be the only system used for control of airborne contaminants. Studies are limited that demonstrate any reduction in SSI with their use.

The use of misting and fogging technologies claim to sanitize/disinfect/sterilize the OR environment within a specific duration of time. A generating unit emits steam, vaporized hydrogen peroxide, or other gaseous oxidating agent. The main use of these units is for terminal cleaning of a room at the end of the day.

Traffic Zones and Control

Designation of specific traffic areas controls separation of clean from dirty areas, segregating clean and sterile supplies from contaminated items, and ensures that only appropriately attired staff enters the operating room.

"Clean areas" includes the operating rooms, scrub sink areas, and the area where sterile supplies are kept.

"Dirty" or "contaminated areas" are the surgical preparation area, anesthesia, lounges, instrument cleaning and processing areas, and offices. Doors between clean and contaminated areas should be kept closed at all times.

Traffic zones are based on the principles of aseptic technique. These zones are categorized as unrestricted, semi-restricted, and restricted zones.

- Unrestricted zone allows personnel in street clothes and may allow mingling with those in surgical attire.
- Semi-restricted zone encompasses the hallways, offices, and supply rooms adjacent to the OR. Surgical attire is required for entrance to this area (i.e., scrubs, hair covering, shoe covers, or designated surgical shoes).
- Restricted zone is the actual OR and surgical scrub area where scrubs, hair covering, shoe covers, and mask are required.

As previously mentioned, the air pressure in the OR is "positive," flowing from inside the room to outside areas so no contaminated air is entering the surgical suite. Limiting the opening of the OR doors maintains this positive pressure. With increased numbers of personnel in the OR, there is a rise in the amount of bacterial shedding, more air turbulence, and the potential for accidental contamination of sterile items.

Transport of Surgical Supplies

Single-use sterile supplies obtained from outside vendors that arrive in corrugated cardboard boxes or other external shipping containers should be taken out of the shipping container before being taken into the semi-restricted zone for storage. These boxes are considered contaminated because they may collect dust, debris, and insects during shipment.

Soiled items from the surgical procedure should be placed in covered containers and taken to the semi-restricted zone until they are reprocessed. For example, instruments should be either sprayed with an enzymatic cleaner or allowed to soak in an enzymatic solution; both should be in covered containers. Contaminated laundry must be placed in a bag and closed so it does not get mixed with clean laundry. Garbage and regulated medical waste from the procedures is collected and securely closed to prevent spillage of the contents. A cart can be used to collect all these items to take them to an area away from the clean or sterile items.

Clean and sterile items only are taken into the OR. Follow the best practice procedures for preparing, packaging, and storing of surgical equipment as described in Chapters 8 and 9. Follow the best practices for high-temperature sterilization described in Chapter 10 and low-temperature sterilization as described in Chapter 11. If sterile packs or peel pouches were taken into the OR in anticipation of use but were not used, they should be removed from the OR and returned to the cabinet or shelf from which they were taken. This facilitates unnecessary accumulation of sterile items in the OR and easier terminal cleaning and disinfection. Also, if sterile items are left in the OR, they could be splashed or inadvertently sprayed with the disinfectant, rendering them contaminated.

Surgical Attire

Surgical attire should be worn in semi-restricted and restricted areas of the facility. AORN states that "the human body is a major source of microbial contamination in this environment;

therefore, scrub clothing is worn to promote a high level of cleanliness and hygiene within the surgical environment."

Attire protocol applies to the surgical team as well as the nonsterile personnel assisting in the surgical area. Surgical attire helps control bacterial shedding; as people move, friction between their bodies and the clothing frees bacteria. Scrubs tops should be tucked into the pants and secured at the waist or fit close to the body (AORN, 2009a).

Surgical scrubs should be donned inside the facility. They should not be worn into the facility from the outside. This practice minimizes the potential for contamination of animal hair or other contaminants from the uncontrolled environment. Scrubs should be changed daily or whenever they become visibly soiled, contaminated with organic material, or wet. Changing as soon as possible helps prevent the potential for cross-contamination. Surgical scrubs should be changed daily and not stored for later use. It has been reported that bacterial colony counts are higher when scrub clothing is removed, stored in a locker, and used again (AORN, 2009a).

Soiled scrubs should be placed in designated containers for laundering. AORN recommends that scrubs worn by the scrubbed-in surgical personnel be laundered by an institution-approved laundry, whether it be in-house or by contract commercial laundry facility. The rationale for this recommendation is limiting the spread of microorganisms from the health care facility, in particular, multidrug-resistant organisms to the community. The home laundering process lacks monitoring to ensure effective killing of these microorganisms. The APIC *Use of Scrubs and Related Apparel in Health Care Facilities* is currently under revision.

Nonscrubbed staff should wear long-sleeved jackets made of the same material as scrubs, snapped or buttoned closed. This prevents bacterial shedding from bare arms onto sterile fields and minimizes the risk of inadvertent contamination by the scrub jacket front flap while handling sterile items.

Fleece is not acceptable in the OR. Fleece tends to produce lint and collect airborne contaminants.

Other garments (e.g., those worn under scrubs) should be contained completely by the surgical attire. For individuals who will be directly involved in the surgical field, the sleeves of the scrub top should be short enough to allow the hands and arms to be scrubbed without getting the sleeves wet.

Each facility can determine the policy for donning of lab coats or other protective attire over the scrubs when they are outside of the surgical environment. The use of lab coats or other cover apparel has been found to have little or no effect on reducing contamination but are used for practical enforcement and cost consideration (AORN, 2009a). Lab coats or cover apparel should be removed before entering a semi-restricted or restricted area because they can be a source of contamination (AORN, 2009a).

Entering the restricted zone of the OR, attire includes head and facial hair coverings, masks, and possibly shoe covers. Hair is a carrier of bacteria. Shedding of hair and dandruff (or in the case of a bald or shaved head, squamous cells or scurf) contaminates the surgical environment (AORN, 2009a). Head covers are designed to minimize microbial dispersal. Beards or other facial hair should be covered completely; this is best accomplished by a hood-style covering. Single-use bouffant or hood-style covers are preferred. Reusable hats or hoods should be laundered after each use. Smaller skullcap-style head covers do not cover sideburns, ears, and hair at the nape of the neck.

Masks should fully cover both mouth and nose and be secured in a manner that prevents venting around the edges of the masks. Masks are worn to filter air and to contain droplets of microorganisms expelled from the mouth and nasopharynx during talking, sneezing, and coughing. Masks should be worn when entering the surgical area. The practice of wearing head coverings and masks anytime in the surgical area should be approved by each facility in the infection control policies.

Masks should be removed by the ties (because the filter portion of the mask harbors bacterial collected from the nasopharynx and mouth) and discarded immediately. Masks should not be left hanging around the neck or tucked into one's pocket for future use.

Shoes worn in the surgical environment should be clean with no visible soiling. Cloth, open-toe, or plastic-type shoes with open holes (e.g., Crocs with open holes) do not provide protection against dropped sharp items or liquids. Shoes constructed of leather with closed toes and low heels offer the best protection and comfort. Shoe covers can be added to facilitate sanitation. Foot attire has no proven significance in reducing the incidence of SSIs (AORN, 2009a). If shoe covers are worn, they should be changed whenever they become torn, wet, or soiled. They should be removed and discarded in a designated container before leaving the surgical area; new shoe covers are donned when returning to the surgery area.

Other recommendations for the surgical personnel include the removal of rings, other jewelry, and watches. Higher bacterial counts have been noted from hands when rings are worn. Items such as earrings could potentially fall into the surgical field if they are not confined by the surgical attire. Necklaces could contaminate the front of a sterile gown if not confined.

AORN recommends that fingernails be kept short, clean, and natural. The subungual region of nails harbors the majority of microorganisms found on the hand. Longer fingernails can cause tearing of surgical or examination gloves and can injure the patient when moving or positioning them. Nail polish that is obviously chipped or worn longer than 4 days is associated with the presence of greater numbers of bacteria and has been associated with infections (AORN, 2009a).

Artificial nails should not be worn because they can harbor organisms and prevent effective hand antisepsis. Fungal growth occurs frequently under artificial nails as a result of moisture becoming trapped between natural and artificial nails.

Maintaining a Sterile Field

Surgical staff participating in the surgical procedures should follow the above protocol for attire, head covering, mask, and footwear. Surgical hand antisepsis is performed using either antimicrobial soap or an alcohol-based hand rub with persistent activity. When performing hand antisepsis using an antimicrobial soap, scrub hand and forearms for the length of time as recommended by the soap manufacturer, generally between 2 and 6 minutes of contact time. When performing surgical hand antisepsis using an alcohol-based surgical product with persistent activity, follow the manufacturer's instruction very carefully. They generally recommend using a fingernail pick to remove any debris from under the fingernail beds prior to application of the product. Some recommend prewashing of the hands and arms with a nonantimicrobial soap, rinsing, then allow hand and arms to completely dry prior to using the alcohol-based hand antisepsis product. After application of the product, it is recommended that the hands and forearms be allowed to dry thoroughly prior to donning sterile gown or gloves.

The following are guidelines for determining the appropriate size gown: the back of the gown should completely cover the surgeon's back, and the sleeve length should prevent exposure of the stockinette cuff outside the gloves. Donning of the surgical gown, followed by closed gloving, is performed away from the main instrument table on another sterile field. The front of the gown is sterile from the level of the sterile field to up to 1–2 inches of the neckline; sleeves are considered sterile from two inches above the elbow to the cuff. The back is never considered sterile. The neckline, shoulders, and underarms are also not considered sterile as they are areas of friction. Refer to Appendix D for the Donning and Removal of a Surgical Gown.

There are two methods of gloving as described by AORN and APIC:

- Closed gloving is the method of donning sterile gloves whereby the scrubbed hands remain inside the cuffs and sleeves of the gown until the cuffs of the sterile gloves are secured over the stockinette cuff of the gown.
- Open gloving is the method of donning sterile gloves whereby the scrubbed hands are advanced through the sleeves and the cuffs of the gown before placing them into the sterile gloves.

The stockinette cuffs collect moisture; therefore, they should be covered by a sterile glove at all times.

If gloves become contaminated, the preferred method of changing contaminated gloves is for one member of the surgical team to glove the other. This technique allows the team member to touch only the outside of the new glove when applying the glove to the other member's hand. This is referred to as "assisted gloving." If assisted gloving is not possible, the open glove method should be used. Performing the closed gloving method would allow the unclean stockinette cuff to be pulled over the scrubbed hands of the surgeon, contaminating them. Once the original sterile gloves are donned, the stockinette cuff of the gown is considered contaminated.

Sterile draping is defined as the art of covering, with sterile barrier materials, the unsterile area immediate to and surrounding the operative site (Church and Bjerke, 2009). The placement of "field drapes" (four quarter drapes) is generally accomplished with the use of huck towels or other disposable, nonabsorbent towels. These towels define the surgical field. Once placed, they should not be readjusted toward the incision site. This would contaminate the site by dragging bacteria into the area. After they are secured with towel clamps, a larger drape is placed over the patient, completely covering the animal and providing a continuous sterile field. The level of the surgical table should be minimally higher than that of the draped patient. Any area below the top surface of either the table or the patient is considered not sterile.

Any items used within a sterile field should be sterile (as opposed to high-level disinfected).

The unscrubbed staff member should introduce the items onto a sterile field by methods that maintain sterility of the field and the item being presented. Packs or peel pouches should be inspected for proper packaging, processing, and integrity prior to opening it.

To present an item wrapped with paper or linen wrap, start by opening the wrapper flap farthest away from you first, then open each side flap, and finally the nearest flap. All wrapper edges should be secured while being handed to the sterile person or to the field. Loose wrapper edges can contaminate the sterile field or the item. The internal indicator should be inspected by the scrubbed person for appropriate color change, verifying the sterilization process.

Peel pouches should be presented to the scrubbed person to prevent contamination of the contents. The edges of the package may curl and the contents may slide over the unsterile edge, contaminating the contents. When presenting any item to the sterile field, the unscrubbed persons should avoid extending their arms over the sterile field. The peel pouch's chevron seal should be opened by grasping the plastic edge with the thumb and fingers of one hand and the paper edge with the thumb and fingers of the other hand; then, with a rolling motion, carefully open the side seals. Keep control of the contents, and allow the scrubbed individual to take the item from the pouch. If there is occasion whereby an item in a peel pouch needs to be placed on a sterile table, carefully open the pouch as previously described but allow the item to lie on one side of the peel pouch; flip the item from the back side of the table onto the sterile field, maintaining control of the peel pouch at all times so it does not contaminate the sterile field. This should never be done directly over a sterile field. Other recommendations for maintaining of surgical field asepsis include the following:

- Prepare the sterile field as close as possible to the time of use. The potential for contamination increases with time. All sterile fields should be visually monitored for breaches of sterility.
- Scrubbed personnel should remain close to the sterile field. They should keep their arms and hands above the level of their waist. Arms should not be folded with hands in the axilla.
- Traffic should be kept to a minimum into and out of the surgical area while a procedure is taking place. Air currents can pick up contaminants shed from personnel and distribute them to the sterile field (AORN, 2009c).
- Unscrubbed personnel should face sterile fields when approaching them; they should not walk between two sterile fields and should be aware of the need for distance from the sterile field.
- When a break in sterile technique occurs, corrective action should be taken immediately for the patient's safety.
- Sterile cables and tubing should be secured to the sterile field with a nonperforating device.

Recommendation for Patient Protection from SSIs

Protecting the patient from SSI includes sterile prep of the surgical site, use of prophylactic antibiotics, and maintaining normal temperatures and glucose levels prior to and during the surgical procedures.

Surgical Prep

Sterile or aseptic technique refers to practices designed to render and maintain areas maximally free from microorganisms. A sterile prep is performed on the surgical patient to render the area being incised, and the adjacent area, as having reduced population of endogenous microorganisms. Proper application method of the antimicrobial agent is crucial. The most common prep agents available are chlorhexidine gluconate (alcohol-based formulation is superior to aqueous-based formulation) and iodophors (povidone-iodine). The choice of a prep agent is based on the procedure. As a general rule, chlorhexidine products are not used around the eyes, in the ears (unless specifically formulated for ear use), or on mucous membranes.

Clipping should be performed just prior to the time of the surgical procedure. Clipping the day before the surgical procedure increases the risk of SSI due to the microbial proliferation from the microscopic nicks and abrasions to the skin which enhances microbial growth. Mechanical clippers are viewed as producing less trauma to the skin than hair removal with a razor. The area being clipped should be large enough to allow for extension of the incision within the sterile field, if necessary. A general guideline is to clip a minimum of 7–8 inches (20 cm) on each side of the incision. Loose hair should be removed with a HEPA-filtered vacuum. Clipping should not be performed in the OR.

Contact time is the critical factor in presurgical skin prep. It follows the same principle as the surgical scrub application to the surgeon's hands prior to a procedure. Manufacturers' recommendations for use as a surgical skin preparation should be followed.

The general guideline for presurgical scrub with chlorhexidine gluconate is to start with the application of the undiluted scrub to the surgical site and swabbing gently with gauze for about 2 minutes to loosen and remove any dirt or organic material. A dry gauze or towel moistened with water can be used to remove the scrub and debris. This is followed by repeated application of the undiluted scrub. Gently swab the scrub around the surgical area, starting at the incision site and proceeding to the periphery. Allow the scrub to remain for a minimum contact time of 5 minutes. This is needed to achieve the maximum benefit of antibacterial activity as well as the great residual effect of the chlorhexidine. At the end of the 5 minutes, use a dry gauze or sterile saline-moistened gauze to remove any remaining soap residue.

Chlorhexidine gluconate is used topically and externally only. Unless specifically formulated for use on mucous membranes or ears, chlorhexidine gluconate should not be used on eyes, ears, or mucous membranes.

Special precautions should be taken when chlorhexidine gluconate scrub is used on cats. Cats will lick at anything that is applied to their fur or skin during grooming. Following a surgical procedure on cats, remove any residual film of the chlorhexidine gluconate from the scrub area as well as the fur surrounding the site with warm water and a towel. Chlorhexidine has been suggested as the cause for adverse reactions to laryngeal/pharyngeal tissues in cats where the surgical scrub had not been thoroughly removed following a procedure. Best practice guidelines would be to rinse the surgical scrub off any patient with warm water and a towel after undergoing a procedure.

Iodophors are used as surgical skin prep in areas where chlorhexidine gluconate cannot be used (around eyes, ears, or mucous membranes) or when the patient has sensitivity to the chlorhexidine. Just as described with chlorhexidine gluconate, iodophor-based scrub should be used at full strength (i.e., in its undiluted form) as recommended by the manufacturer. It should be applied and allowed to remain in contact with the skin surface for the time period recommended by the manufacturer to obtain the desired outcome (generally about 5 minutes). Wipe off the remaining soap residue with sterile gauze saturated with water. The area can then be "painted" with an iodophor solution and allowed to dry before draping the patient.

Prophylactic Antibiotics

Appropriate administration of prophylactic antibiotics can help prevent SSIs. The CDC and American Society for Health System Pharmacists have collaborated to produce comprehensive guidelines concerning administration of prophylactic antibiotics (Church and Bjerke, 2009). Their guidelines include the following:

- Choice of the antimicrobial agent should be safe, inexpensive, bactericidal, and will cover the most probable contaminants expected with the procedure.
- Time the administration of the antimicrobial so that the greatest concentration present in serum and tissues is at bactericidal levels when the skin is first incised.
- Therapeutic levels of the antimicrobial should be maintained until a few hours after the incision is closed.

Maintaining Patient Temperature

Patients are placed at an increased risk for SSI if the core body temperature is not maintained during a surgical procedure. Hypothermia results in lowered tissue oxygenation caused by dermal vasoconstriction, reduced blood flow to surgical sites, and impaired immune function. At induction of anesthesia, there is a redistribution of body heat. Active measure for maintaining normal core temperatures include warmed inspired gases, warmed intravenous fluids, forced air warming blanket, and water recirculation heating pad. Prewarming the patient during preoperative radiograph and during the surgical prep can help in maintaining the patient's temperature.

Glucose Control

For patient with diabetes, medical complications and SSIs are more common. Paying close attention to serum glucose levels is recommended throughout the entire perioperative period. Hypoglycemia requiring treatment also occurs postoperatively. Patients with poorly controlled diabetes are at greater surgical risk overall, and if an elective surgical procedure can be postponed until the patient is better controlled, better surgical outcomes will be achieved.

Environmental Cleaning of the Operating Room

Most surgical infections develop from bacteria entering the incision site during the surgical procedure. To reduce the potential for infection, it is important to reestablish a clean environment after each surgical procedure. Cleaning and disinfection of the surgical area is performed at the beginning of the day, between each patient, at the end of the day, weekly, and monthly. Cleaning involves the removal of organic materials (e.g., blood, urine, feces). Disinfection refers to the application of a chemical agent that reduces the number of microorganisms on the inanimate surfaces. Follow the dilution and contact time recommended by the disinfectant manufacturer.

Daily Routine for Cleaning and Disinfection

All horizontal surfaces in the operating room (e.g., lights, tables, stools) should be damp-dusted before the first scheduled case of the day. This is done using an EPA-registered hospital disinfectant that has been freshly made that morning in accordance with the manufacturer's dilution recommendation. This helps to reduce the airborne contamination that can travel on dust and lint.

After each surgical procedure, put on a pair of exam gloves and collect all the instruments; place them in a bin with an enzymatic solution made in the proper dilution or use a commercially prepared spray-on enzymatic foam. Collect all waste that was generated and place in the appropriate disposal container. Place contaminated linens in a laundry bag. Disconnect and clean suction unit and remove suction jar for cleaning and disinfection. (Note that scrub sinks should not be used for cleaning of instruments or as a place to dispose of body fluids.) Clean and disinfect the instrument and surgical patient tables, heating pad and insulating mat, kick buckets, and IV stand bases, as well as any surface that is visibly contaminated with blood or body fluids. The general rule is to start with the cleanest surface (instruments table), then continue with the patient table. Next clean and disinfect items closer to the floor, and lastly the floor itself. Visibly soiled areas of the floor should be cleaned and disinfected using a cloth and disinfectant solution (or mop bucket of freshly made disinfectant solution and a clean mop head that is used only in the OR). For the floor end-of-procedure cleaning, only a 3- to 4-foot perimeter around the surgical field needs to be cleaned and disinfected. Check to see if any fluid has accumulated under the base of the surgical patient table.

If another procedure is to follow immediately, the sterile instruments should not be opened until the OR is completely disinfected and all instruments, wastes, towels, and linens from the previous patient are removed. If the OR has multiple procedures occurring simultaneously, care should be taken to minimize contamination and aerosolization of dust and lint.

Terminal Cleaning at the End of Each Day

At the end of the day, the OR should be terminally cleaned. This includes cleaning and disinfecting beginning at the highest level (i.e., ceiling fixtures) and progressing downward to the tables, and lastly the floors.

- Surgical lights and other fixed or ceiling-mounted equipment
- All furniture, stools, chairs, step-stools, kick buckets, wheels or casters on gurneys, carts, or other movable equipment
- Horizontal surfaces, including cabinet tops and handles, fixed shelving, x-ray view boxes, and countertops
- Telephones, keyboards, and monitors
- Any commonly touched surfaces (e.g., light switches, door handles, table-adjustment handles)
- All anesthetic monitoring equipment (pulse oximeters, blood pressure cuffs, EKG leads, dopplers) according to the device manufacturers' recommendations
- Scrub areas and scrub sinks

Wet vacuuming the floors with an EPA hospital disinfectant is the optimal procedure for reducing the number of microorganisms, dust, and any organic debris that may be present in the surgical area. A mop-and-bucket method, if used incorrectly, can actually spread contamination. If mops are used, the mop head should be freshly laundered, placed in a freshly made dilution of the EPA-registered hospital disinfectant, and then wrung out prior to mopping the floor. Use a second bucket with clean (tap water) rinse water; the mop is placed in the bucket with the rinse water, "rinsed," and wrung out prior to being dipped back into the disinfectant solution. This releases some of the organic material that was accumulated in the mop; it helps keep the organic load of the disinfection solution to a minimum. This mop and bucket should only be used in the surgical area. At the end of the mopping, the mop head should be laundered and dried. Any equipment used in the cleaning and disinfection process also needs to be cleaned, have disinfectant agent applied for the appropriate contact time, rinsed, and allowed to dry before storage.

The anesthesia or surgical preparation area should also have a written protocol for cleaning and disinfection between patients and at the end of the day. If gurneys are used to transport patients (or any other items that have wheels or casters), special attention should be paid to removing loose patient hair clippings from the gurney, shelf (if applicable), wheels, and the floor around the gurney. This prevents hair from being transported into the surgery room via any horizontal surface, wheels, and staff feet. Once the patient leaves the preparation area, the area can be further cleaned and disinfected. The clipper blades should be cleaned of hair and disinfected between each patient use. The clipper handpiece should be wiped off with a rag moistened with soap and warm water to remove any organic material or hair, allowed to dry, then wiped off with an alcohol-soaked gauze and allowed to dry.

Weekly or Monthly Schedule of Cleaning

A weekly or monthly schedule of cleaning and disinfecting surgical areas and adjacent areas should be performed. A clean environment will reduce the number of microorganisms present. A schedule can be established by visually assessing the area and noting the frequency of use and degree of contamination. Weekly/monthly cleaning and disinfection schedules require, at a minimum, that you do the following:

- Remove any movable equipment and thoroughly clean and disinfect the walls, floor, and ceiling.
- Clean return ventilation and heating grills or air conditioning equipment.
- Remove the contents of shelves in supply cabinets to allow cleaning and disinfection of the shelves.
- Empty supply or utility carts of their contents to allow cleaning and disinfection of the carts.
- Clean and disinfect all storage areas.
- Clean and disinfect the fluid-warming cabinets, refrigerators, and microwaves.
- Clean adjacent rooms including anesthesia/surgical preparation rooms, recovery areas, locker room/lavatories, and lounges.
- Clean and disinfect paper towel dispensers.
- Check the supply of surgical hand scrub at the scrub sinks and other soap dispensers. If the scrub sink is foot- or knee-operated and contains tubing and a spout, the soap supply should be removed and warm tap water is flushed through the tubing and spout to keep hand scrub from building up and obstructing the flow of scrub soap or becoming a reservoir for microorganisms.
- Check the level of product in general hand soap dispensers. These dispensers should not be "topped off" because they can become contaminated and serve as a reservoir for microorganisms (AORN, 2009e). They should be allowed to empty, be thoroughly cleaned and disinfected, and be allowed to dry before refilling. Optimally, they should be a style that contains no reservoir. When the soap is empty, the container can be disconnected and a new container placed for use.

Table 14.2 is a summary of cleaning frequency for items in the OR.

Strict attention to the surgical environment and surgical personnel can minimize contamination during surgery. A correlation has been noted between the number of people, their movements, and the number of airborne bacteria in the surgical area.

Summary

Comprehensive infection control policies and procedures for maintaining a surgical environment should be developed and reviewed periodically to keep current with surgical techniques and technologies. Training sessions for new employees should include review of the policies and procedures. It is of moral conscience that every member of the surgical team be vigilant in assuring the sterility of all surgical items and the surgical field.

INFECTION CONTROL PRACTICES FOR ANESTHESIOLOGY

Anesthesia equipment used in induction, intubating, and maintaining a patient during a surgical procedure is exposed to potentially infectious materials through direct contact with patient's skin, mucous membranes, secretions, and blood. Because it is impossible to know which equipment has become contaminated, all equipment should be cleaned and disinfected or sterilized. This includes items such as the anesthesia machine system, ancillary instruments, and medical devices used while maintaining the anesthetized patient. Intubation and mechanical ventilation alter and bypass first-line defense mechanisms and increase the risk of aspiration and infection (Kane,

Table 14.2 Summary of Cleaning Activities

Cleaning and disinfecting activity	End of procedure	Daily	Weekly or monthly, depending on use
Damp-dusting all horizontal surfaces		x	
Collection of instruments & place in bin of enzymatic cleaning solution	x		
Collect all waste generated	x		
Collect contaminated linens	x		
Disconnect; clean and disinfect suction jar	x		
Clean and disinfect instrument table	x	x	
Clean and disinfect surgical patient table, insulating mat, heating pad	x	x	
Clean and disinfect kick bucket and IV stand bases	x	x	
Clean and disinfect the floor	x	x	
Clean and disinfect the scrub sinks		x	
Surgical lights and other ceiling mounted fixtures		x	
Clean and disinfect all furniture, stools, chairs		x	
Clean and disinfect wheels on gurneys, carts, or other movable equipment		x	
Clean and disinfect all horizontal surfaces (countertops)		x	
Clean and disinfect cabinet tops, shelving, x-ray view boxes		x	
Clean and disinfect phones, keyboards, monitors		x	
Clean and disinfect all commonly touched surfaces		x	
Remove any movable equipment; clean and disinfect walls, floor, and ceiling in that area			x
Clean and disinfect return ventilation and heating grills or air conditioning equipment			x
Remove the content of shelves of supply cabinets to allow cleaning and disinfection of the shelves and any bins or containers			x
Empty the contents of supply or utility carts of contents to allow cleaning and disinfection of the carts, including wheels			x
Clean and disinfect all storage areas, including removal of items from shelving to clean items			x
Thoroughly clean adjacent rooms in a similar manner as described for the operating room to include anesthesia/surgical preparation room, recovery area, patient holding area			x
Clean and disinfect paper towel dispenser and refill as necessary			x
Check the supply of surgical hand scrub and flush with warm water (if applicable)			x
Check the level of product in general hand soap dispensers; clean and disinfect exterior surface			x

2009). Risk of infection also increases with the length of time a patient is on a mechanical ventilator and when leakage around an endotracheal tube cuff allows pools of secretions to be aspirated. Routes of transmission of pathogens associated with anesthetized patients include airborne droplet nuclei (device generated) or direct or indirect contact with contaminated hands and equipment. Employing standard infection control practices and meticulous hand hygiene practices is essential for the protection of all patients.

The American Society of Anesthesiologists recommends following the Spaulding Classification System to categorize the various equipment and its risk classification.

Critical risk items are those that enter sterile body cavities or the vascular systems. These must be sterile at the time of use on a patient. Examples include needles, catheters, tubing, and stopcocks.

Semi-critical risk items are those that come in contact with mucous membranes. These, ideally, should be sterile, but it is acceptable that this category of equipment undergo exposure to a high-level disinfection process. Examples include laryngoscope blades, reusable temperature probes, esophageal stethoscopes, breathing circuits and connectors, and breathing masks or "cones." Once these items are used, they should be rinsed to remove blood and secretions as soon as possible. Endotracheal tubes removed from the patient should have the ties removed, the exterior of the tube and the lumens flushed with water, then be allowed to soak in an enzymatic detergent solution until they can be further cleaned. Once they are thoroughly cleaned, rinsed, and allowed to dry, they should undergo either sterilization by steam, ethylene oxide, or a high-level disinfectant. Always check with the manufacturer of each item to see what the recommended methods of sterilization or high-level disinfection are. Some examples of liquid chemical high-level disinfectants are glutaraldehyde, hydrogen peroxide, or OPA. Refer to Chapter 11 for further information on low-temperature chemical disinfectants/sterilants. Semi-critical items should be stored in a clean location to minimize the risk of contamination or damage (AORN, 2009f).

Noncritical devices are those items that touch the patient's intact skin or do not touch the patient directly. These include blood pressure cuffs and tubing, pulse oximeter probes and cables, electrocardiogram (ECG) leads and cables, and the exterior of these items and the exterior surfaces of the anesthesia machine or other monitoring equipment. These items are cleaned and disinfected with an intermediate- to low-level disinfectant. Reusable laryngoscope handles are included in this category and should be cleaned and undergo low-level disinfection between each patient (AORN, 2009f). Examples of this class of disinfectants are sodium hypochlorite, quaternary ammonium compounds (QAC), and alcohols. Refer to Chapter 7 for further information on chemical disinfectants. Table 14.3 is a summary of anesthesia equipment according to the Spaulding Classification System.

Maintaining Anesthesia Equipment

Based on the Spaulding Classification System, all anesthesia equipment should undergo regular, routine cleaning and disinfection. Refer to the manufacturer's recommendation of each specific piece of equipment and follow their guidelines. Table 14.4 is a summary of some common anesthesia equipment with the cleaning and disinfecting recommendations by their specific manufacturers.

The Anesthesia Machine

Each distinctive part of the anesthetic machine requires different levels of disinfection/sterilization depending on its use.

Table 14.3   Anesthetic Equipment According to the Spaulding Classification System

Spaulding Classification System	Equipment	Sterilization/Disinfection
Critical	Needles, catheters, IV tubing, stopcocks	Sterilization by steam, ethylene oxide, vaporized hydrogen peroxide
Semicritical	Laryngoscope blade, stylets, reusable temperature probes, masks (cones), breathing circuits, and connectors	Sterilization preferred, otherwise high-level disinfectant
Noncritical	Blood pressure cuffs, ECG leads and cables, pulse oximeter sensors and cables, reusable laryngoscope handles	Intermediate- to low-level disinfectant

The horizontal exterior surface of the machine should be wiped down with a low-level disinfectant in between each patient as well as all the commonly touched dials and knobs. At the end of each day, the exterior surfaces should be terminally cleaned and disinfected with a low-level disinfectant. At least once a week, the items stored in drawers should be removed and the drawers and items should both be cleaned with a disinfectant. When gas cylinders are used, before being brought into the OR, they should be cleaned with water and detergent, then disinfected with a low-level disinfectant (Dorsch and Dorsch, 1999).

As a general guide, only the components between the common gas outlet and the patient require sterilization (Sharn Inc., 2009) Routine sterilization of the internal components of the anesthesia machine (gas outlets, gas valves, pressure regulators, flow meters, and vaporizers) are not necessary (ASA, 1999). The patient circuit contains all components that directly communicate with the patient's respiratory system. These include the CO_2 absorber and canister(s); inhalation and exhalation check valves; the breathing circuit; the adjustable pressure limiting (APL) or pop-off valve; rebreathing bag; bag to ventilator switch; and, if present, the ventilator bellows and either head or base of the bellows system.

The CO_2 absorbent canister should be disassembled, cleaned, and disinfected/sterilized according to the instructions of each manufacturer. The canisters should be cleaned during routine changing of the absorbent to remove absorbent residue from the canister chamber and the gasket surface. The absorbent should be changed weekly or when the absorber has changed color. The absorbent canister dust cup should be checked periodically and emptied. The screen should be checked for build-up of a gummy film produced by the absorbent.

Plastic domes on check valves should be unscrewed and the valve disc removed. Clean with a detergent solution and sterilize according to the manufacturer's instructions.

The pop-off valve on reusable absorbers cannot be immersed in a liquid solution (Sharn Inc., 2009). Immersion can trap liquids in the valve and impair its function. The exterior surface should be cleaned with a cloth moistened with water and detergent and allowed to dry. Follow the manufacturer's recommendations for sterilization.

The reservoir bag should be removed and cleaned with water and detergent. Allow the bag to dry, then sterilize according to the manufacturer's recommendations. Generally they can be steam sterilized, but this causes the rubber to deteriorate. They can be sterilized with ethylene oxide, but once reattached to the machine, it should be filled and emptied a few times before being used on a patient.

The ASA guidelines for cleaning and sterilization of the ventilator bellows and bellows head/base state that they should be "cleaned and sterilized at regular intervals" (ASA, 1999).

Table 14.4 Examples of Cleaning and Disinfection of Anesthesia Equipment

Equipment	Components	Cleaning agent	Disinfecting agent	Frequency	Comments
Narkomed 2B	Painted, plated, or plastic surfaces		Soft cloth moistened with diluted disinfectant cleaner.		Do not allow liquid to enter the interior of the machine
	Ventilator bellow assembly and ventilator relief valve (inspiratory and expiratory)	Mild detergent solution followed by a distilled water rinse, drip dry assembly			
	Rubber goods: hoses, breathing bags, or other components of the breathing system	"Follow Hospital Procedures" (Clean, rinse, dry)	"Follow Sterilizer manufacturer's instructions"		
	Respiratory volume monitor sensor	"Run distilled water through the housing; do NOT immerse the senor. Dry the sensor with a hose drying unit or allow to dry overnight"	"Sterilize with ethylene oxide and allow proper aeration"	Lubricate the sensor bearings after 2 months or 30 EO cycles.	Do not steam sterilize
	Breathing pressure pilot line	Clean with a mild detergent solution and rinse with water. Allow to dry thoroughly.	"Sterilize with ethylene oxide and allow proper aeration"		
	Oxygen sensor capsule and sensor housing		"Sterilize with ethylene oxide and allow proper aeration"		Do not steam sterilize sensor assembly
	Absorbent canister	Clean surfaces with a mild detergent		"Frequently"	
	Dust cup	Clean surfaces with a mild detergent			

Medex-Medfusuion 3500	Exterior surfaces	"Follow your institution's guidelines for cleaning and disinfection of devices. Use a mild detergent mixed with water. For best results, clean by spraying cleaner directly onto a soft cloth then wiping surfaces dry."	10% bleach solution diluted with water, 70% isopropyl alcohol, and surface disinfectants compatible with plastic materials.	Do not use organic solvents (acetone), QACs, strong acids or bases. Never spray cleaning or other fluids directly into openings on the bottom of the pump.
i-STAT	Display	Clean the display screen with a soft, dry tissue.		
	Case	Clean the case using a gauze pad moistened with mild, nonabrasive cleaner; detergent; soap and water; or alcohol. Rinse using another gauze pad moistened with water and dry.	Decontaminate analyzer whenever a specimen is spilled on the analyzer. Wear gloves. Prepare 1:10 solution of sodium hypochlorite; soak a few gauze pads in solution, squeeze to remove excess solution. Soften, then remove any dried blood with gauze pads soaked in solution; do not scrape. Repeat this procedure, rinse surface with gauze pads moistened with tap water, and dry.	Do not immerse the analyzer

(Continued)

Table 14.4 *(Continued)*

Equipment	Components	Cleaning agent	Disinfecting agent	Frequency	Comments
Datex 3800 Pulse Oximeter	Oximeter: display panel	"Use a cotton swab moistened with 70% isopropyl alcohol and gently wipe panel."			Use cleaning solution sparingly; do not soak or immerse the monitor in any liquid.
	Oximeter: outer surface	"Use a soft cloth dampened with a mild soap and water solution or 70% isopropyl alcohol, quaternary ammonia, 3% H_2O_2 in water, 100:1 bleach or Cidex plus activator."			
	Sensor	Refer to the instructions for the sensor.			Dependent on the type of sensor used.
Datex Portable Bedside Capnograph	Exterior surfaces	"Dampen a cloth with commercial, nonabrasive cleaner and wipe the top, bottom, and front surfaces lightly."			Do not spray or pour any liquid directly on the monitor or its circuits.

Narkomed 2B Operator's Manual; Drager Medical, Telford, PA.
Medfusion Syringe Pump, Model 3500, Revision 2 Operator's Manual, page 66; Medex Smith Medical, Dublin, OH.
iSTAT Model, Section 6: Routine Care, Troubleshooting & Technical Information, Revision May 1997; Abbott Laboratories, Abbott Park, IL.
Datex 3800 Pulse Oximeter Operator's Manual, Section 4: Cleaning, page 4-1; Datex-Ohmeda, Madison, WI.
Datex Portable Bedside Capnograph, Model Operator's Manual, Maintenance Section: Cleaning, page 54; Datex-Ohmeda.

Sharn, Inc. recommends that the ventilator bellows and bellows head/base are a part of the patient circuit and should be sterilized between uses unless bacterial filters are used to protect the inspiratory, expiratory, and ventilator limbs of the circuit (Sharn Inc., 2009). Each facility should determine, according to the risk of potential contamination by contagious organisms, whether to sterilize the bellows and bellows head/base after each patient or at regular intervals. Always follow the manufacturer's guidelines for proper disassembly, cleaning, disinfecting, or sterilization of each component.

General instructions include the following:

- Clean the bellows with cold water and a detergent, dry, and gas sterilize and aerate according to the bellows manufacturer.
- Wash the bellows housing with a mild detergent solution and thoroughly rinse with cold distilled water. Dry with a soft, lint-free cloth. The bellows exteriors are exposed only to the driving gas, not the gas exhaled by the patient. If there is a leak or tear in the bellows, the housing will need to be sterilized by the manufacturer because it has been exposed to gas exhaled by the patient.
- Wash the pressure-sensing tube with a detergent and water solution. Rinse with cold distilled water and allow the tube to dry completely.
- Clean the exterior surface of the base with warm water and detergent solution. The driving gas outlet is normally only exposed to oxygen so it does not need to be cleaned. Rinse the base with distilled water to remove any detergent residue. Do not immerse the base; it can trap liquids, which will impair its performance.
- Wash the interface manifold (if present) between the ventilator and machine with a mild detergent solution and rinse with cold water to remove any detergent residue. Allow the interface manifold to dry before processing according to the manufacturer's recommendations.

After sterilization or cleaning, check all rubber parts for swelling, stickiness, holes, cracking, or any other signs of deterioration or damage. Reassemble the bellows according to the manufacturer's recommendations.

Attachments to the Patient

The breathing tubes used on patient are corrugated; this makes the tubes difficult to clean and disinfect. After use on a patient, the tubing should be rinsed with tap water to prevent drying of any film or debris within these corrugations. They should be allowed to soak in a bin of water and detergent until further cleaning can take place. Cleaning with a brush is not effective due to the length of the tube and all the ridges. The tube can be placed in an ultrasonic cleaner to remove any debris from the corrugations. An alternate method is to pour clean a detergent solution in one end of the tube and agitate in a see-saw manner. The tube is emptied and rinsed thoroughly with tap water, then allowed to dry. Chemical disinfection can be carried out by immersion of the tube into a liquid agent. It is important that the tube be introduced into the solution vertically, making sure there are no air pockets and the tube is completely filled inside.

The "Y" piece should be removed from the breathing tubing and rinsed with tap water. It can easily be scrubbed with a brush and soap solution to remove any residue or debris. It should then be rinsed and allowed to dry for further processing by a liquid chemical agent or ethylene oxide.

Bain circuits should be disassembled and cleaned, rinsed, dried, and processed as described for other parts of the patient circuit.

Any adaptor used in the breathing circuit should be cleaned and sterilized according the manufacturer's recommendations. They are generally easily cleaned by placing in a solution of water and soap, scrubbed, rinsed, and allowed to dry. They can be disinfected by liquid chemical agent or sterilized.

Patient Care Items

Any items used in the process of anesthetizing of the patient need to be cleaned and be disinfected according to the Spaulding classification system. A few of these items include a thermometer, stethoscope, clippers, blood gas analyzers, pulse oximeter, ECG clips, laryngoscope with the appropriate size blades to name a few. The use of thermometer covers on digital probles are recommended as the area between the tip and adjoining plastic is difficult to clean. Even with the use of a cover, the thermometer should be cleaned with water and a detergent, followed by wiping it with alcohol. Stethoscope bells should be wiped off with alcohol after examining each patient. The clipper blades used to clip an area so a catheter can be placed should undergo cleaning and disinfection after each patient. Minimally, a disinfectant clipper spray should be used. To aid in the cleaning process, a "blade wash" may be used to assist in freeing the hair from the area between the blade and the clipper base. Clipper blades should be replaced on a routine basis as a dull blade can cause nicks or irritation in the skin. This can set up the area for bacterial contamination.

The blood gas analyzer, pulse oximeter, or capnograph should be cleaned and disinfected according to manufacurer's recommendations. Not following their specific guidelines can damage the unit. The sensors used can be damaged by water or the use of unsuitable chemicals.

ECG lead cables should be wiped down after use on each patient according to the manufacturer's recommendations. They can become contaminated directly from blood or body fluids from the patient or indirectly from the staff handling the patient while attaching them. The clips that attach to the patient should also be cleaned after each patient. Conductive gel can build up on them if they are not routinely changed after each patient. They should be cleaned then low-level disinfectant.

The reusable laryngoscope handles should be cleaned and disinfected between patients; these handles become contaminated during the process of establishing an airway. The blades should be removed from the handle, and the exterior surfaces of the reusable handle should be wiped with a cloth soaked with warm water and detergent to remove any organic material. It should then be rinsed with a cloth soaked with warm water and allowed to dry. The exterior surfaces can then be disinfected with an alcohol-soaked gauze. The blade should be cleaned to remove organic debris prior to being exposed to a sterilant or high-level disinfectant.

Use of Multidose Vials

The use of multiple-dose vials (MDVs) is very common in the veterinary field, especially for anesthetic agents. Their use is based on convenience, ability to adjust dosages based on a patient weight, and cost-effectiveness. However, contamination of these vials and subsequent injection into a patient can occur. Every time a needle pokes through the rubber stoppers of an MDV, there is potential for inadvertent injection of microorganisms to the remaining contents of the vial from the rubber stopper or contaminated needle and syringe (Sabino, 2006). During several outbreak investigations in the human health care setting by the CDC, MDVs of propofol were found to be contaminated with microorganisms *Staphylococcus aureus, Moraxella osleoensis,*

Candida albicans, Enterobacter agglomerans, and *Serratia marcesens* (Chiarello, 2010). MDVs of dextrose and heparinized saline had also been implicated in *Enterobacter cloacae, Pseu-domonas aeruginosa,* and *S. marcesens* bloodsteam infectons (Chiarello, 2010). The risk of contamination increases with the number of withdrawals from the vial and whether aseptic technique was used by personnel. Injection of environmental air into the vial prior to extraction, duration of use, storage conditions (temperature, sun exposure), and whether or not the MDV contained preservatives can all be contributing factors in contaminating MDVs.

There are steps that can be taken to reduce the risk of contamination and safely use MDVs. The first consideration is to use smaller volume containers; this would decrease the number of withdrawals from the vial. Ideally, persons handling the MDV would perform hand washing or use alcohol-based hand sanitizer prior to withdrawing medication. This is typically not the case, but staff should be aware that there is a great potential for contamination in an environment or situation with higher levels of organic debris. The rubber stoppers (top of the vials) should be swabbed with 70% isopropyl alcohol before inserting a needle into the vial. Only a sterile needle and syringe should be used to access the MDV. Do not reuse a syringe even if the needle is changed (Siegel et al., 2007). The manufacturer's guidelines for storage temperature and exposure to light should be followed to ensure the efficacy of the drug. The expiration date of the medication should be honored. The leftover contents of single-use vials should not be "pooled" for later use; these ampules or vials generally do not contain preservatives. Keep MDVs in an area where they will not be exposed to inadvertent contamination by spray or spatter by the patient. If there is any question as to the sterility of the contents of a MDV, it should be discarded.

Environmental Concerns

The anesthesia area is generally located fairly close to surgical suites; therefore, it is important to keep this area cleaned and disinfected. This is where clipping and surgical prep are performed, creating a lot of loose fur and hair. This should be vacuumed with a unit that contains a HEPA filter to minimize aersolization of dust and particles. There should be a designated "clean area" adjacent to where the patient is anesthetized for prepared equipment to be used in catheterization, intubation, and monitoring the patient as well as a "dirty or contaminated area," where used devices are placed. These areas should be clearly defined so items will not be used on another patient before they have been appropriately cleaned and disinfected or sterilized.

The cleaning and decontamination area for anesthetic equipment should be separate from other areas. Signs indicating where dirty equipment is to be placed should be prominently displayed. The sinks used should be large enough to contain the largest devices that need to be cleaned. There should be enough sink area to facilitate concurrent soaking, washing, and rinsing of equipment. It is not recommended to soak items in a sink that is also used for hand washing. That will allow further dilution of the soak basin solution as well as more organic materials to be added. There should be attached counters or work surfaces to accommodate drying of the items prior to appropriate disinfection or sterilization processing. It is highly recommended that the cleaning and disinfection/sterilization of anesthetic equipment be delegated to a well-trained individual who understands the principles of containment of contamination and disinfection and sterilization process (Dorsch and Dorsch, 1999).

The anesthesia room should be cleaned and disinfected as previously described for the surgical area.

Summary

Tracheal intubation bypasses the patient's first-line airway defense mechanism, increasing the risk of aspiration and subsequent infection of the lungs. Contaminated condensate in the ventilator circuit can also be passed to the patient. Devices used in intubation can be contaminated and indirectly pass organisms from one patient to another. The hands of staff members can transfer organisms to patients.

Development of comprehensive infection control policies and procedures for care and maintaining anesthesia equipment it essential; it should be and reviewed periodically to keep current with new techniques and technologies. Training sessions for all employees on new equipment is vital for patient care. New employees should have extensive training on all of the anesthetic equipment and devices, including their cleaning, disinfection, and sterilization.

SPECIAL CONSIDERATIONS FOR THE DENTISTRY AND "DIRTY SURGERY" AREAS

Veterinarians and technicians can be exposed to a wide variety of microorganisms via blood and oral/respiratory secretions when performing routine dental procedures, oral surgery, or draining of abscesses. Sources for microbial cross-contamination and infections exist during treatment from hands and any instruments used. Spatter from the patient's mouth when using the ultrasonic scalers during a dental prophy or flushing a dirty contaminated open skin wound on a patient aerosolizes many bacteria that can affect other patients nearby. Making staff aware of the biologic hazards and creating an effective infection prevention program based on the routes of potential microbial transmission allow for the safety of staff and patients. Droplet or airborne route of transmission creates more of a challenge because contamination can be spread by inhalation of the organisms, items becoming contaminated then serving as fomites, or can be spread simply by the staff not washing their hands. This section will focus on mainly the dental procedures but can be generally applied for any "dirty" procedure that is performed.

Environmental Aspects

The area of the facility that is designated to perform dental procedures should be separate from where aseptic surgical procedures are performed. Dental procedures produce thousands of aerosolized microorganisms; therefore, they should not be performed near surgical areas or areas where critically ill patients are housed. The walls, ceiling, floor, and counters should be made from impervious materials that can withstand frequent chemical applications from the cleaning and disinfection process.

The room should allow sufficient free space to allow ease in movement of patients, equipment, and staff. It should be free of clutter or any unnecessary equipment and supplies. This facilitates easier daily cleaning and disinfection of the room.

The room should be adequately ventilated to reduce the bacterial aerosols, fumes of chemicals used in x-ray developing, or products used in restorative procedures. It should be exhausted to the outside and not recirculated within the facility (Deeprose, 2007).

Environmental surfaces within the room can be divided into two categories: the clinical contact surfaces and the housekeeping surfaces (CDC, 2003). The housekeeping surfaces (e.g., floors, walls) have a limited risk of disease transmission; therefore, they can be decontaminated with less frequency than the clinical contact surfaces. The clinical contact surfaces can be directly contaminated from patient material, either directly by spray or spatter or by contact with the doctor's or technician's gloved hands.

Housekeeping Surfaces

The housekeeping surfaces require actual physical removal of microorganisms and soils by wiping or scrubbing, followed by application of an EPA-registered detergent/disinfectant. The floors and sinks should be cleaned and disinfected daily. The cleaning and disinfection of the walls should be performed on a weekly basis to prevent build-up of a large organic load. Whenever the floor or wall is visibly contaminated, it should be promptly cleaned and disinfected. A schedule of thorough room cleaning and disinfection (such as described in the previous section) should be developed and implemented.

Clinical Contact Surfaces

Frequently touched surfaces can serve as reservoirs of microbial contamination. Transmission of microorganisms occurs when the surface is contaminated directly from aerosolized bacteria from the spray or spatters from the patient or indirectly by contaminated hands or instruments, then subsequently transferred to other environmental surfaces or to the mouth of the patient. A majority of the aerosolized bacteria from power scaling occurs within a 3-foot radius of the patient's head (Kessel, 2000). Examples of this type of surface includes light handles, countertops, switches on dental equipment, drawer handles, faucet handles, pens, computers, doorknobs, and phones or pagers. Barrier protection of the surface and equipment can prevent some contamination but is particularly effective for those that are difficult to clean (CDC, 2003). Barriers can be as simple as clear plastic wrap, bags, or other impervious material covering the surfaces. The barrier is discarded after each patient, and the covered surface is examined for any inadvertent contamination. These barriers should be removed while the staff member is still gloved. After gloves are removed, the staff member should wash his/her hands with soap and water. Thorough cleaning and disinfection with an EPA-approved disinfectant should be performed daily for these surfaces.

If barriers are not used, the surfaces should be cleaned and disinfected after each patient with the facility-approved EPA disinfectant. It is recommended to check with the manufacturer of the dental equipment regarding material compatibility with the disinfectant the facility uses.

At the end of the day, all surfaces of the equipment used, patient table, chairs, stools, heating pads, etc. are to be cleaned and disinfected following the infection control protocol established by the facility and the manufacturer's recommendations for each piece of equipment.

Staff Safety

Aerosolized bacteria, viruses, and potentially fungi can affect the staff members performing the dental procedures (Molinari, 2003). Inhalation of aerosolized bacteria can cause nose, throat, and lung infections; direct contact with spatter, foreign bodies (calculi or teeth), or even fractured burrs can enter the eyes; and direct contact with lacerated, abraded, or cracked skin can serve as a means of transmission.

Dental staff should all be trained in appropriate radiographic techniques, including proper protection, appropriate exposure setting, methods of reducing exposure to the central beam, and processing techniques.

Dental staff should be following state and federal regulations regarding handling of contaminated sharp and regulated biohazardous waste materials. Sharps containers should be placed close to where they are generated to avoid sharp-related accidents. Examples of items to be placed in the sharps containers are needles, files, burrs, and no longer useful scalers, probes, and curettes.

Correct posture, appropriate hand positioning, and the use of ergonomic furniture should be used to reduce immediate discomfort and reduce the risk of long-term musculoskeletal disorders (Deeprose, 2007).

Hand hygiene is essential. Follow good hand washing techniques and appropriate use of alcohol hand sanitizers. Use lotions that are compatible with latex gloves to keep hands from drying out. Petroleum-based lotions can weaken the latex and increase permeability. Fingernails should be keep short to facilitate cleaning under and round them (this area harbors a majority of microorganisms) and prevents the fingernails from puncturing holes in the gloves. If nail polish is worn, it should be freshly applied and show no signs of chipping. Jewelry should be removed as it can harbor microorganisms. Artificial nails or extenders should not be worn; they make putting on gloves more difficult, cause them to tear more easily, and have been implicated in multiple outbreaks in fungal and bacterial infections (CDC, 2003).

Personal Protective Equipment (PPE) Barrier Protection

Primary PPE used in dentistry settings includes gloves, masks, protective eyeware or face shields, and protective clothing. All PPE should be removed before leaving the dentistry area.

Gloves should be worn whenever examining or performing a dental procedure. These can be in the form of either examination gloves or surgical gloves. Gloves should be changed when they are torn or punctured and should be used for only one patient. Wearing gloves does not eliminate the need for hand washing. There can be small defects in the glove material, allowing for bacterial contamination of the hands. Bacteria can grow rapidly in the moist environment underneath the gloves; therefore, prompt removal of torn gloves and immediate hand washing and thorough drying should be performed prior to donning another pair of gloves.

Surgical masks should be worn during dental procedures. This protects against microorganisms generated with greater than 95% bacterial filtration efficiency (for particles 3–5 microns in diameter) and protects from large particle droplet spatter (CDC, 2003). The mask's outer surface will become contaminated with droplets from the spray of the patient's oral fluids or from touching the mask with your contaminated fingers. When a mask is removed due to excess moisture generated during normal exhalation or fluid spray on the outside, it should be handled by the strings, not the actual mask that covers the mouth and nose.

A majority of surgical masks are not National Institute for Occupational Safety and Health (NIOSH) certified as respirators (CDC, 2003). There are a few designated as surgical N95 respirator that do meet the requirements and are certified NIOSH respirators. These masks refer to the ability to filter 1–micron particles in the unloaded state with a filter efficiency of greater than 95%, given the flow rate of ≤ 50 liters/minute, the average flow rate of normal human breathing (CDC, 2003). These should be used when there is a risk of airborne transmission of a disease process.

Eye protection should be routinely used to prevent eye injury or infection from sprays, broken or loose burs, or even calculus cracked off a tooth. Safety glasses with side shields or goggles are one option. The disadvantage of these is they can fog up when worn with a surgical mask. Another option is a clear face shield mounted on a headband. This may be an easier style for staff that wears regular eyeglasses. The other benefits of wearing the full face shield is that it protects your face from flying debris and it will not fog up with use. With either system, airborne particles can still enter your eyes because you are in a cloud of bacteria during the procedure. There are also styles of disposable face shields that are connected to the surgical mask.

Wearing of disposable surgical caps and a dedicated jacket or smock will help reduce transfer of microorganisms to other areas of the facility or to the next patient. The smock or jacket should cover the arms, and the front neck and chest portion of the individual performing the procedures. These protective garments should be removed before leaving the dental area. Hand washing should be performed after PPE and smocks.

Appropriate footwear that protects the feet against spillage and other substances should be worn. They should be easily cleaned and have nonskid soles.

Patient Safety

The patient that comes in for a dental prophy generally has a foul-smelling, dirty mouth. The patient needs to have "protection" to undergo this procedure. The gingival will most likely be traumatized during the procedure, causing bleeding. Bleeding signifies an opening into the circulatory system; if blood comes out, bacteria can enter the animal's vascular system. Antibiotics should be administered so they are in the patient's bloodstream at the beginning of the procedure. Injectable antibiotics are preferred for this reason. Subcutaneous or intramuscular antibiotics take up to an hour if they are normothermic; oral antibiotics need to be administered several hours prior to the procedure. The antibiotic of choice should be broad spectrum to cover both gram-positive and gram-negative bacteria.

Patients need to be anesthetized for the procedure. They will be intubated with an endotracheal (ET) tube for the procedure. An appropriately inflated, cuffed ET tube will eliminate inhalation of aerosolized microorganisms or fluid packed with bacteria. This also helps protect the individual performing the dental prophy from anesthetic gas leaks from the breathing circuit.

The patient's eyes need to be lubricated well with an ocular product to protect them from bacterial contamination absorption through the cornea and conjunctival surfaces as well as preventing the cornea from drying out while anesthetized.

Prior to ultrasonic scaling, the patients' teeth should be rinsed with an oral antiseptic. This will kill many bacteria on contact and will reduce the live bacterial aerosolization up to about 90%. Chlorhexidine gluconate or diacetate at a 0.1% or 0.2% concentration is very effective (Kessel, 2000). Betadine solution and sanguinaria extract (Viadent mouthwash) can also be used, but they both can stain as they are aerosolized.

Dental Equipment Cleaning and Disinfection

Dental equipment used in patient care is categorized using the Spaulding Classification System, the same system used for all other medical and surgical equipment and devices used. This classifies the equipment by the potential risk for infection associated with their use. The categories are labeled critical, semicritical, and noncritical (CDC, 2003). In review, critical items pose the greatest risk of transmitting infection and should be sterilized. Semicritical items touch mucous membranes or nonintact skin and have a lower risk of disease transmission. If these items are heat-tolerant, they should be sterilized. If the item is heat-sensitive, it should be processed

Table 14.5   Examples of Dental Equipment According to the Spaulding Classification System

Classification	Description	Dental instrument	Relative risk of disease	Reprocessing recommended
Critical	Penetrates tissue and contact sterile systems	Hand instruments Cutting instruments Burs, files, needles, handpieces, scaler tips	High	Sterilization Single-use disposable
Semicritical	Contacts mucous membranes or nonintact skin	Hand instruments, mouth props, poly prophy angles, rubber dams, framework	Intermediate	Heat sterilization Chemical sterilization Single-use disposable
Noncritical (intraoral contact)	May contact skin or mucous membrane	Impressions, prostheses, and other apparatus	Low	Thorough rinsing by EPA intermediate-level disinfectant
Noncritical (no intraoral contact)	Contacts unbroken skin	Blood pressure cuffs, face masks	Low	Low-level disinfection Removable covers
Clinical contact	Contact with clinical personnel	Dental unit surface Laboratory equipment x-ray equipment	Low	Low-level disinfection Removable covers
Housekeeping surfaces	Rarely contacts personnel or patients	Floors, walls	Minimal	Low-level disinfectant

minimally by a high-level disinfectant. Noncritical patient care items pose the least risk of transmission of infection; contacting only intact skin, they can be low-level disinfected with an EPA-registered hospital disinfectant. Table 14.5 is a sampling of items used in the dental area and their corresponding Spaulding Classification Category.

Dental unit waterlines can become colonized with microorganisms, including bacteria, fungi, and protozoa (CDC, 2003). These lines can become covered by a layer of biofilm on the interior surfaces of the waterline tubing, which serves as a reservoir that can amplify the number of free-floating microorganisms in water used for dental treatment. Also, patient material (e.g., oral microorganisms, blood, and saliva) can enter the dental water system during patient treatment (CDC, 2003). There is a potential risk for retraction of oral fluids into internal compartments of high- and low-speed handpieces and ultrasonic scaling tips. Restricted physical access limits the cleaning of this compartment. Subsequent intraoral expulsion of these materials to the next patient can occur. Dental devices that are connected to the dental water system, including ultrasonic scalers and headpieces, should be operated to discharge water and air for a minimum of 20–30 seconds after each patient. This will physically flush out patient material that may have entered the air, turbine, or waterlines. Refer to the manufacturer's recommendations for specific guidelines for each individual piece of equipment.

All dental hand instruments are heat-tolerant and should undergo the same cleaning and sterilization process described previously for surgical instruments (Chapters 8–10).

Summary

Individuals who perform dental procedures and the patients can be exposed to a wide variety of microorganisms through blood and other oral or respiratory secretions. The patient's mouth is full of bacteria; aerosolization from dental handpieces and ultrasonic scaling devices leads to droplet spatter, which contains large amounts of bacteria. Recognizing the potential routes for microbial transmission is fundamental in the establishment of appropriate infection control policies and procedures. Policies for instituting respiratory precaution protocols and limiting the possibility of direct or indirect transmission via equipment, instrument, or staff hands should be implemented and reviewed periodically. The proper use of barrier protection for the staff plays a vital role in preventing inadvertent transmission. Initial and continual training of individuals who will be performing dental procedure will ensure the highest level of safety for both the individual staff member and patients.

REFERENCES

[ASA] American Society of Anesthesiologists. 1999. *Recommendations for Infection Control for the Practice of Anesthesiology, 2nd ed.* Available at: http://www.asahq.org/publicationsAndServices/infectioncontrol.pdf. ASA, Ridge Park, IL.

[AORN] Association of periOperative Registered Nurses. 2009a. *Perioperative Standards and Recommended Practices.* RP: Surgical Attire. Recommendation I–VII. AORN, Denver, CO, pp 299–303.

AORN. 2009b. *Perioperative Standards and Recommended Practices.* RP: Maintaining a Sterile Field. Recommendation I–VII. AORN, Denver, CO, pp 317–322.

AORN. 2009c. *Perioperative Standards and Recommended Practices.* RP: Traffic Patterns. Recommendation I–VI. AORN, Denver, CO, pp 327–330.

AORN. 2009d. *Perioperative Standards and Recommended Practices.* RP: Safe Environmental Care. Recommendation V. AORN, Denver, CO, pp 418–420.

AORN. 2009e. *Perioperative Standards and Recommended Practices.* RP: Environmental Cleaning. Recommendation I–XI. AORN, Denver, CO, pp 439–451.

AORN. 2009f. *Perioperative Standards and Recommended Practices.* RP: Cleaning, Handling and Processing Anesthesia Equipment. Recommendation I–VIII. AORN, Denver, CO, pp 569–574.

Bartley J, Olmsted R. 2009. Chapter 104: Heating, ventilation, and air conditioning. *Association for Infection Control and Epidemiology (APIC) Text, 3rd ed.* APIC, Washington, DC.

[CDC] Center for Disease Control. 2003. Guidelines for infection control in dental health-care settings. *MMWR* 52(RR-17):1–66.

Chiarello LA. 2010. Study on multidose vials and disposable medical equipment, in *Report to the Governor and New York State Legislature New York State Public Health Law 239-b*, pp 1–24.

Church NB, Bjerke NB. 2009. Chapter 45: Surgical services. *Association for Infection Control and Epidemiology (APIC) Text, 3rd ed.* APIC, Washington, DC.

Deeprose J. 2007. Operator safety and health considerations, in C Tutt, J Deeprose, D Crossley, eds., *BSAVA Manual of Canine and Feline Dentistry, 3rd ed.* BSAVA, Gloucester, pp 56–66.

Dorsch J, Dorsch S. 1999. Equipment care and planning, in *Understanding Anesthesia Equipment, 4th ed.* Williams & Wilkins, Baltimore, MD, pp 973–1006.

Fossum TW. 2007. Chapter 3: Surgical facilities, equipment, and personnel, in *Small Animal Surgery.* Mosby, St. Louis, MO, pp 15–18.

Fossum TW. 2007. Chapter 4: Care and maintenance of the surgical environment, in *Small Animal Surgery.* Mosby, St. Louis, MO, pp 19–21.

Holmstrom SE, et al. 2004. Chapter 13: General health safety and ergonomics in the veterinary dental workplace, in *Veterinary Dental Techniques for the Small Animal Practitioner, 3rd ed.* Saunders, Philadelphia, PA, pp 637–654.

Kane C. 2009. Respiratory care services, in *Association for Infection Control and Epidemiology (APIC) Text, 3rd ed.* APIC, Washington, DC.

Kessel ML. 2000. Performing the Dental prophy, safety and health considerations, in *Veterinary Dentistry for the Small Animal Technician.* Blackwell Publishing, Ames, IA, pp 81–99.

Molinari JA. 2003. Infection control: its evolution to the current standard precautions. *J Am Dental Assoc* 134: 569–574.

Molinari JA, Harte JA. 2009. Chapter 50: Dental services. Dental Infection Control. *Association for Infection Control and Epidemiology (APIC) Text, 3rd ed.* APIC, Washington, DC.

Organization for Safety and Asepsis Procedures (OSAP). 2000. Environmental Surface Disinfection. Reprinted from *Monthly Focus* #6, 1998. Annapolis: OSAP Research Foundation in *The Dental Assistant.* November/December 2000, pp 4–10.

Sabino CV, Weese JS. 2006. Contamination of multiple-dose vials in a veterinary hospital. *Can Vet J* 47: 779–783.

Sharn, Inc. 2009. Infection control procedures for anesthesia equipment, in *Professional Anesthesia Handbook.* Available at: http://www.sharn.com/images/pdf/proaneshandbook.pdf. Sharn, Inc., Tampa, FL.

Siegel JD, et al. 2007. *Guideline for Isolation Precautions: Preventing Transmission of Infectious Agents in Healthcare Settings.* CDC, Atlanta, GA.

U.S. Department of Health and Human Services. 1999. Hospital Infection Control Practices Advisory Committee. National Center for Infectious Diseases. Centers for Disease Control and Prevention. Guideline for the Prevention of Surgical Suite Infection. Hospital Infections Program. Public Health Service.

Appendix A
Medical Term Reference Information

Medical terminology is the language for the health care industry. Medical equipment and supplies often derive their names from medical terms. Some basic understanding of the basic elements of the terms can help you unravel the most complex word.

A majority of medical terms come from Latin or Greek origin. A word may consist of one to four elements:

Root or base component: this is the core of the word; it may indicate a disease, process, or body part.

Prefix component: this comes before the root element; it alters or modifies its meaning.

Suffix component: this is one or two syllables attached to the end of a root element, which alters or varies its meaning. A suffix may relate to a diagnosis, operative procedure, or symptom.

Combining vowels: usually *a, i,* or *o* to make the words easier to pronounce; a vowel is usually deleted from a combining form when the next letter that follows is also a vowel.

On the next few pages is just a sampling of some commonly used suffixes, prefixes, and root elements of medical terms. It is far beyond the scope of this book to include all terms that one will encounter in the medical field.

Table A.1 Common Root Terms

Root	Definition	Example of term	Explanation
Aden	Gland	Adenoma	Tumor of a gland
Aer	Air	Aerobic	An organism that lives in the presence of air
Arth	Joint	Arthritis	Inflammation of a joint
Bronch	Bronchus	Bronchitis	Inflammation of the bronchus
Card	Heart	Electrocardiogram	Graphic record of the heart
Cephal	Head	Cephalic	Pertaining to the head
Chol	Bile	Cholecyst	Gallbladder
Cost	Rib	Intercostals	Pertaining to the space between ribs
Crani	Skull	Craniotomy	Surgical opening into the skull
Cysto	Sac or bladder	Cystoscope	Instrument to examine the bladder
Cyto	Cell	Erythrocyte	Red blood cell
Derma	Skin	Dermal	Pertaining to the skin
Enter	Intestine	Enteritis	Inflammation of the intestines
Gastro	Stomach	Gastrointestinal	Pertaining to the stomach and intestines
Glyco	Sweet	Glycemia	Sugar in the blood
Hem or Hemat	Blood	Hematoma	Blood tumor

Veterinary Infection Prevention and Control, First Edition. Edited by Linda Caveney and Barbara Jones with Kimberly Ellis.
© 2012 John Wiley & Sons, Inc. Published by John Wiley & Sons, Inc.

Table A.1 (Continued)

Root	Definition	Example of term	Explanation
Hepato	Liver	Hepatitis	Inflammation of the liver
Herni	Rupture	Herniorrhaphy	Surgical repair of hernia
Histo	Tissue	Histology	Study of tissue
Hydro	Water	Hydrocyst	Sac containing watery fluid
Hyster	Uterus	Hysterectomy	Excision of the uterus
Lapro	Abdomen	Laprotomy	Incision into the abdomen
Leuko	White	Leukocyte	White blood cell
Lip	Fat	Lipemia	Fat in the blood
Lith	Ston	Lithiasis	Presence of stones
Masto	Breast	Mastectomy	Removal of a breast
My	Muscle	Myocardium	Heart muscle
Nephr	Kidney	Nephrosclerosis	Hardening of the kidney
Oculo	Eye	Oculomotor	Movement of the eye
Ophthalmo	Eye	Ophthalmoscope	An instrument to look into the eye through the pupil
Osteo	Bone	Ostertome	An instrument to cut into bone
Pneumo	Lung, air	Pneumococcus	Microorganism causing pneumonia or other infections
Pyo	Pus	Pyogenic	Pus forming
Rhino	Nose	Rhinoscope	Instrument to look into the nose
Trachea	Windpipe	Tracheotomy	Incision into the trachea
Tuber	Swelling, node	Tubercle	Small lesion produced by *Mycobacterium tuberculosis*
Vaso	Vessel	Vasoconstriction	Narrowing of a blood vessel
Viser	Organ	Visceral	Pertaining to an organ

Table A.2 Common Prefix Components

Prefix	Meaning	Example	Definition
a-, an-	Without	Anerobic	Organism that grows in the absence of air
ab-	Away from	Abnormal	Away from the norm
ad-	Toward	Addiction	Toward dependence on a drug
ante-	Before	Antepartum	Before onset of labor
anti-	Against	Antiseptic	Substance that inhibits growth or kills microorganisms
bi-	Two, both	Biconvex	Having two convex surfaces
co-, con-	Together	Congenital	Born with, hereditary
contra-	Against, opposite	Contraindicated	Condition antagonistic to a type of treatment
dys-	Bad, difficult, or painful	Dysplasia	Abnormality of development
ec-, ect-	Out, outside	Ectropion of eyelid	Eversion of the eyelid margin
en-	In	encephalopathy	Any disease of the brain
epi-	Upon, in addition to	Epidermis	Outer layer of the skin
ex-	Out, away from	Exacerbation	Aggravation of symptoms
hemi-	Half	Hemiplegia	Paralysis of one side of the body
hyper-	Above, excessive	Hyperacidity	Exess of acid in the stomach
hypo-	Beneath, below	Hypoglycemia	Low blood sugar
inter-	between	Interarticular	Situated between articular surfaces
intra-	Within	Intracordial	Within the heart
iso-	Equal	Isocellular	Composed of the same kinds of cells

Table A.2 (Continued)

Prefix	Meaning	Example	Definition
mono-	One	Monocyte	Single cell
neo-	New	Neonatal	newborn
pan-	All	Panarthritis	Inflammation of all joints
para-	Beside, near	parathyroid	Area near the thyroid
peri-	Around, about	Pericardium	Double membranous sac enclosing the heart
post-	After, behind	Postpartum	After childbirth
pre-	Before, in front of	Precancerous	Before development of cancer
pro-	Forward, in front of	Prognosis	Prediction of probable disease outcome
retro-	Behind, backward	Retroperitoneal	Located behind the peritoneum
sub-	Under, beneath	Subcostal	Beneath the ribs
supra-, super-	Above, superior	Suprapelvic	Located above the pelvis
sym-, syn-	With, together	Syndrome	A set of symptoms that occur together
trans-	Across, over	Transaction	Incision across the long axis

Table A.3 Common Suffix Components

Suffix	Definition	Example	Explanation
-algia	Pain	Myalgia	Muscle pain
-centesis	Puncture for aspiration	Thoracentesis	Aspiration of the chest
-cide	Kill	Germicide	Destruction of germs
-cise	Cut	Excise	To cut out
-ectomy	Surgical removal	tonsillectomy	Removal of tonsils
-emia	Blood	Hyperglycemia	High blood sugar
-genic	Origin	Osteogenic	Originating in the bones
-graphy	Drawing	Cardiography	Recording of the heart's movements
-itis	Inflammation	Arthritis	Inflammation of the joints
-lysis	Breaking down	Hemolysis	Breaking down of red blood cells
-ology	Study of	Bacteriology	Study of bacteria
-oma	Tumor	Carcinoma	Malignant tumor
-oscopy	Examination	Bronchoscopy	Examination of the bronchi with a scope
-osis	Condition	Dermatosis	Condition of the skin
-ostomy	Creation of an artificial opening	Colostomy	Creation of an opening into the colon
-otomy	Incision	Gastrotomy	Incision into the stomach
-penia	Decrease	Leukopenia	Abnormal decrease of white blood cells
-pexy	Fixation	Gastropexy	Fixation of the stomach to the abdominal wall
-plasty	Surgical correction	Hernioplasty	Surgical repair of a hernia
-rrhage	Flow	Hemorrhage	Uncontrolled flow of blood
-rrhaphy	To suture	Myorrhaphy	Suture of torn muscle
-rrhea	Flow	Diarrhea	Frequent liquid fecal material
-rrhexis	Rupture	Myorrhaphy	Rupture of a muscle
-stenosis	Abnormal tightening	Arteriostenosis	Condition of narrowing of the arteries

Appendix B
Common Concentrate Dilutions

Dilution Ratio	Spray Bottle		Quart/Liter		Gallon		5 Gallon	
	24 oz	682 ml	32 oz	946 ml	128 oz	3785 ml	640 oz	18927 ml
1:8	2 $^1/_2$ oz	75 ml	3 $^1/_2$ oz	105 ml	14 $^1/_2$ oz	430 ml	71 oz	2100 ml
1:12	1 $^3/_4$ oz	52 ml	2 $^1/_2$ oz	73 ml	9 $^3/_4$ oz	292 ml	49 $^1/_4$ oz	1456 ml
1:20	1 oz	30 ml	1 $^1/_2$ oz	45 ml	6 oz	180 ml	31 oz	930 ml
1:32	$^3/_4$ oz	22 ml	1 oz	30 ml	4 oz	120 ml	20 oz	600 ml
1:48	3/8 oz	11 ml	$^3/_4$ oz	22 ml	3 oz	90 ml	15 oz	450 ml
1:64	1/3 oz	10 ml	$^1/_2$ oz	15 ml	2 oz	60 ml	10 oz	300 ml
1:128	1/5 oz	6 ml	$^1/_4$ oz	7.4 ml	1 oz	30 ml	5 oz	150 ml
1:256	1/10 oz	3 ml	1/8 oz	3.4 ml	$^1/_2$ oz	15 ml	3 oz	90 ml

Veterinary Infection Prevention and Control, First Edition. Edited by Linda Caveney and Barbara Jones with Kimberly Ellis.
© 2012 John Wiley & Sons, Inc. Published by John Wiley & Sons, Inc.

Appendix C
Table of Disease Transmission and Disinfection Guidelines

Veterinary Infection Prevention and Control, First Edition. Edited by Linda Caveney and Barbara Jones with Kimberly Ellis.
© 2012 John Wiley & Sons, Inc. Published by John Wiley & Sons, Inc.

Disease	Organism	Transmission by:	Zoonotic (Y/N)	Comments	Disinfection
Actinobacillus spp.	A. suis, A. equuli, A. pleuropneumoniae Gram-negative rod	Direct contact with infected animals and fomite	Can be, through bite from infected animal, generally species-specific	Found on mucous membranes, oral cavity, and upper respiratory tract of animals; doesn't live long in environment	Killed with cleaning and regular disinfectants (QAC Roccal D-Plus, Nolvasan)
Avian influenza	Orthomyxoviridae virus family Enveloped virus	Direct contact with bird feces or respiratory secretions of infected bird, fomite	Yes	Virus can live in environment	Killed with cleaning and aldehydes, sodium hypochlorites (bleach), oxidizing agents (Trifectant), phenols (Tek-Trol)
Blastomycosis	Blastomyces dermatiditis – Fungal organism	Inhalation of airborne spores from contaminated soil in wooded areas	Yes	Can't be transmitted from animal-to-animal or animal-to-person	Killed with cleaning and 1% sodium hypochlorite, phenols, formaldehyde, glutaraldehyde
Bordatella (kennel cough)	*Bordatella bronchiseptica* Gram-negative bacteria	Direct contact, airborne of respiratory secretions, fomite	Can be, but rare	Can survive in the environment	Easily killed with cleaning and regular disinfectants QAC (Roccal D-Plus, Kennelsol), oxidizing agents (Virkon-S)
Brucellosis	*Brucellaceae* family Gram-negative bacteria	Direct contact by oral ingestion, direct contact, or aerosol exposure to infected animal body fluids, fomite	Yes	Can survive in the environment	Easily killed with cleaning and regular disinfectants QAC (Roccal D-Plus, Nolvasan), sodium hypochlorites (bleach), oxidizing agent (Trifectant)
Bubonic plague (plague)	*Yersinia pestis* Gram-negative bacteria	Vector-borne transmission –bites from infected rat fleas	Yes	Handling of infected tissues is means of transmission	Killed with cleaning and regular disinfectants QAC (Roccal D-Plus, Nolvasan)

Disease	Agent	Transmission	Zoonotic	Notes	Disinfection
Campylobacteriosis	*Campylobacter jejuni* Gram-negative bacteria	Direct contact with sick animal, ingestion of fecal-contaminated feed or water or fomite	Yes	People can also get it from raw or undercooked meats or milk	Killed with cleaning and oxidizing agent (Trifectant, Virkon S)
Canine parvovirus	*Parvoviridae* virus family Nonenveloped virus	Ingestion of the feces of an infected animal (fecal–oral transmission), fomite	No	Animals shed gigantic amounts of virus in stool, hardy in the environment	Killed with cleaning and, sodium hypochlorites (bleach), oxidizing agent (Virkon-S), phenol (Tek-Trol)
Canine influenza	*Orthomyroviridae* virus family Enveloped virus	Airborne spread by respiratory secretions, fomite	No	All dogs susceptible to this, no vaccine	Killed with cleaning and oxidizing agent (Trifectant) or sodium hypochlorites
Cat scratch fever	*Bartnella henselae* Gram-negative bacteria	Direct contact; being licked, bitten, or scratched by an infected cat	Yes	Cats are carriers, not ill, transmitted between cats by fleas	Easily killed with cleaning and regular disinfectants QAC (Roccal D-Plus, Nolvasan), sodium hypochlorites (bleach)
Cheyletiella (walking dandruff)	*Cheyletiella* mites	Direct contact with infected animals, fomite	Can be, but rare	Can live off animal for several days	Killed with thorough cleaning and regular disinfectants (QAC)
Chlamydiosis (psittacosis)	*Chlamydia psittaci* (intracullular parasite; gram-negative)	Direct contact with infected birds, inhaling dried dropping or respiratory secretions from infected birds	Yes	Wear gloves, mask, and eye protection when cleaning cages or area of infected birds	Alcohol hand sanitizer does not kill; can use oxidizing agent (Trifectant), 1:100 sodium hypochlorites (bleach) solution
Clostridium difficile	*Clostridium difficile* toxins Anaerobic spore-forming, gram-positive rod	Ingestion of spores, fecal–oral transmission	Yes		Difficult to kill spores, resistant to most disinfectants; 1:10 sodium hypochlorites (bleach) can be effective

(Continued)

Disease	Organism	Transmission by:	Zoonotic (Y/N)	Comments	Disinfection
Clostridium perfringes	Clostridium perfringes toxins Anaerobic spore-forming, gram-positive rod	Ingestion of spores, fecal–oral transmission	Yes	Can be found in soil	Difficult to kill spores, resistant to most disinfectants; 1:10 sodium hypochlorites (bleach) can be effective
Cryptosporidiosis	Protozoa, cryptosporidium	Ingestion of contaminated food or water with protozoa shed from feces of infected animal, fomite	Yes	From oocysts, difficult to rid the area	Resistant to chemical disinfection
Dermatophytosis (ringworm)	Microsporum family Trichophyton family (fungi)	Direct contact or airborne contact with infected hairs or skin scales	Yes	Infective spores can remain viable for several months to years in the environment	Mechanical removal of shed skin and hairs then cleaning and regular disinfectant (QAC)
Enterobacter	Enterobacter cloacae Enterobacter aerogenes Gram-negative bacteria	Direct contact with fecal-contaminated equipment, fomite, ingestion of contaminated food (fecal–oral transmission)	Yes	Routinely found in the environment	Easily killed by cleaning and regular disinfectants (QAC)
Enterococcus	Enterococcus faecalis, Enterococcus faecium Gram-positive bacteria	Direct contact with feces of infected animal; endogenous is soil, food, water, and plants; ingestion of contaminated food	Yes	Part of normal GI flora	Easily killed by cleaning and regular disinfectants (QAC)
Equine viral arteritis	Arteriviridae virus family, enveloped virus	Direct or indirect contact with aerosolized respiratory tract secretions or tissues, fomite, venereal transmission	No		Easily killed by cleaning and regular disinfectants (QAC)

Disease/pathogen	Transmission	Zoonotic	Environmental survival	Disinfection
E. coli *Escherichia coli* Gram-negative bacteria	Direct contact with feces of infected animal, ingesting contaminated food, fomite (fecal–oral transmission)	Yes	Can remain in feces and soil for over 2 months	Easily killed by cleaning and regular disinfectants
FeLV, (feline leukemia virus)	Retrovirus family Enveloped virus	Direct contact with saliva and nasal secretions, also urine and feces of infected cat	No	Doesn't survive long outside the cat's body	Easily killed by cleaning and regular disinfectants (QAC)
FIP, (feline infectious peritonitis virus)	Coronavirus family Enveloped virus	Direct contact with saliva and feces, inhalation or ingestion from infected cat, fomite	No	Can survive for weeks in the environment	Easily killed by cleaning and regular disinfectants (QAC)
FIV, (feline immunodeficiency virus)	Lentivirus Retrovirus family Enveloped virus	Bite wounds from an infected cat	No		Easily killed by cleaning and regular disinfectants (QAC)
Foot-and-mouth disease	Picornaviridae virus family Nonenveloped virus	Transmission by direct and indirect contact with infected animals and infectious aerosols, fomite	No	Stable in the environment, can spread infectious aerosols by wind over long distances	Killed with cleaning and disinfecting with oxidizing agents (Trifectant) or sodium hypochlorites (bleach)
FURTD, feline upper respiratory tract disease	Feline calicivirus (FVC) Nonenveloped virus and feline herpesvirus (FHV-1) Enveloped virus	Aerosol droplets of respiratory and nasal secretions of infected cats, fomite	No	Alcohol hand sanitizers are not effective, against calicivirus wash hands with soap and water	Killed with cleaning and disinfecting with oxidizing agents (Trifectant) or sodium hypochlorites (bleach)
Giardia	Protozoa, giardia intestinalis	Direct contact with infected feces, ingestion of contaminated food, water, soil or surface that has been contaminated by infected feces	Yes	Can survive in the environment for a long time	Killed with cleaning and regular disinfectants (QAC)

(Continued)

Disease	Organism	Transmission by:	Zoonotic (Y/N)	Comments	Disinfection
Herpes virus (avian, bovine, caprine, equine, canine, feline)	Herpesviridae virus family Enveloped virus	Inhalation of aerosolized virus, for equine-direct contact with aborted foal, fomite	No	Highly contagious	Easily killed with cleaning and regular disinfectants (QAC)
Influenza virus (avian, equine, swine)	Orthomyxoviridae virus family Enveloped virus	Airborne- spread by inhalation of the aerosolized virus	No		Easily killed with cleaning and regular disinfectants (QAC)
Leptospirosis	Leptospira bacteria Gram-negative bacteria	Direct contact with urine of infected animals, contact with contaminated water (ingestion) or soil (can enter through cuts in skin or mucous membranes)	Yes	Can survive in water or soil for weeks to months; wear gloves when handling infected animals; caution with blood or body tissue	Easily killed with cleaning and regular disinfectants (QAC)
Lyme Disease	Borrelia burgdorferi Gram negative bacteria	Indirect by bite from infected tick	Yes		Heat-sensitive Easily killed with cleaning and regular disinfectants (QAC)
Mange (scabies) Human scabies Canine scabies Feline scabies	Sarcoptes scabiei var. hominis Sarcoptes scabiei var. canis Notoedres cati	Direct contact with mites, highly contagious, fomite	Yes *Note mites are species specific, are self-limiting	Don't survive for long periods in the environment; wear gloves and protective clothing	Use insecticides, wash bedding in hot water and hot dryer
MRSA, methicillin-resistant Staphylococcus aureus	Staphylococcus aureus Gram-positive bacteria	Direct contact with contaminated hands, aerosolization of organism from colonized patient, fomite	Yes	Generally causes skin infections and deep SSI; wounds should be covered	Easily killed with cleaning and any regular disinfectants ({QAC-Kennelsol, Roccal D-Plus}, Tek-Trol, Virkon S, sodium hypochlorite)

MRSI, methicillin-resistant *Staphlococcus intermedius* *Staphlococcus intermedius* Gram-positive bacteria	Direct contact with contaminated hands, aerosolization of organism from colonized patient, fomite		Generally causes skin infections and deep SSI; wounds should be covered	Easily killed with cleaning and any regular disinfectants ({QAC-Kennelsol, Roccal D-Plus}, Tek-Trol, Virkon S, Sodium Hypochlorite)
Pseudomonas aeruginosa Gram-negative bacteria	Opportunistic bacteria, occurs in compromised patients	Yes	Generally found in the environment	Easily killed by hospital disinfectants (QAC), except Nolvasan is NOT effective
Rabies Rhabdoviridae virus family Enveloped virus	Direct contact by bite of an infected animal's saliva, rarely by inhaling aerosolized virus or exposure to infected brain or spinal cord fluid	Yes	Does not survive for long periods in environment except in cool dark areas	Avoid contact, killed with cleaning and regular disinfectants (QAC)
Rhodococcus *Rhodococcus equi* Gram positive bacteria	Direct contact with feces of infected animal, ingesting contaminated feed (fecal/oral route), fomite, can be inhaled in contaminated dusty areas.	Can be an opportunistic infection in immunocompromised	Found in soil on endemic farms	Killed with cleaning and regular disinfectants (QAC)
Ringworm: See Dermatophytosis				
Rotavirus foal diarrhea	*Reoviridae* virus family, Nonenveloped virus	Direct contact with contaminated feces, fomite (fecal/oral route)	No	Resistant to iodophors, QAC, and sodium hypochlorite; highly contagious	Killed with cleaning and disinfection with phenolic disinfectant (Tek-Trol)

(Continued)

Disease	Organism	Transmission by:	Zoonotic (Y/N)	Comments	Disinfection
Salmonella	*Salmonella arizonae* Salmonella Gp B,C1,C2 Gram-negative bacteria	Direct contact with animals or objects contaminated by fecal material from infected animal, fomite (fecal/oral route)	Yes	Reptiles carry salmonella bacteria and shed these bacteria in feces	Easily killed with cleaning and regular disinfectants (QAC)
Strangles	*S. equi* Gram-positive bacteria	See Streptococcosis			
Streptococcosis	*S. equi, S. canis, S. pyogenes* Gram-positive bacteria	Direct contact with wound infections to open wounds, burns or bites, aerosols of wound secretions, fomite	Can be, but rare	Cause of necrotizing fascitis	Easily killed with cleaning and regular disinfectants (QAC)
Toxoplasmosis	*Toxoplasma gondii* protozoa	Direct (oral) contact with oocysts that are shed in feces of infected cats, inhale as aerosols, or contact with contaminated soil	Yes, mainly with compromised immune system or pregnant	Highly resistant, can remain in environment 18 months in water or warm, moist soils	Destroyed within 10 minutes by temperature over 150°F
Viral encephalitis (in horses) EEE, WEE, VEE	*Togaviridae* virus family Enveloped virus	Vector borne transmission by mosquitos, birds are the primary reservoir host	No direct transmission between affected animal and human	Control is through ridding the area of mosquito breeding sites	Related virus killed with cleaning and regular disinfectants (QAC)
West Nile fever	*Flaviviridae* virus family enveloped virus	Vector-borne transmission by mosquitos, birds are the primary reservoir host	No direct transmission between affected animal and human	Control is through ridding the area of mosquito breeding sites	Related virus killed with cleaning and regular disinfectants (QAC)

Appendix D
Donning and Removal of a Surgical Gown

The surgical gown is folded so that, when it is unwrapped for donning, the inside of the gown is accessible. The outside should not be touched with the scrubbed hands; it will then be considered contaminated.

Procedure for Closed-Cuff Method of Donning

With one hand, pick up the entire folded gown from the wrapper by grabbing inside the layers of the gown. Step back from the table.

Hold the gown by the inside of the gown's neck and shoulder area. Shake to unfold, being careful that it does not touch either your body or other unsterile area.

Grab the inside shoulder seam and open the gown with the armhole openings facing you.

Slide your arms into the sleeves of the gown, keeping your hands at shoulder level and away from your body.

A nonsterile person can assist by grasping from the inside of the shoulders and positioning the gown over your shoulder or by grabbing the ties at the neck and lifting upward, therefore allowing you to slide your arms further into the sleeves. Do not allow any part of your hands to protrude from the sleeve cuff.

The ties at the neck are secured. Some gowns are secured at the neck by means of Velcro closure, others by snaps. Once this area is secured, the ties at the waist level are secured. Generally, the left side of the back of the gown has a tie; the right side tie is found inside the gown attached to the right side gown seam. These are tied at the back of the gown.

Closed-Cuff Gloving

Open the inner package containing the gloves; pick up the left-hand glove by the folded cuff edge with the right sleeve-covered hand.

Place the glove on the left gown sleeve, palm down, with the glove fingers pointing toward your left elbow. The palm of your left hand inside the gown sleeve should be facing upward toward the palm of the glove.

Place the glove's rolled cuff edge proximal to the seam that connects the sleeve to the gown cuff. Grab the bottom rolled cuff edge of the glove with your left thumb and index finger (through the gown sleeve).

Grab the uppermost edge of the glove's cuff with the right hand. Be sure the fingers of the left hand do not get exposed while doing this.

Continue to stretch the glove's cuff with the right hand over the left sleeve cuff being held by the left thumb and index finger. This will cover the opening of the left gown sleeve cuff.

Using the right sleeve–covered hand, grab both the left glove cuff and sleeve cuff seam and pull the glove onto the hand. Pull any excess gown sleeve from underneath the cuff of the glove.

Using the left gloved hand, put on the right glove in the same manner as described for the left hand. When completed, the gown cuffs are totally covered by the glove cuff.

Veterinary Infection Prevention and Control, First Edition. Edited by Linda Caveney and Barbara Jones with Kimberly Ellis. © 2012 John Wiley & Sons, Inc. Published by John Wiley & Sons, Inc.

Tying the gown at waist level is achieved with the assistance of an unscrubbed individual. This procedure is done one of two ways. Generally with disposable gowns, there is a paper "tab" securing the both ends of the waist level ties. With a reusable gown, the ties are tied together in a bow-tie fashion. Each procedure will be described.

*Disposable Gowns

The gowned person will take hold of the paper tab that holds the ties together with the right hand and pull it away from the gown front.

With the left hand, grab the loop of the left side of the secured tie and pull to free the tie from the tab. Do not let go of the tie.

With the right hand holding the tab, hand the unscrubbed person the tab. The unscrubbed person will be careful not to touch the ties that remain in the tab or the hand of the gowned person.

The unscrubbed person will remain still holding the tab while the gowned person will turn counter-clockwise. The gowned person will grab the tie remaining in the tab and tie the ties at waist level.

*Reusable Gowns

The gowned person will untie the gown ties and lean slightly forward. This will allow the unscrubbed person to grap the distal end of the tie that is connected to the back portion of the gown.

The gowned person will stand still while the unscrubbed person will move to the back of the gowned person.

The gowned person will lean slightly forward so the unscrubbed person can grab the other gown tie.

The unscrubbed person will ties the both gown ties in a bow-tie fashion toward the back of the gowned person.

Removal of Surgical Attire

The gowned person will untie the front waist ties.

The unscrubbed person unties the neck and inside waist ties.

The gowned person will grab the gown at the shoulders and pull the gown forward and down over the arms and gloved hands.

Holding the arms away from the body, fold the gown so the outside of the gown is folded in.

Discard the gown in the appropriate waste container or if reusable, into a linen hamper.

Grab the outer surface of one glove at the cuff edge with the other gloved hand and pull off the glove. Place the fingers of the exposed hand inside the cuff of the glove on the other hand. Pull off the glove. Each glove will end up with the outside in.

Index

Note: Page numbers followed by f and t indicates figure and table respectively.

Veterinary Infection Prevention and Control, First Edition. Edited by Linda Caveney and Barbara Jones with Kimberly Ellis.
© 2012 John Wiley & Sons, Inc. Published by John Wiley & Sons, Inc.